Case Studies in Dentistry

Case Studies in Dentistry

Editor: Gabrielle Bennett

AMERICAN
MEDICAL PUBLISHERS
www.americanmedicalpublishers.com

AMERICAN
MEDICAL PUBLISHERS
www.americanmedicalpublishers.com

Cataloging-in-Publication Data

Case studies in dentistry / edited by Gabrielle Bennett.
p. cm.
Includes bibliographical references and index.
ISBN 979-8-88740-595-7
1. Dentistry. 2. Oral medicine. 3. Teeth. I. Bennett, Gabrielle.
RK51 .D46 2023
617.6--dc23

American Medical Publishers,
41 Flatbush Avenue,
1st Floor, New York,
NY 11217, USA

ISBN 979-8-88740-595-7 (Hardback)

Contents

Preface ... IX

Chapter 1 **Concentrated Growth Factor: A Novel Platelet Concentrate for Revascularization of Immature Permanent Teeth – A Report of Two Cases** ... 1
M. S. Nivedhitha, Benoy Jacob and Aishwarya Ranganath

Chapter 2 **Unusual Site for a White Nodule on the Palatine Tonsil: Presentation, Differential Diagnosis and Discussion** ... 9
Ashwag Yagoub Aloyouny

Chapter 3 **CBCT Evaluation and Conservative Management of a Large Periapical Lesion Associated with Dens Invaginatus Type II** ... 13
Laïla Azzahim, Nisrin Bassim and Faïza Abdallaoui

Chapter 4 **Novel Management for Severe Odontogenic Maxillary Sinusitis Based on Pathophysiology** ... 17
Yoshio Ohyama, Masaru Ogawa and Satoshi Yokoo

Chapter 5 **Long-Term Follow-up after Conservative Surgical Treatment of Odontogenic Myxoma: A Case Report and Literature Review** ... 20
Hitoshi Sato, Yuji Kurihara, Sunao Shiogama, Kotaro Saka, Yuya Kurasawa, Masakatsu Itose, Atsutoshi Yaso and Tatsuo Shirota

Chapter 6 **Acemannan Induced Bone Regeneration in Lateral Sinus Augmentation Based on Cone Beam Computed Tomographic and Histopathological Evaluation** ... 26
Hai Anh Trinh, Van Viet Dam, Wijit Banlunara, Polkit Sangvanich and Pasutha Thunyakitpisal

Chapter 7 **Prelacrimal Window Approach in the Management of Odontogenic Maxillary Sinusitis from Dental Foreign Body** ... 31
Saikrishna Ananthapadmanabhan, Anthony Noor and Niranjan Sritharan

Chapter 8 **Mental Nerve Paraesthesia: A Report of Two Cases Associated with Endodontic Etiology** ... 37
Neeta Patel, Akshayraj Langaliya, Shikha Kanodia, Aravind Kumbhar, Aastha Buch, Aarshvi Shah, Himani Bhatt, Drashti Panchal, Sharan Shah and Jinali Shah

Chapter 9 **A Case Series of Psychological Stress Evaluation as a Risk Factor for Oral Lichen Planus** ... 45
Irna Sufiawati, Ani Megawati, Muhammad Al Farisyi and I. Nyoman Gede Juwita Putra

Chapter 10 **Maxillary Fungal Osteomyelitis Mimicking and Treated as Endodontic Pathosis** ... 54
Sarang Suresh Hotchandani, Feroze Ali Kalhoro, Priya Rani Harjani and Mahwish Memon

Chapter 11 **Clinicoradiographic Features and Histopathologic Variations of Intraosseous Lipoma: Report of a Case and Review of the Literature** 62
Saede Atarbashi-Moghadam, Ali Lotfi, Mohammad Mehdizadeh and Fazele Atarbashi-Moghadam

Chapter 12 **Management of 3 Avulsed Permanent Teeth: Case Report of a 3- Year Follow-up** 67
Soukaina El Kharroubi, Sofia Drouri, Bouchra Doumari, Sara Dhoum and Hafsa El Merini

Chapter 13 **Unusual Variant of Unicystic Ameloblastoma with CEOT-Like Areas: A Rare Case Report with Review of Literature** 73
Venkata Ramanand Oruganti, Shylaja Sanjeevareddygari, Manay Srinivas Munisekhar, Sharath Kumar Reddy Eppalapalli, Raghu Vamshi Vishwakarma, Kiran Kumar Ganji, Kiran R. Halkai and Rahul Halkai

Chapter 14 **Clinical and Immunohistochemical Features of Oral Angioleiomyoma: A Comprehensive Review of the Literature and Report of a Case in a Young Patient** 78
Amerigo Giudice, Francesco Bennardo, Caterina Buffone, Ylenia Brancaccio, Francesca Maria Plutino and Leonzio Fortunato

Chapter 15 **An Atypical Case of Oral Squamous Cell Carcinoma of Mandibular Alveolus** 87
Seba Abraham, Bhagyalekshmi Mallika, Arunima Reshma and ReejaMol Mohammed Kassim

Chapter 16 **A Rare Case of Orthograde Retrieval of Extruded Instrument following Periapical Tissue Healing** 93
Ahmed Elhakim and Tarek Mohamed Abd El-Wahab

Chapter 17 **Management of Edentulous Microstomia Patient: A Case Report and Classification System** 97
Maria S. Abbasi, Naseer Ahmed, Adil Bin Irfan, Samar Al-Saleh, Tariq Abduljabbar and Fahim Vohra

Chapter 18 **Piezosurgery-Assisted Surgical Treatment in Impacted Canine Transmigration** 102
Matheus Francisco Barros Rodrigues, Layla Louise de Amorim Rocha, Rodrigo da Franca Acioly, Cristofe Coelho Lopes da Rocha and Daniel do Carmo Carvalho

Chapter 19 **Esthetic Rehabilitation using Magnet-Retained Cheek Plumper Prosthesis** 105
Alisha Rewari, Nupur Dabas, Reshu Sanan, Shefali Phogat, Sumit Singh Phukela and Monika Vigarniya

Chapter 20 **New Approach in the Management of Vertical Root Fracture with the Help of Biodentine and CBCT** 109
H. C. Baranwal, Nidhi Singh, Neeraj Kumar, Riya Garg, Jyoti Yadav and Richik Tripathi

Chapter 21 **Endodontic Management of Maxillary Second Molar Tooth with a Single Root and Single Canal** 115
Neelam Mittal, Vijay Parashar and Prasad Suresh Patel

Chapter 22 **Bilateral Atypical Facial Pain Caused by Eagle's Syndrome** 118
V. Anuradha, Ravi Sachidananda, Satish Kumaran Pugazhendi, Preeti Satish and Romir Navaneetham

Chapter 23 **Delayed Epistaxis which was Developed after Orthognathic Surgery with Le Fort I Osteotomy and Managed by Endoscopic Cauterization** 122
Yuya Kurasawa, Hitoshi Sato, Ryogo Katada, Takanobu Inada, Tatsuo Shirota and Toshikazu Shimane

Chapter 24 **Genetic Risk of Talon Cusp: Talon Cusp in Five Siblings** 127
Nuha Abdel-Rahman Elmubarak

Chapter 25 **Long-Term Follow-up of SAPHO Syndrome for 15 Years Led to a Diagnosis of Temporomandibular Joint Pain and Trismus** 136
Koki Takamatsu, Hitoshi Sato, Takashi Moriya, Arisa Yasuda, Takaaki Kamatani and Tatsuo Shirota

Chapter 26 **Early Creeping Attachment Noted after Mandibular Labial Frenuloplasty** 142
P. Stylianou, N. Soldatos, E. K. Edmondson, N. Angelov and R. Weltman

Chapter 27 **Oral Lichenoid Reaction: An Uncommon Side Effect of Rituximab** 146
Amerigo Giudice, Francesco Liborio, Fiorella Averta, Selene Barone and Leonzio Fortunato

Chapter 28 **An Uncommon Case of Plasma Cell Mucositis of the Tongue in a Young Man** 149
Alessandro Antonelli, Fiorella Averta, Federica Diodati, Danila Muraca, Ylenia Brancaccio, Chiara Mignogna and Amerigo Giudice

Chapter 29 **Closure of Orocutaneous Fistula using Submandibular Gland as a Pedicled Flap** 157
Erol Cansiz, Emine Deniz Gozen and Murat Yener

Chapter 30 **Parosmia, Dysgeusia and Tongue Features Changes in a Patient with Post-Acute COVID-19 Syndrome** 161
Aliaa Abdelmoniem Bedeir Eita

Chapter 31 **Maxillomandibular Transverse Osteodistraction: A Multidisciplinary Case Report with 30-Month Follow-up** 166
G. Turatti, A. Bruni, M. Savoini, M. Giordano and G. Gerbino

Chapter 32 **Facial Emphysema following Closure of Oroantral Fistulae** 177
Muhammad Aiman Mohd Nizar and Syed Nabil

Chapter 33 **Mouthwash with Active Oxygen (blue®m) Reduces Postoperative Inflammation and Pain** 181
Bruna Marca Mattei, Soraia A. W. Imanishi, Grasieli de Oliveira Ramos, Paloma Santos de Campos, Suyany Gabriely Weiss and Tatiana Miranda Deliberador

Chapter 34 **High Submandibular Anteroparotid Approach for Open Reduction and Internal Fixation of Condylar Fracture** 187
Kamichika Hayashi, Takeshi Onda, Hirona Honda, Mitsuru Takata, Hiroyuki Matsuda, Hidetoshi Tamura and Masayuki Takano

Chapter 35 **Management of Intracanal Separated File Fragment in a Four-Rooted Mandibular Third Molar** 196
Benoy Jacob, Anjaneyulu K., Aishwarya Ranganath and Riluwan Siddique

Permissions

List of Contributors

Index

Preface

Dentistry is a vital and specialized field within the medical profession that focuses on the diagnosis, treatment, and prevention of oral health conditions. It plays an important role in the maintenance and improvement of oral health. Some of the oral health issues which are treated within this field are tooth decay, gum diseases, malocclusion and oral infections. It also deals with restoring damaged teeth through procedures such as fillings, crowns, and dental implants. Some of the important specialized areas within this field are orthodontics, periodontics, endodontics, oral and maxillofacial surgery, prosthodontics, pediatric dentistry, and oral pathology. This book provides comprehensive insights into the field of dentistry. From theories to research to practical applications, case studies related to all contemporary topics of relevance to this field have been included herein. The book will prove to be immensely beneficial to students and researchers in this field.

After months of intensive research and writing, this book is the end result of all who devoted their time and efforts in the initiation and progress of this book. It will surely be a source of reference in enhancing the required knowledge of the new developments in the area. During the course of developing this book, certain measures such as accuracy, authenticity and research focused analytical studies were given preference in order to produce a comprehensive book in the area of study.

This book would not have been possible without the efforts of the authors and the publisher. I extend my sincere thanks to them. Secondly, I express my gratitude to my family and well-wishers. And most importantly, I thank my students for constantly expressing their willingness and curiosity in enhancing their knowledge in the field, which encourages me to take up further research projects for the advancement of the area.

Editor

Concentrated Growth Factor: A Novel Platelet Concentrate for Revascularization of Immature Permanent Teeth—A Report of Two Cases

M. S. Nivedhitha, Benoy Jacob, and Aishwarya Ranganath

Department of Conservative Dentistry and Endodontics, Saveetha Institute of Medical and Technical Sciences, No. 162, Poonamalle High Road, Chennai, 600077 Tamil Nadu, India

Correspondence should be addressed to M. S. Nivedhitha; nivea16@hotmail.com

Academic Editor: H. Cem Güngör

This article elucidates the utilization of a novel platelet concentrate-concentrated growth factor (CGF) for rapid and successful healing outcome in regenerative endodontics. This case report focusses on two cases: 23-year-old and 21-year-old patients with incomplete root formation and periapical lesion. Case 1 and case 2 are classified as stage IV and stage II, respectively, in accordance with Cvek's classification of open apex and had varied outcomes. The extent of open apex, root dentin thickness, and lesion were assessed using periapical radiograph and CBCT. Revascularization procedure was carried out after obtaining patient consent. Following bleeding induction, CGF was prepared, placed, and condensed using pluggers in the root canal space, followed by the placement of mineral trioxide aggregate (MTA) up to the level of CEJ. At 1-year follow-up, apical closure with increased root dentin thickness and reduced periapical radiolucency was evident.

1. Introduction

The developing dentition is perpetually subjected to various mechanical or biological insults pertaining to trauma, caries, and diverse developmental anomalies [1]. There has been tremendous research aimed at the management of nonvital immature anterior permanent teeth to reestablish the pulp-dentin complex. Since the nonvital tooth is devoid of blood supply, the root fails to develop and is subjected to fracture in the long run. Cvek in 1992 classified five stages of root development according to the width of the apical foramen and length of the root where he described teeth with wide divergent apical opening estimated to be less than half, half, two-thirds, nearly completed, and finally teeth with closed apical foramen and completed root development [2].

Revascularization or revitalization is widely described as the restoration of vascularity to a tissue or organ with the sole purpose of reestablishing the pulp-dentin complex, thereby contributing to repair and continued development of the necrotic immature permanent anterior teeth with respect to periapical healing, increase in root dimensions, and closure of the apical foramen [3].The current concept in regenerative endodontics primarily stems from the pioneering work done by Dr. B.W. Hermann wherein the meticulous application of calcium hydroxide for vital pulp therapy was described [4]. The judicious use of calcium hydroxide had gained acceptance worldwide and was also enlisted as the material of choice in apexification procedures before the advent of MTA [5]. However, the conventional endodontic approaches described above failed to offer any benefits as far as continued root development and thickening of root dentinal walls were concerned. As a result, a high incidence of root fracture could be elicited in such cases as reported by Andreasen et al. [6].

Reynolds et al. evaluated a revascularization protocol for rejuvenating the pulp-dentin complex in necrotic immature permanent teeth and reported a case of connective tissue formation in root canals following routine pulpectomy procedure [7]. Rule and Winter further strengthened the concept when pulpal bleeding was induced to revitalize a nonvital immature mandibular premolar [8]. This frank attempt tasted remarkable success when continued root formation and apical closure were detected. The concept of this "induced bleeding" technique has fast gained popularity over the years and catapulted regenerative endodontics into the limelight as an alternative to conventional root canal therapy when all else failed.

In recent years, various attempts have been made to regenerate the lost pulp which involved incorporation of popular platelet concentrates such as platelet-rich plasma (PRP) and platelet-rich fibrin (PRF). While the former suffers from few shortcomings pertaining to cost, handling, tedious centrifugation, and purification procedures, the latter scores over it in terms of simplicity and cost; the use of bovine thrombin and anticoagulants are also avoided [9]. Apart from the conventional platelet concentrates, CGF has been suggested as an ideal biomaterial as it releases growth factors that induces cell migration and proliferation and chemotactic activity on inflammatory cells and stimulates angiogenesis and tissue remodelling [10]. However, a comprehensive search of the literature revealed the absence of any publication regarding the use of CGF in pulp revitalization, thereby making it a novel platelet concentrate for application in regenerative endodontics. For describing the case reports, we have followed the checklist given in CARE guidelines (http://www.care-statement.org/) [11].

2. Case Presentation

2.1. Case Report 1. A 23-year-old male patient reported to the Department of Conservative Dentistry and Endodontics with chief complaint of broken teeth and pain in the upper front tooth region. There was no contributing medical history. Past dental history revealed traumatic injury 14 years back associated with sharp pain on biting. Intraoral clinical examination revealed fracture of 11 and 12 (Figure 1(a)). Both the teeth were sensitive to percussion and palpation. Cold test was carried out using refrigerant spray (Coltene/Whaledent, Switzerland), and electric pulp testing (Gentle Pulse™ Pulp Vitality Tester, Parkell, USA) showed no response when compared with the control teeth. Periapical radiograph revealed loss of crown structure in 11, immature roots in 12, and radiolucency in the periapical area of 11 and 12 (Figure 1(b)). CBCT (Dentsply Sirona, Orthophos XG 3D) was taken at standardized settings (90 kV, 6 mA, 5 ∗ 5.5 cm, 160 μm, 14 s). The lesion extent measured 4.84 ∗ 5.59 ∗ 9.35 mm (Figure 1(g)). Apical diameter measured 1.96 mm (Figure 1(k)). The root dentin thickness at coronal third was 1.62 ∗ 1.80 mm, middle third was 1.59 ∗ 1.46 mm, and apical third was 1.23 ∗ 1.03 mm (Figure 1(i)).

Based on these findings, the diagnosis made was pulpal necrosis with symptomatic apical periodontitis in 11 and 12. Revascularization protocol was applied for 12, and endodontic therapy was carried out in 11 with placement of intracanal medicament for three weeks (Figures 1(c)–1(f)). No adverse events were reported during the follow-up periods. Intraoral periapical radiograph and CBCT at 12-month follow-up revealed marked closure of the apex in 12 and decreased extent of periapical lesion in 11 and 12. The lesion extent measured 4.00 ∗ 4.07 ∗ 8.96 mm (Figure 1(h)). The root dentin thickness at coronal third was 1.90 ∗ 2.21 mm, middle third was 1.59 ∗ 1.80 mm, and apical third was 1.28 ∗ 1.30 mm (Figures 1(j)–1(l)).

Livewire segmentation using OSIRIX version 9.5 (PIXMEO, Geneva, Switzerland) was done to delineate the lesion from healthy bone. Preoperative and postoperative volume calculations were 0.1012cm^3 and 0.0824 cm^3, respectively (Figures 2(a) and 2(b)). The lesion reduction size was found to be 18.57%.

2.2. Case Report 2. A 21-year-old male patient reported to the Department of Conservative Dentistry and Endodontics with chief complaint of discoloured and broken teeth in the upper front tooth region. Patient revealed a history of trauma 9 years back. Clinical examination revealed discoloured and fractured 21 with sinus opening and pus discharge (Figure 3(a)). On radiographic examination, incomplete root formation was evident in 21 with radiolucency in the periapical region (Figure 3(b)). The lesion extent in CBCT was measured to be 5.41 ∗ 4.29 ∗ 9.92 mm (Figure 3(g)). The root dentin thickness at coronal third was 2.70 ∗ 2.20 mm, middle third was 1.77 ∗ 1.83 mm, and apical third was 1.19 ∗ 1.26 mm (Figure 3(i)). Apical diameter measured 2.66 mm (Figure 3(k)). Based on these findings, a diagnosis of chronic apical abscess in 21 was made. Revascularization protocol was followed in 21 (Figures 3(c)–3(f)). No adverse events were reported by the patient during the follow-up periods. Intraoral periapical radiograph and CBCT at 12-month follow-up revealed increased root dentin thickness in 21. The lesion extent in CBCT was measured to be 4.00 ∗ 3.89 ∗ 8.98 mm (Figure 3(h)). The root dentin thickness at coronal third was 2.90 ∗ 2.23 mm, middle third was 2.26 ∗ 1.84 mm, and apical third was 1.84 ∗ 1.47 mm (Figure 3(j)). Apical diameter measured 1.96 mm (Figure 3(l)).

Preoperative and postoperative volume calculations were 0.0675cm^3 and 0.0541 cm^3, respectively (Figures 2(c) and 2(d)). The lesion reduction size was found to be 19.85%.

2.3. Common Treatment Protocol. Prior to the revascularization procedure, informed consent was obtained from the patient. On the first visit, teeth were isolated with a rubber dam, followed by access cavity preparation with endo access bur (Dentsply Maillefer, Switzerland) and working length determination using a #80 K-file (Mani, Inc., Japan) radiographically. The canals were irrigated using a 30-gauge side-vented needle with 20 ml of 1.5% sodium hypochlorite (VIP, Vensons, India) followed by saline rinse prior to the placement of calcium hydroxide (RC Cal, Prime dental products, India) as intracanal medicament for three weeks. For temporary sealing of the access cavity, zinc oxide eugenol was used. On the second visit, the patients were asymptomatic. 2% lignocaine (Lignox, India) without vasoconstrictor was administered. The medicament was flushed out of the root canal with copious amount of 0.9% saline (AcuLIFE, India). The root canal was then irrigated with 10 ml of 17% EDTA (Canalarge, Ammdent, India). Following this, the canals were dried with paper points, bleeding was induced using #80 K-file to a length of 2 mm beyond the working length, and the bleeding was made to fill the root canal. A

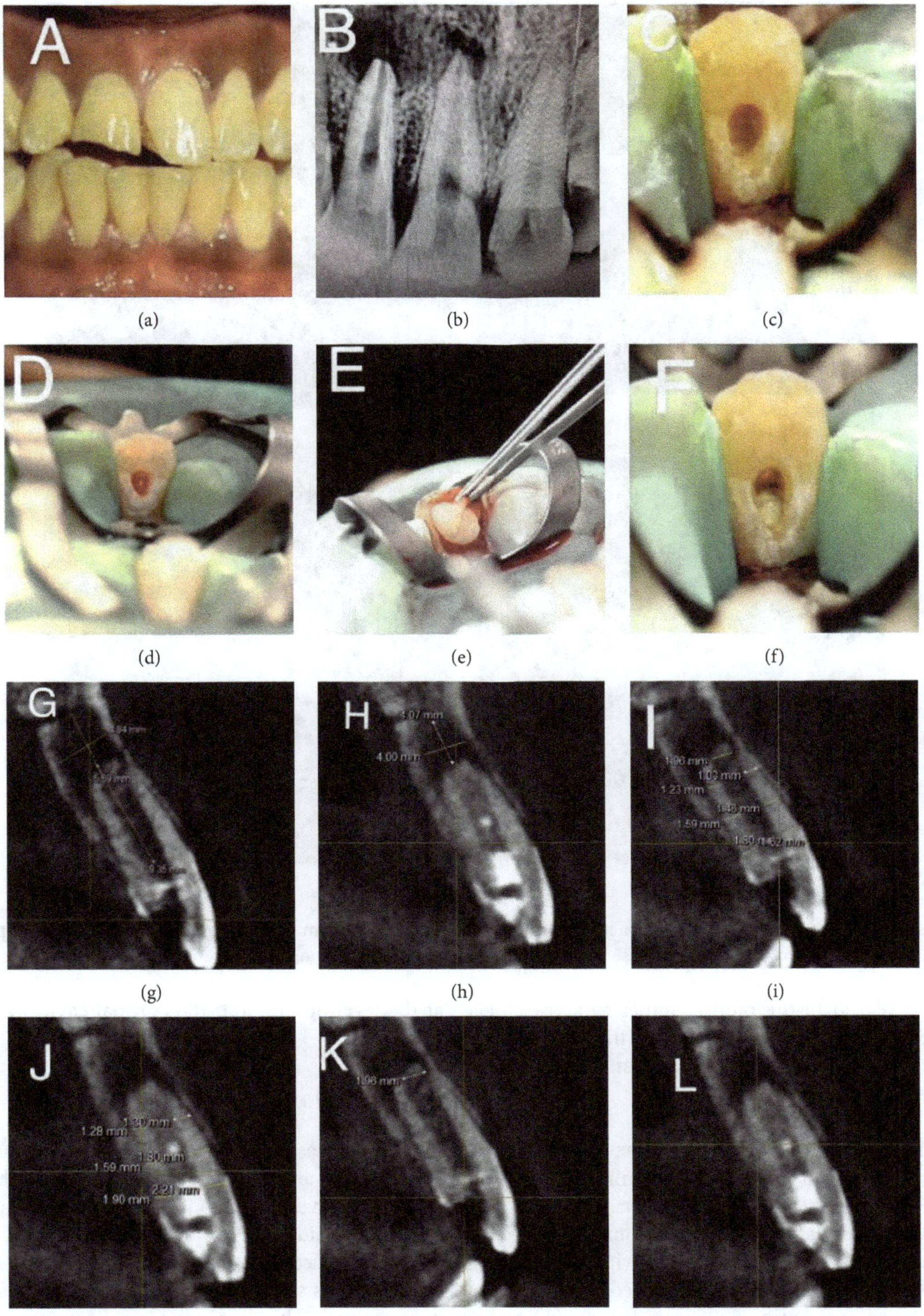

Figure 1: Preoperative clinical, revascularization procedure and radiographic images—IOPA and CBCT images (case report 1). (a) Pre-op clinical photograph showing fractured of 11 and 12. (b) Preoperative IOPA showing the periapical lesion involving the apices of 11 and 12 and immature roots of 12. (c) Access opening done in 12. (d) Bleeding induced in 12 for revascularization. (e) Placement of CGF in the root canal space. (f) MTA plug of 3 mm placed at the level of CEJ in 12. (g) Pre-op CBCT image showing the extent of lesion in sagittal slice. (h) Post-op CBCT image showing the extent of lesion in sagittal slice. (i) Pre-op CBCT showing the root dentin thickness measurement in sagittal slice. (j) Post-op CBCT showing the root dentin thickness measurement in sagittal slice. (k) Pre-op CBCT showing the apical diameter measurement in 12. (l) Post-op CBCT showing the apical diameter in 12.

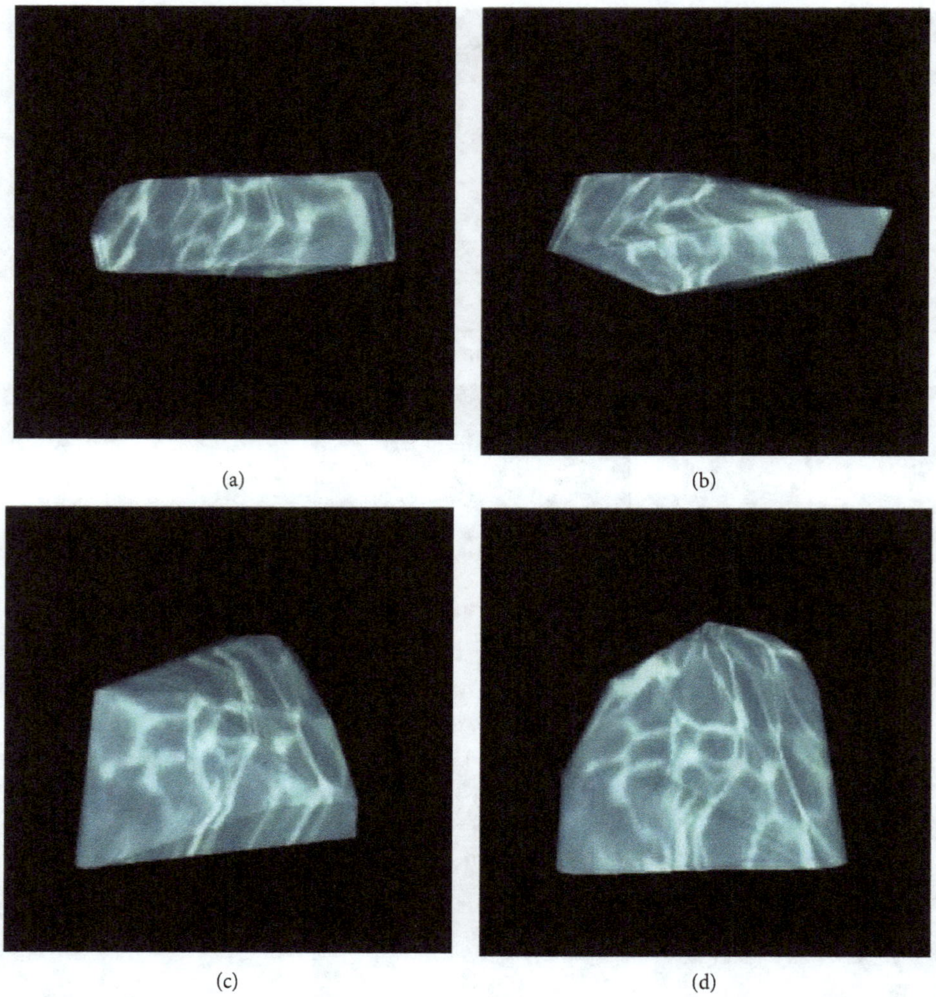

FIGURE 2: Preoperative and postoperative volume calculations to delineate the lesion from healthy bone. Case report 1: (a, b) preoperative and postoperative volume calculations, respectively. Case report 2: (c, d) preoperative and postoperative volume calculations, respectively.

cotton pellet was placed in the pulp chamber to allow clot formation. The protocol thus followed was in accordance with the guidelines proposed by the American Association of Endodontists (AAE).

2.4. Preparation of Concentrated Growth Factor. Two disposable 10 ml nonanticoagulant tubes and a matching centrifuge device (MEDIFUGE, Silfradent SRL, S. Sofia, Italy) were used. 10 ml of intravenous blood sample from the patient was obtained and placed in centrifuge tubes without anticoagulants; accelerated for 30 seconds; centrifuged at 2700 rpm for 2 min, 2400 rpm for 4 min, 2700 rpm for 4 min, and 3000 rpm for 3 min; and decelerated for 36 secs to stop. At the end of the automated preprogrammed cycle, the centrifuge tube encompassed a concoction of four different layers; the uppermost or the 1st layer contained serum, the 2nd layer was composed of a fibrin buffy coat, the 3rd layer constituted the much needed growth factors, and lastly, the lowermost or the 4th layer was occupied by the red blood cells. The fibrin gel containing the concentrated growth factor was separated from the red blood cells. The CGF obtained was packed into the canals to the level of cementoenamel junction. 3 mm MTA (MTA Angelus Brazil) plug was placed at the level of CEJ, and the coronal cavity was sealed using composite.

3. Discussion

The present case report most notably focused upon achieving revitalization at a flourishing rate, made possible by incorporating the novel autologous platelet concentrate (CGF), well within the guidelines proposed by the AAE. CGF was introduced by Sacco in 2006. As "concentrated" as it seems to be, CGF does stand out from its predecessors by the way it is concocted. This is ascribed to its unique centrifugation technique which depends upon varied time intervals and centrifugation speeds, finally churning out a much concentrated, thicker, and elongated fibrin matrix [12]. In a comparative study, it was claimed that CGF indeed had an upper hand over PRP and PRF in terms of cell proliferation and osteoblastic differentiation as well as a richer growth factor content [13].

In recent years, CGF has carved a niche for itself in terms of sinus ridge augmentation procedures, implant surgeries, and surgical endodontics as reported by Sohn et al., Qiao et al., Ying et al., and Sureshbabu et al., eliciting predictable

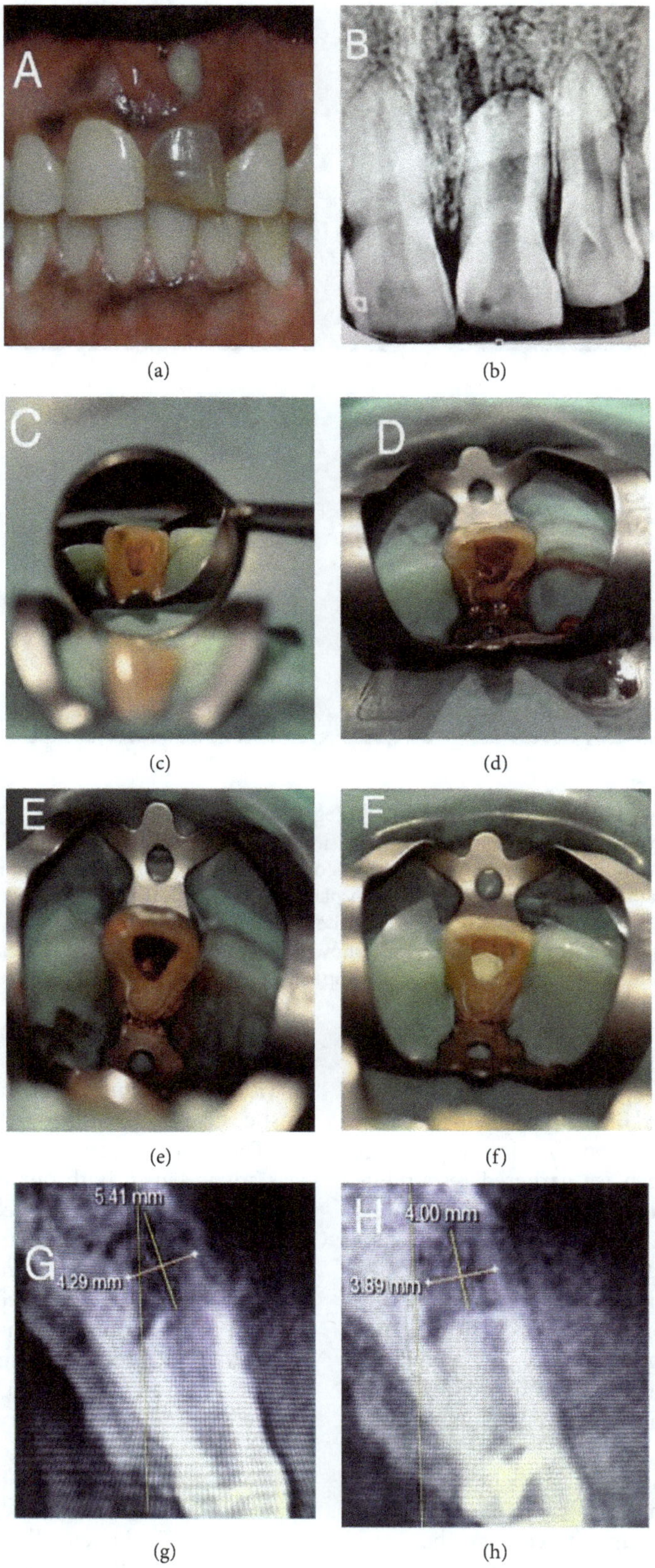

(a) (b) (c) (d) (e) (f) (g) (h)

Figure 3: Continued.

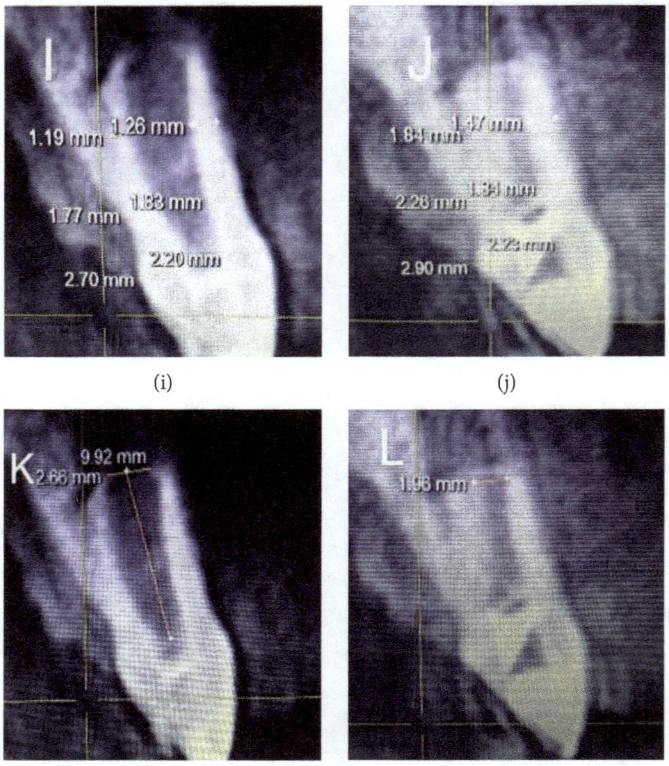

(i) (j) (k) (l)

Figure 3: Preoperative clinical, revascularization procedure and radiographic images—IOPA and CBCT images (case report 2). (a) Pre-op clinical photograph showing discoloured and fractured 21 with sinus opening and pus discharge. (b) Preoperative IOPA showing periapical lesion involving the apices of 21 and open apex. (c) Access opening done in 21. (d) Bleeding induced in 21 for revascularization. (e) Placement of CGF in root canal space. (f) MTA plug of 3 mm placed at the level of CEJ in 21. (g) Pre-op CBCT image showing the extent of lesion in sagittal slice. (h) Post-op CBCT image showing the extent of lesion in sagittal slice. (i) Pre-op CBCT showing the root dentin thickness measurement in sagittal slice. (j) Post-op CBCT showing the root dentin thickness measurement in sagittal slice. (k) Pre-op CBCT showing the apical diameter measurement in 21. (l) Post-op CBCT showing the apical diameter in 21.

and positive clinical impact in ridge augmentation and accelerated healing of intrabony defects, lateral cysts, and periapical pathologies, respectively [14–18]. In our recently published case report, we focused on the conspicuous coalescence of CGF and bone graft (sticky bone) to intercept a large periapical bony lesion, for which we garnered resounding success in stemming the repair and regenerative process [14]. Additionally, in our previously published clinical case presentation of two cases, we had implemented CGF as a scaffold in the surgical endodontic treatment procedures with great effect and were able to elicit successful healing outcomes [18]. Furthermore, Hong et al. reviewed the potential application of CGF and concluded that the autologous platelet concentrate could be a promising biomaterial in regenerative endodontics [19].

In case 1, routine IOPAR revealed a slight anatomical variation at the apex of 12 with periapical lesion which was followed by two parallax radiographs to confirm the same. Since periapical radiographs being a two-dimensional imaging modality, we could not ascertain as to whether the said tooth had a closed apical foramen and also could not assess the extent of the lesion in 11 and 12. In case 2, a single periapical radiograph confirmed the presence of blunderbuss canal with periapical lesion in 21. In both cases, the extent of lesion and apical diameter along with root dentin thickness had to be verified and measured with the aid of CBCT. According to AAE guidelines, CBCT scan with a small field of view is recommended in clinical research trials for diagnostic accuracy [20].

The use of anaesthetic solution without a vasoconstrictor was advocated in both our cases which was well in accordance with a study conducted by Petrino et al. [21]. It was reported that several attempts were made to induce bleeding into the canal space when anaesthetic solution containing a vasoconstrictor was employed. Jung et al. suggested that the induction of bleeding into the root canal provides stem cells that can induce dentin formation [22]. Similarly, in both our cases, bleeding was induced using a #80 K-file instrumented 2 mm beyond the working length. According to Wang et al., the outcome of revascularization procedure improved with the inclusion of blood clot in the root canal space which resulted in a process of repair rather than revitalization [23]. To that end, the autologous platelet concentrate has been effectively deployed in these cases as scaffold materials to compensate for the lack of formation of high-quality blood clots.

Rodella et al. demonstrated that growth factors TGF-ß1 and VEGF were found in abundance which according to the literature are highly essential for stimulating cell proliferation, matrix rehabilitation, and angiogenesis [24]. Based on an immunohistochemical analysis, the aforesaid study also confirmed the existence of circulating CD34+ cells in CGF and RBC layers which again is crucial for the revascularization process [25].

Disinfection is of prime importance in enhancing the predictability of regenerative endodontic procedures. According to Ruparel et al., Galler, and Segura-Egea et al., the use of antibiotics in regenerative endodontics should be avoided [26–28]. Althumairy et al. stated that disinfection with calcium hydroxide leads to a greater survival of SCAP cells as opposed to antibiotic pastes [29]. Irrigants are selected based on both their bacteriostatic or bactericidal properties and the ability to sustain the survival of stem cells. The chelating effect of 17% EDTA promoted the release of dentin-derived growth factors which in turn regulates the survival and differentiation of stem cells, whereas 2% chlorhexidine proved to be cytotoxic with no viable cells [30].

The biological mechanism of regeneration depends on the "self-renewal" [31] capacity of the stem cells of apical papilla (SCAP), capable of differentiating into odontoblast-like cells ultimately resulting in the formation of dentin-like tissue [32]. While treating nonvital immature permanent teeth, the preservation of SCAP promotes continuous formation of the root to its completion [33] Induced bleeding into the root canal space triggers higher concentration of mesenchymal stem cells (MSCs) from the apical papilla [34] that may not be sufficient for the formation of pulp-dentin complex; hence, autologous platelet concentrate as scaffold serves as a reservoir of growth factors, thus aiding in the regenerative process [35].

Histologic confirmation of dental pulp with an intact odontoblastic layer and restoration of a functional pulp is a pinnacle in regenerative treatment goals; therefore, further objective should be targeted at histological evaluation of viable pulp tissue [36]. The limitation of these case presentations is that it is not proved that true pulp-dentin complex regeneration has occurred for which histological examination is required. The effect of CGF in regenerative endodontics could be well established by randomized clinical trials and longer follow-up periods.

4. Conclusion

Although evidence concerning the implementation of CGF in revascularization procedures is scarce, however, based on available and limited data, it does deliver phenomenal success in diverse oral surgical applications (described earlier). In this case presentation, CGF was utilized with great effect as a fibrin-rich block, progressively releasing the much noteworthy growth factors to bring about a rapid and successful healing outcome. At one-year follow-up, CBCT assessment confirmed marked apical closure in case 1, increased root dentin thickness in case 2, and complete reduction in size of the periapical lesion in both cases. All things considered, CGF holds substantial promise for use in revascularization techniques to enhance the repair and regenerative process in a manner most beneficial in terms of all-round satisfactory healing of the immature permanent tooth.

Acknowledgments

The authors would like to acknowledge Dr. Sri Prakash for the skillful support rendered for CGF preparation.

References

[1] M. Cvek, "Prognosis of luxated non-vital maxillary incisors treated with calcium hydroxide and filled with gutta-percha. A retrospective clinical study," *Dental Traumatology*, vol. 8, no. 2, pp. 45–55, 1992.

[2] B. P. Mathew and M. N. Hegde, "Management of non vital immature teeth–case reports and review," *Endodontology*, vol. 18, pp. 18–22, 2010.

[3] P. E. Murray, F. Garcia-Godoy, and K. M. Hargreaves, "Regenerative endodontics: a review of current status and a call for action," *Journal of Endodontia*, vol. 33, no. 4, pp. 377–390, 2007.

[4] R. Chandki, M. Kala, P. Banthia, and R. Banthia, "From stem to roots: tissue engineering in endodontics," *Journal of Clinical and Experimental Dentistry*, vol. 4, no. 1, pp. e66–e71, 2012.

[5] T. Jeeruphan, J. Jantarat, K. Yanpiset, L. Suwannapan, P. Khewsawai, and K. M. Hargreaves, "Mahidol study 1: comparison of radiographic and survival outcomes of immature teeth treated with either regenerative endodontic or apexification methods: a retrospective study," *Journal of Endodontia*, vol. 38, no. 10, pp. 1330–1336, 2012.

[6] J. O. Andreasen, B. Farik, and E. C. Munksgaard, "Long-term calcium hydroxide as a root canal dressing may increase risk of root fracture," *Dental Traumatology*, vol. 18, no. 3, pp. 134–137, 2002.

[7] K. Reynolds, J. D. Johnson, and N. Cohenca, "Pulp revascularization of necrotic bilateral bicuspids using a modified novel technique to eliminate potential coronal discolouration: a case report," *International Endodontic Journal*, vol. 42, no. 1, pp. 84–92, 2009.

[8] D. C. Rule and G. B. Winter, "Root growth and apical repair subsequent to pulpal necrosis in children," *British Dental Journal*, vol. 120, no. 12, pp. 586–590, 1966.

[9] S. Mirkovic, T. Djurdjevic-Mirkovic, and T. Puskar, "Application of concentrated growth factors in reconstruction of bone defects after removal of large jaw cysts: the two cases report," *Vojnosanitetski Pregled*, vol. 72, no. 4, pp. 368–371, 2015.

[10] E. Borsani, V. Bonazza, B. Buffoli et al., "Biological characterization and in vitro effects of human concentrated growth factor preparation: an innovative approach to tissue regeneration," *Biologie et Médecine*, vol. 7, no. 5, p. 1, 2015.

[11] J. J. Gagnier, the CARE Group, G. Kienle et al., "The CARE guidelines: consensus-based clinical case reporting guideline development," *Journal of Medical Case Reports*, vol. 7, no. 1, 2013.

[12] P. G. Robey, M. F. Young, K. C. Flanders et al., "Osteoblasts synthesize and respond to transforming growth factor-type beta (TGF-beta) in vitro," *The Journal of Cell Biology*, vol. 105, no. 1, pp. 457–463, 1987.

[13] D. M. Dohan Ehrenfest, N. R. Pinto, A. Pereda et al., "The impact of the centrifuge characteristics and centrifugation protocols on the cells, growth factors, and fibrin architecture of a

leukocyte-and platelet-rich fibrin (L-PRF) clot and membrane," *Platelets*, vol. 29, no. 2, pp. 171–184, 2018.

[14] N. M. Sureshbabu, A. Ranganath, and B. Jacob, "Concentrated growth factor – surgical management of large periapical lesion using a novel platelet concentrate in combination with bone graft," *Annals of Maxillofacial Surgery*, vol. 10, no. 1, pp. 246–250, 2020.

[15] D. S. Sohn, J. W. Moon, Y. S. Moon, J. S. Park, and H. S. Jung, "The use of concentrated growth factors (CGF) for sinus augmentation," *Journal of Oral Implantology*, vol. 38, no. 1, pp. 25–38, 2009.

[16] J. Qiao, J. Duan, Y. Zhang, Y. Chu, and C. Sun, "The effect of concentrated growth factors in the treatment of periodontal intrabony defects," *Future Science OA*, vol. 2, no. 4, article FS136, 2016.

[17] X. Ying, Y. Chen, N. Luo, L. Shi, Y. Tong, and J. Zhang, "The use of concentrated growth factors and autogenous bone for periodontal soft tissue augmentation and bone regeneration: a case report," *Electronic Journal of Biology*, vol. 13, no. 3, pp. 269–273, 2017.

[18] N. Malli Sureshbabu, K. Selvarasu, M. Nandakumar, and D. Selvam, "Concentrated growth factors as an ingenious biomaterial in regeneration of bony defects after periapical surgery: a report of two cases," *Case Reports in Dentistry*, vol. 2019, Article ID 7046203, 6 pages, 2019.

[19] S. Hong, L. Li, W. Cai, and B. Jiang, "The potential application of concentrated growth factor in regenerative endodontics," *International Endodontic Journal*, vol. 52, no. 5, pp. 646–655, 2019.

[20] M. I. Fayad, M. Nair, M. D. Levin et al., "AAE and AAOMR joint position statement: use of cone beam computed tomography in endodontics 2015 update," *Oral Surgery, Oral Medicine, Oral Pathology, Oral Radiology*, vol. 120, no. 4, pp. 508–512, 2015.

[21] J. A. Petrino, K. K. Boda, S. Shambarger, W. R. Bowles, and S. B. McClanahan, "Challenges in regenerative endodontics: a case series," *Journal of Endodontia*, vol. 36, no. 3, pp. 536–541, 2010.

[22] I. Jung, S. Lee, and K. Hargreaves, "Biologically based treatment of immature permanent teeth with pulpal necrosis: a case series," *Journal of Endodontia*, vol. 34, no. 7, pp. 876–887, 2008.

[23] X. Wang, B. Thibodeau, M. Trope, L. M. Lin, and G. T.-J. Huang, "Histologic characterization of regenerated tissues in canal space after the revitalization/revascularization procedure of immature dog teeth with apical periodontitis," *Journal of Endodontia*, vol. 36, no. 1, pp. 56–63, 2010.

[24] L. F. Rodella, G. Favero, R. Boninsegna, A. Borgonovo, R. Rezzani, and F. Santoro, "TGF-beta1 and VEGF after fresh frozen bone allograft insertion in oral-maxillo-facial surgery," *Histology and Histopathology*, vol. 25, no. 4, pp. 463–471, 2010.

[25] L. F. Rodella, G. Favero, R. Boninsegna et al., "Growth factors, CD34 positive cells, and fibrin network analysis in concentrated growth factors fraction," *Microscopy Research and Technique*, vol. 74, no. 8, pp. 772–777, 2011.

[26] N. B. Ruparel, F. B. Teixeira, C. C. Ferraz, and A. Diogenes, "Direct effect of intracanal medicaments on survival of stem cells of the apical papilla," *Journal of Endodontia*, vol. 38, no. 10, pp. 1372–1375, 2012.

[27] K. M. Galler, "Clinical procedures for revitalization: current knowledge and considerations," *International Endodontic Journal*, vol. 49, no. 10, pp. 926–936, 2016.

[28] J. J. Segura-Egea, K. Gould, B. H. Şen et al., "European Society of Endodontology position statement: the use of antibiotics in endodontics," *International Endodontic Journal*, vol. 51, no. 1, pp. 20–25, 2018.

[29] R. I. Althumairy, F. B. Teixeira, and A. Diogenes, "Effect of dentin conditioning with intracanal medicaments on survival of stem cells of apical papilla," *Journal of Endodontia*, vol. 40, no. 4, pp. 521–525, 2014.

[30] E. G. Trevino, A. N. Patwardhan, M. A. Henry et al., "Effect of irrigants on the survival of human stem cells of the apical papilla in a platelet-rich plasma scaffold in human root tips," *Journal of Endodontia*, vol. 37, no. 8, pp. 1109–1115, 2011.

[31] H. Egusa, W. Sonoyama, M. Nishimura, I. Atsuta, and K. Akiyama, "Stem cells in dentistry–part I: stem cell sources," *Journal of Prosthodontic Research*, vol. 56, no. 3, pp. 151–165, 2012.

[32] W. Sonoyama, Y. Liu, D. Fang et al., "Mesenchymal stem cell-mediated functional tooth regeneration in swine," *PLoS One*, vol. 1, no. 1, article e79, 2006.

[33] G. T.-J. Huang, W. Sonoyama, Y. Liu, H. Liu, S. Wang, and S. Shi, "The hidden treasure in apical papilla: the potential role in pulp/dentin regeneration and bioroot engineering," *Journal of Endodontia*, vol. 34, no. 6, pp. 645–651, 2008.

[34] T. W. Lovelace, M. A. Henry, K. M. Hargreaves, and A. Diogenes, "Evaluation of the delivery of mesenchymal stem cells into the root canal space of necrotic immature teeth after clinical regenerative endodontic procedure," *Journal of Endodontia*, vol. 37, no. 2, pp. 133–138, 2011.

[35] K. M. Hargreaves, A. Diogenes, and F. B. Teixeira, "Treatment options: biological basis of regenerative endodontic procedures," *Pediatric Dentistry*, vol. 35, no. 2, pp. 129–140, 2013.

[36] M. Torabinejad and H. Faras, "A clinical and histological report of a tooth with an open apex treated with regenerative endodontics using platelet-rich plasma," *Journal of Endodontia*, vol. 38, no. 6, pp. 864–868, 2012.

2

Unusual Site for a White Nodule on the Palatine Tonsil: Presentation, Differential Diagnosis and Discussion

Ashwag Yagoub Aloyouny

Basic Dental Sciences Department, College of Dentistry, Princess Nourah Bint Abdulrahman University, Riyadh, Saudi Arabia

Correspondence should be addressed to Ashwag Yagoub Aloyouny; ayaloyouny@pnu.edu.sa

Academic Editor: Vlaho Brailo

Introduction. Palatine tonsils are part of the mucosa-associated lymphoid tissue, located in the oropharyngeal region. Although these tissues protect the body from foreign intruders, they are more prone to infections due to their anatomical structure and location. For instance, the differential diagnosis of a white lesion on the palatine tonsil can range from benign to malignant lesions. Oral lymphoepithelial cysts commonly arise as painless, yellowish nodules on the floor of the mouth and the ventral or lateral surface of the tongue. *Case Presentation.* This paper presents a rare case of an unusual site of a lymphoepithelial cyst (LEC) in the oral cavity. The lesion was located in the tonsil of a 20-year-old woman with a chief complaint of a painless, white lump in the back of the mouth for nine months. *Discussion.* The differential diagnosis of a white lesion on the palatine tonsil is caused by several factors, such as bacterial, viral, and fungal infections; trauma; stones; cysts; abscess; or cancer. In this case, both the clinical presentation and extra- and intraoral examinations were highly associated with LEC. Oral LEC etiopathogenesis is uncertain, and several theories have been proposed to discuss the causes of LEC. In addition, oral LEC could be monitored without surgical intervention if the nodule is asymptomatic. *Conclusion.* We emphasize the importance of a thorough clinical examination of oral and oropharyngeal lesions, which are usually neglected.

1. Introduction

The palatine tonsil is a component of the posterior oropharynx lymphoid tissue ring called Waldeyer's ring. The location of the palatine tonsil makes it more amenable to bacterial infections and cyst formation [1].

The differential diagnosis of a white lesion on the palatine tonsils encompasses benign and malignant lesions. Benign lesions are more common in this location, including oral lymphoepithelial cysts (LECs), tonsilloliths, and lipomas and infectious entities such as tonsillitis, strep throat, infectious mononucleosis, oropharyngeal candidiasis, and peritonsillar abscess [2]. It could also include benign lesions that have a potential for malignant transformation such as papilloma. Moreover, although malignant lesions rarely arise from the palatine tonsils, they are not excluded from the differential diagnosis list [3].

LECs are rare, benign, developmental, and nonodontogenic cysts. They may develop in any area of the body, which consists of lymphoid tissues. Usually, they are less than 1 cm in size. Oral LEC has a high occurrence on the floor of the mouth and in the lateral and ventral tongue. It affects females more than males (2 : 1) at any age [2].

The phenomenon of oral LECs in the palatine tonsils is very unlikely. Additionally, very few reported cases in the literature present oral LECs in the tonsils. Herein, we present a rare case of an oral LEC that appeared in the left palatine tonsil and discuss its resolution without intervention.

The work has been reported in line with the SCARE criteria [4].

2. Case Report

A 20-year-old woman visited the oral medicine clinic for evaluation of a nine-month history of a painless, white lesion at the back of the mouth. She believed that the lesion started as a pinhead size and then grew in size over time until it reached the present size. She did not recall any trauma or surgery in the area of the white patch. Her medical and dental histories were noncontributory. She denied taking any over-the-counter or prescribed medications, such as antibiotics or steroids. In addition, genetic problems, family medical history, and social history were unremarkable. Furthermore, the lesion was worrisome, which had a negative impact on daily life. Extraoral clinical examination was not significant. Routine laboratory blood test results were normal. The patient denied a history of fever, fatigue, body rashes, stuffy nose, headache, earaches, stiff neck, hoarseness, sore throat, coughing, sneezing, difficulty chewing or swallowing, halitosis, lymphadenopathy, and difficulty breathing. She also denied having hemoptysis and an unexplained weight loss in the last few weeks. Intraoral inspection revealed a 0.5 cm, asymptomatic, light yellow-white hued, smooth, raised, soft on palpation, movable, well-circumscribed, unilateral, localized submucosal nodule, exhibiting no exudate arising from the normal-sized left palatine tonsil (Figure 1). Radiographic interpretation of orthopantomograph showed normal anatomical structures and no signs of radiopacities in the left palatine tonsil region.

The differential diagnoses of the white lesion on the palatine tonsil, in this reported case, included tonsillar cyst, tonsilloliths, tonsillitis, papilloma, lipoma, strep throat, infectious mononucleosis, oropharyngeal candidiasis, and peritonsillar abscess.

In this case, the distinct clinical appearance, features, and clinical examination highly indicated an LEC. The patient was assured that the clinical appearance of the white lump in the tonsil was highly associated with the diagnosis of a benign nodule called an oral lymphoepithelial cyst. She was also provided with information regarding the possible treatment options and associated outcomes.

The ideal management for the white lesion on the palatine tonsil is to excise the lesion along with the whole tonsil. Therefore, an oral medicine specialist recommended performing a left palatine tonsillectomy. However, the surgical procedure of the affected palatine tonsil was not an option from the patient's side. Notably, the patient was anxious and worried about the surgical procedure and its consequences. Therefore, she refused to proceed with the surgical option. Because the nodule was asymptomatic and based on the lesion size (5 mm) and the patient's decision, the lesion was monitored regularly for an eight-month period. One-month, two-month, three-month, six-month, and eight-month follow-up periods were scheduled to monitor the lesion. The nodule did not change in size or color during this period. Surprisingly, the lesion ruptured and resolved spontaneously without any conventional or surgical intervention (Figure 2). At the one- and two-year follow-up, there were no signs of lesion recurrence.

3. Discussion

The posterior oropharynx contains a lymphoid tissue ring called Waldeyer's ring, which mainly involves the palatine tonsils, pharyngeal adenoid tonsils, Eustachian tonsils, and lingual tonsils. These lymphoid tonsils have special anatomical structures and locations, which make them more susceptible to bacterial infections and cyst formation [1].

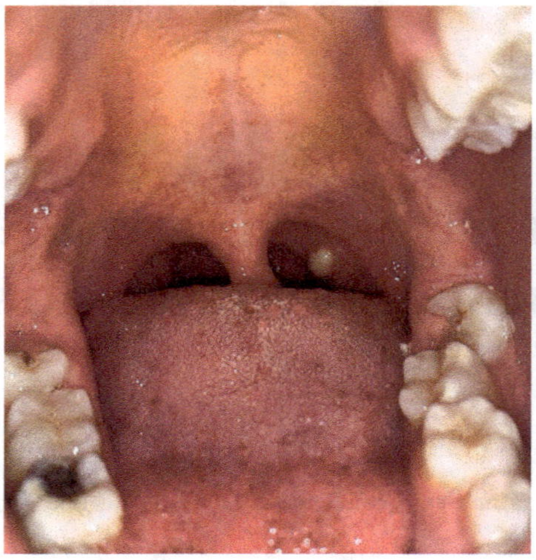

Figure 1: Clinical presentation of a 0.5 cm, yellow nodule with intact mucosa arising from the left palatine tonsil.

The differential diagnosis of a white lesion on the palatine tonsil includes tonsillar cysts or oral LECs, tonsilloliths, papillomas, lipomas, tonsillitis, strep throat or streptococcal pharyngitis, infectious mononucleosis, peritonsillar abscess, oropharyngeal candidiasis, and palatine cancers [5].

Tonsilloliths or tonsil stones are unilateral, painful, and hard on palpation and consist of calcium deposits in the lymphoid tissue crypts. These stones occur due to the accumulation of mucus, bacteria, and food particles, which are accompanied by dysphagia, halitosis, and otalgia [6]. Papilloma is not uncommon, benign, exophytic, cauliflower-like verrucous lesion that is characterized by a unique appearance and possesses finger-like projections on the rough surface of the lesion [7]. Lipomas are very rare to develop in the palatine tonsil, and there are few documented cases in the English literature [8].

Bacterial infections of the palatine tonsils, such as tonsillitis and strep throat or streptococcal pharyngitis, are contagious and usually caused by *Streptococcus pyogenes*. Bacterial infections commonly occur along with many symptoms such as fever, fatigue, sore throat, headache, and difficulty swallowing. If left untreated, it could progress to a peritonsillar abscess. Viral infections of the palatine tonsils, such as infectious mononucleosis or mono, are characterized by bilateral, white-yellowish pus covering both swollen tonsils. Infectious mononucleosis is caused by a contagious virus called the Epstein-Barr virus. Bacterial and viral infections commonly occur along with many symptoms such as fever, fatigue, sore throat, headaches, and difficulty swallowing [9].

Patients with a suppressed body immune system are at a high risk of oropharyngeal candidiasis. It is the most common type of fungal infection in the oral cavity and is usually caused by *Candida albicans*. Low body immunity could be caused by uncontrolled diabetes, long-term use of antibiotics, or steroid medications. The diagnosis of the infection can be confirmed by collecting throat swab samples and culture from the site of the white patches or lesions [9].

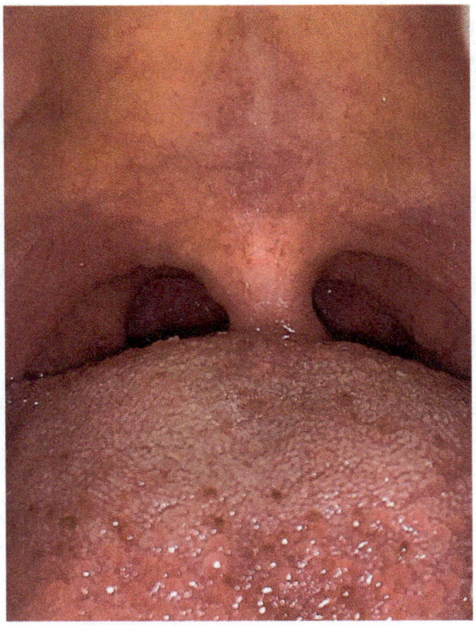

Figure 2: At eight-month follow-up visit, the yellow nodule in the left palatine tonsil completely disappeared.

In our case, the patient was in a very good health condition and did not complain of any abnormal signs or symptoms; the nodule had a distinct clinical appearance and was highly associated with LEC. LEC is an uncommon developmental, nonodontogenic cyst that was first described as a branchial cleft cyst in 1962 by Gold [10].

Yang et al. [2] studied the most common sites of oral LECs out of 120 reported cases. The study illustrated that 70.7% of oral LECs were encountered on the floor of the mouth, followed by the lateral surface (10.7%) and then the ventral surface of the tongue (7.3%). This study did not report any cases of palatine tonsils. Sykara et al. [11] collected data from 26 published cases, only two of which were in the palatine tonsils.

The pathogenesis of oral LEC is controversial, and many theories have been proposed to discuss the etiology of LEC. However, the most accepted theory was proposed by Knapp. He believed that oral LECs are pseudocysts that develop from submucosal lymphoid tissue aggregates on the floor of the mouth, ventral tongue, and soft palate [12].

Histopathological evaluation of oral LEC demonstrates a thick cystic cavity composed of parakeratinized stratified squamous epithelial lining filled with viscous fluid and desquamated keratin. The cystic wall is infiltrated by lymphocytes organized as germinal centers [13].

Oral LEC can be managed either conservatively or surgically based on the medical history, lesion size, lesion location, and patient discomfort. For instance, patients who have asymptomatic, small oral LECs can be monitored periodically. These small-sized oral LECs may rupture and disappear without surgical procedures. In the present case, the lesion was painless, approximately 0.5 cm in its greatest dimension, and the patient refused any intervention, but follow-up visits were conducted to monitor the lesion. The lesion disappeared after eight months of periodic follow-up visits [14]. Furthermore, for patients who complain of a large-sized lesion that causes dysphagia or risk of airway obstruction, surgical removal is indicated to avoid life-threatening conditions and improve patient quality of life.

4. Conclusion

The incidence of oral LEC in the palatine tonsils is uncommon. Based on the lesion size and the symptoms reported by the patient, oral LEC may be managed only with follow-up and clinical intraoral examination. In addition, oral LECs can resolve spontaneously without any kind of intervention.

5. Patient Perspective

The patient was assured that the lesion was benign and small in size and could resolve without intervention. The resolution of the lesion improved her self-confidence.

Consent

Written informed consent was obtained from the patient for publication of this case report and accompanying images. A copy of the written consent is available for review by the Editor-in-Chief of this journal on request.

Acknowledgments

This research was funded by the Deanship of Scientific Research at Princess Nourah Bint Abdulrahman University through the Fast-track Research Funding Program.

References

[1] N. Meegalla and B. W. Downs, "Anatomy, head and neck, palatine tonsil (faucial tonsils)," *Treasure Island (FL)*, Ashwag Yagoub Aloyouny, 2021.

[2] X. Yang, A. Ow, C. Zhang et al., "Clinical analysis of 120 cases of intraoral lymphoepithelial cyst," *Oral Surgery, Oral Medicine, Oral Pathology and Oral Radiology*, vol. 113, no. 4, pp. 448–452, 2012.

[3] G. Kumar, R. Sharma, D. Pal, and Geeta, "Various spectrum of lesion in palatine tonsil underwent for tonsillectomy in tertiary care center: a two years retrospective study," *International Journal of Otorhinolaryngology and Head and Neck Surgery*, vol. 6, no. 7, p. 1331, 2020.

[4] R. A. Agha, T. Franchi, C. Sohrabi, G. Mathew, and A. Kerwan, "The scare 2020 guideline: updating consensus surgical case report (scare) guidelines," *International Journal of Surgery*, vol. 84, pp. 226–230, 2020.

[5] M. Gottlieb, B. Long, and A. Koyfman, "Clinical mimics: an emergency medicine-focused review of streptococcal pharyngitis mimics," *The Journal of Emergency Medicine*, vol. 54, no. 5, pp. 619–629, 2018.

[6] M. Mesolella, M. Cimmino, M. Di Martino, G. Criscuoli, L. Albanese, and V. Galli, "Tonsillolith. Case report and review

of the literature," *Acta Otorhinolaryngol Ital*, vol. 24, no. 5, pp. 302–307, 2004.

[7] H. Mortazavi, Y. Safi, M. Baharvand, S. Rahmani, and S. Jafari, "Peripheral exophytic oral lesions: a clinical decision tree," *International Journal of Dentistry*, vol. 2017, Article ID 9193831, 19 pages, 2017.

[8] C.-P. Wang, P.-C. Kwan, and C.-Y. Ho, "Lipoma of the palatine tonsil," *Journal of the Formosan Medical Association*, vol. 106, no. 8, pp. 673–675, 2007.

[9] E. A. Sykes, V. Wu, M. M. Beyea, M. T. W. Simpson, and J. A. Beyea, "Pharyngitis: approach to diagnosis and treatment," *Canadian Family Physician*, vol. 66, no. 4, pp. 251–257, 2020.

[10] C. Gold, "Branchial cleft cyst located in the floor of the mouth: report of a case," *Oral Surgery, Oral Medicine, and Oral Pathology*, vol. 15, no. 9, pp. 1118–1120, 1962.

[11] M. Sykara, P. Ntovas, E. M. Kalogirou, K. I. Tosios, and A. Sklavounou, "Oral lymphoepithelial cyst: a clinicopathological study of 26 cases and review of the literature," *Journal of Clinical and Experimental Dentistry*, vol. 9, no. 8, pp. e1035–e1043, 2017.

[12] M. J. Knapp, "Pathology of oral tonsils," *Oral Surgery, Oral Medicine, and Oral Pathology*, vol. 29, no. 2, pp. 295–304, 1970.

[13] A. Buchner and L. S. Hansen, "Lymphoepithelial cysts of the oral cavity: a clinicopathologic study of thirty-eight cases," *Oral Surgery, Oral Medicine, and Oral Pathology*, vol. 50, no. 5, pp. 441–449, 1980.

[14] J. G. L. Castro, G. M. Ferreira, E. F. Mendonça, and L. A. Castro, "A rare occurrence of lymphoepithelial cyst in the palatine tonsil: a case report and discussion of the etiopathogenesis," *International Journal of Clinical and Experimental Pathology*, vol. 8, no. 4, pp. 4264–4268, 2015.

3

CBCT Evaluation and Conservative Management of a Large Periapical Lesion Associated with Dens Invaginatus Type II

Laïla Azzahim, Nisrin Bassim, and Faïza Abdallaoui

Faculty of Dentistry of Rabat, Mohamed V University, Rabat, Morocco

Correspondence should be addressed to Laïla Azzahim; dr.azzahim.laila@gmail.com

Academic Editor: Sreekanth Kumar Mallineni

This case report illustrated the conservative management of an invaginated type II tooth with a large periapical lesion. This dental malformation is characterized by the complexity of root canal anatomy, which when associated with a periapical lesion complicates the performance of conventional endodontic treatment, hence resulting to the difficulty of obtaining the optimal disinfection of the root canal system, which is an essential element for the success of any endodontic treatment. In the present case report, clinical and radiographic examinations were supplemented by CBCT examination to identify the root canal configuration and the extension of the periapical lesion. Conservative orthograde endodontic treatment was performed by combining mechanical and chemical action. Additionally, active nonsurgical decompression was performed and the follow-up visits revealed a favorable outcome.

1. Introduction

Dens invaginatus (DI), also known as dens in dente, is a dental malformation found mostly in the permanent dentition and has been reported to affect 0.3% to 10% of the population [1]. According to the most widely accepted theory, it results in an invagination of the enamel organ into the dental papilla prior to the calcification of dental tissues [2]. The maxillary lateral incisor is the most commonly affected tooth [3]. The root canal system is characterized by anatomic complexity. Thus, the diagnosis and treatment planning are considered difficult [4].

This case report showed the importance of the use of Cone Beam Computer Tomography (CBCT) evaluation to facilitate the exploration and accessibility of the complicated root canal system of the invaginated tooth. In addition, it demonstrated that the use of the orthograde conservative approach alone allowed the healing of the periapical lesion despite the complexity of the root canal anatomy and the wide extension of the periapical lesion.

2. Case Presentation

A 34-year-old male patient, with good general health, was referred for endodontic treatment of the maxillary lateral right incisor (tooth #12). The patient had priorly received an endodontic treatment by a general practitioner. The patient had been complaining of pain associated with recurrent palatal swelling on the right side of the palate for 6 months. There was no history of trauma.

The extraoral examination revealed no abnormalities. The intraoral examination showed tooth #12 as a "rice-shaped tooth," a palatal swelling on the right side (Figure 1), and a fistula in the alveolar mucosa, proximally to the apical area of tooth #12. Response to pulp sensitivity test was negative, while both vertical and horizontal percussions were positive. There was no increased tooth mobility or probing depth. Palpation at the level of palatal swelling was painful and allowed drainage of pus from the vestibular fistula (Figure 2).

The radiographic examination showed the presence of DI; the invagination extended from the crown to the root

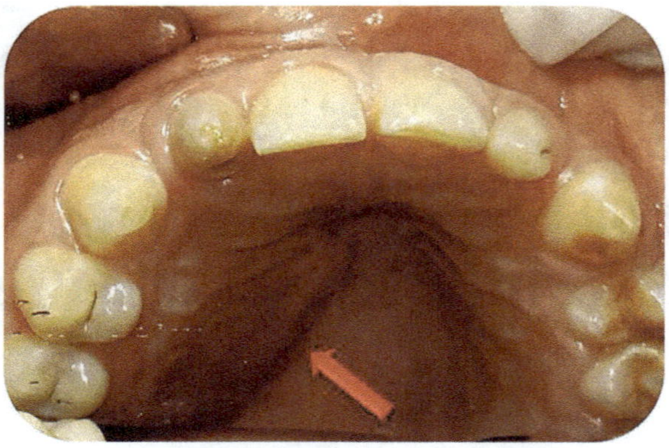

FIGURE 1: Preoperative photograph showing a palatal swelling on the right side.

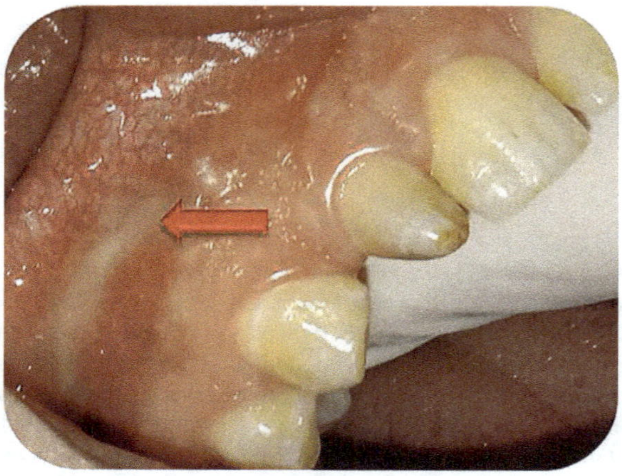

FIGURE 2: Drainage of pus from the vestibular fistula proximal to the apical area of tooth #12.

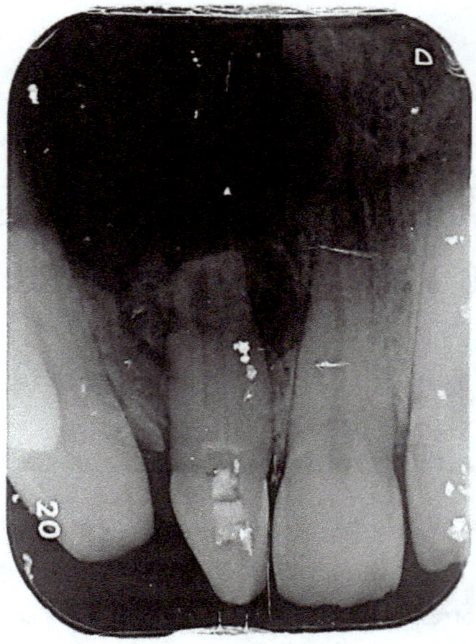

FIGURE 3: Preoperative radiograph showing a complex root canal configuration corresponding to that of type II DI associated with a large extending periapical image in relation to tooth #12.

apex, associated with a radiolucent lesion in the periapical area of tooth #12 (Figure 3). Cone Beam Computer Tomography (CBCT) scan showed the presence of type II invagination communicating with the root canal and revealed a large periapical radiolucency related to tooth #12 (Figures 4 and 5). The diagnosis was chronical apical periodontitis related to tooth #12 with an infected DI type II. The treatment plan was to perform an orthograde endodontic treatment.

After obtaining the patient's informed consent, a rubber dam was applied, the access cavity was modified, and the root canal and the invagination were located. The working length was measured using an apex locator and confirmed with an X-ray examination. Both the canal and the invagination were instrumented through a crown-down technique using manual instruments. In order to overcome the lack of mechanical instrumentation in the presence of complex root canal anatomy, all attention has been paid to chemical disinfection. Irrigation used was 2.5% Sodium Hypochlorite (NaOCl) for a total time of 30 minutes for the root canal and the invagination. NaOCl was conveyed into the canal using an irrigation syringe with a side outlet needle, the solution was renewed regularly. To improve disinfection, sonic activation was used with the EndoActivator sonic device (Dentsply Sirona) for 30 seconds. NaOCl irrigation was alternated with 17% Ethylene Diamine Tetra acetic Acid (EDTA) gel to dissolve inorganic substances. The active nonsurgical decompression with an irrigation syringe was performed with the objective of aspirating as much as possible the intracanal serosities. Then, the intracanal dressing with calcium hydroxide ($Ca(OH)_2$) paste was placed for 2 weeks. The access cavity was sealed with a temporary restorative material. Two weeks later, the tooth was asymptomatic. Since the intracanal serosities did not dry up, the intracanal medication was renewed. After a month, the tooth became asymptomatic and the canal dry. Then, root canal filling was performed by a lateral condensation technique associated with thermomechanical compaction using gutta-percha cones and the access cavity was restored using a laminate technique (glass ionomer cement-light-cured composite resin).

Clinical and radiographic control sessions were carried out at 6, 12, and 18 months after the treatment. During the follow-up period, no signs and symptoms related to the concerned tooth were reported by the patient and bone neoformation was noticed in the periapical area (Figure 6).

3. Discussion

The endodontic management of DI is a challenge due to the complexity of the root canal anatomy. Several classifications of DI have been proposed; the most commonly used one was proposed by Oehlers [5]. According to this classification, there are 3 types of invagination [5, 6].

(i) Type I shows an invagination limited to the crown

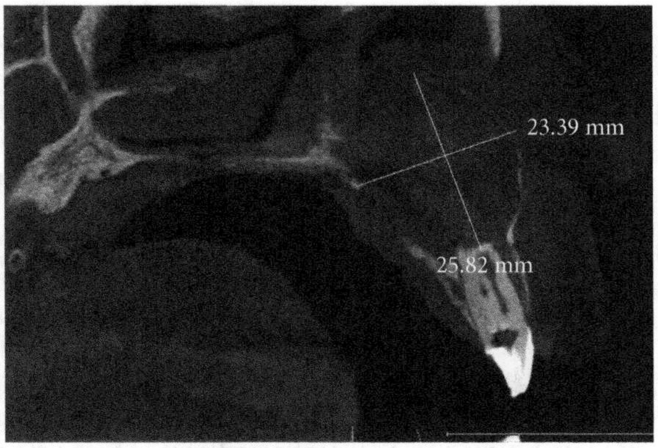

FIGURE 4: CBCT sagittal section confirmed that it is a type II DI, showing a wide radiolucent periapical image measuring 25.82 mm × 23.39 mm communicating with the nasal cavity.

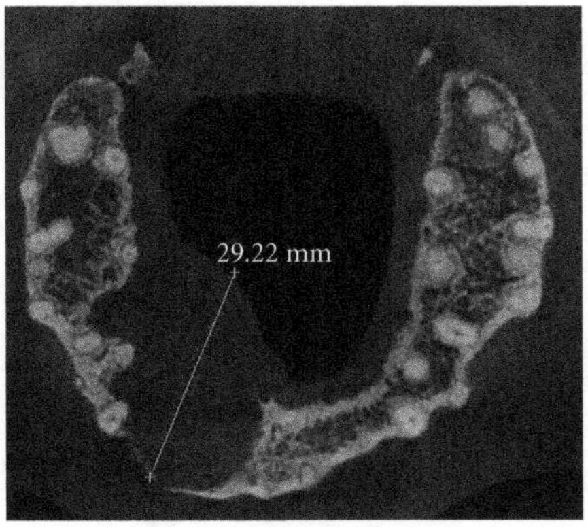

FIGURE 5: CBCT axial section showing the rupture of the internal and external bony cortices caused by the extension of the periapical lesion.

(ii) Type II extends below the cementoenamel junction, ends as a blind sac, and may or may not have communication with the pulp

(iii) Type III extends through the root and perforates the apical (type IIIa) or lateral area (type IIIb), without any immediate communication with the dental pulp [5]

When this complicated canal configuration (type II or III) is associated with an extensive periapical lesion, nonsurgical endodontic treatment is difficult to perform, but it must be considered before any surgical treatment [3]. The use of CBCT as an auxiliary tool is recommended for the diagnosis and the treatment planning of teeth with such developmental anomalies [7].

Root canal can be instrumented with manual or rotary files while it is recommended to shape the invagination with manual instruments to prevent the occurrence of instrumental fractures with rotary files within the invagination since the surface is predominantly covered by enamel and has varying shapes [4]. The use of XP-endo Finisher was also reported to shape the root canal in a maxillary lateral incisor presenting type II [8]. In the present case, both the root canal and the invagination were shaped with hand NiTi endodontic instruments according to the crown-down concept. It is important to increase the chemical disinfection alternating abundant 2.5% NaOCl irrigation and EDTA gel to compensate for the insufficient mechanical instrumentation due to the complex canal anatomy [9]. NaOCl has bactericidal, solvent effect for organic material and lubricating action [10]. The use of ultrasound is essential in optimizing disinfection [8] and can also be supplemented with $Ca(OH)_2$ medication [11]. Although this medication is currently controversial, its use in this case was justified by the presence of abundant serosities and the need to alkalize the inflammatory medium created by the periapical reaction of the deep periodontium, in addition to its antibacterial, hemostatic, and osteogenic properties [11]. Another molecule that can be used in intracanal medication is the 2% chlorhexidine gel. It has a bactericidal action on bacteria resistant to $Ca(OH)_2$ by remanence effect for at least two weeks, but its parietal elimination is difficult [12].

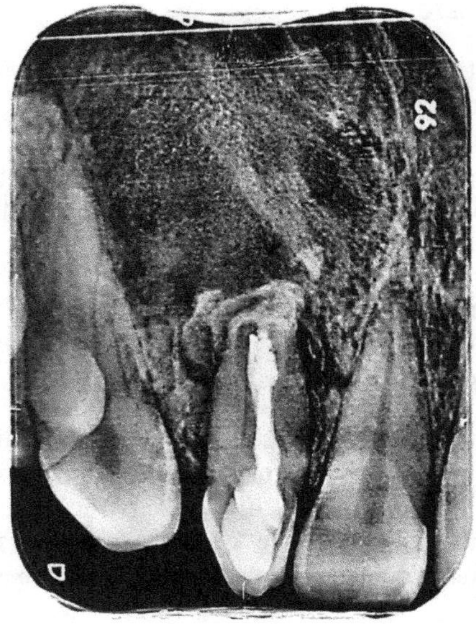

FIGURE 6: 18-month follow-up radiograph showing signs of bone neoformation.

The success of endodontic therapy can be judged clinically by the absence of symptoms (pain, infection, and fistula) and radiographically by the decrease in bone lesion size, osteoformation, and reconstitution of the lamina dura [13]. The presented case was followed up clinically and radiographically for 18 months, indicating the absence of clinical symptoms associated with regression of the radiolucent image size, which was considered a success of endodontic orthograde therapy. Indeed, studies have shown that 90% of periapical lesions show signs of healing after 1 year when the majority of lesions heal at 2 years, but in some cases, the disappearance of the lesion can take 4 to 5 years. Generally, the success of endodontic treatment is judged during the first year of follow-up [13].

3.1. The Clinical Relevance. The importance of combining mechanical action with chemical disinfection has been widely proven to eradicate endodontic infection and can be effective without resorting to endodontic surgery which is mutilating to periapical tissue even with complex anatomy.

4. Conclusion

In the light of the findings of the present case report, three points need to be stressed:

(i) The presence of a complex root canal anatomy does not systematically justify the use of apical surgery

(ii) Orthograde endodontic treatment is the first-line treatment for the management of large extended periapical lesions. Only if this fails, other options should be considered

(iii) The mechanical instrumental action is limited by the presence of a complex root canal anatomy. To compensate for this limitation of mechanical action, contact time of the chemical solution should be extended and more molecules should be added

References

[1] A. Abu Hasna, D. M. T. Ungaro, A. A. P. de Melo et al., "Non-surgical endodontic management of dens invaginatus: a report of two cases," *F1000Research*, vol. 8, no. 8, p. 2039, 2019.

[2] A. Alani and K. Bishop, "Dens invaginatus Part 1: classification, prevalence and aetiology," *International Endodontic Journal*, vol. 41, no. 12, pp. 1123–1136, 2008.

[3] P. Zhang and X. Wei, "Combined therapy for a rare case of type III dens invaginatus in a mandibular central incisor with a periapical lesion: a case report," *Journal of Endodontia*, vol. 43, no. 8, pp. 1378–1382, 2017.

[4] K. Bishop and A. Alani, "Dens invaginatus. Part 2: clinical, radiographic features and management options," *International Endodontic Journal*, vol. 41, no. 12, pp. 1137–1154, 2008.

[5] F. A. Oehlers, "Dens invaginatus (dilated composite odontome): I. Variations of the invagination process and associated anterior crown forms," *Oral Surgery, Oral Medicine, and Oral Pathology*, vol. 10, no. 11, pp. 1204–1218, 1957, contd.

[6] N. G. de Oliveira, M. T. da Silveira, S. M. Batista, S. R. M. Veloso, M. V. Carvalho, and R. M. C. Travassos, "Endodontic treatment of complex dens invaginatus teeth with long term follow-up periods," *Iran Endod Journal*, vol. 13, no. 2, pp. 263–266, 2018.

[7] V. Mehta, A. Raheja, and R. K. Singh, "Management of dens in dente associated with a chronic periapical lesion," *BML Case Reports*, vol. 11, 2015.

[8] E. A. Rodrigues, F. G. Belladonna, G. De-Deus, and E. J. Silva, "Endodontic management of type II dens invaginatus with open apex and large periradicular lesion using the XP-endo Finisher: a case report," *Journal of Clinical and Experimental Dentistry*, vol. 10, no. 10, pp. e1040–e1044, 2018.

[9] C. S. Teixeira, M. C. Felippe, and W. T. Felippe, "The effect of application time of EDTA and NaOCl on intracanal smear layer removal: an SEM analysis," *International Endodontic Journal*, vol. 38, no. 5, pp. 285–290, 2005.

[10] C. E. Radcliffe, L. Potouridou, R. Qureshi et al., "activity of varying concentrations of sodium hypochlorite on the endodontic microorganisms Actinomyces israelii, A. naeslundii, Candida albicans and Enterococcus faecalis," *International Endodontic Journal*, vol. 37, no. 7, pp. 438–446, 2004.

[11] C. Sathorn, P. Parashos, and H. Messer, "Antibacterial efficacy of calcium hydroxide intracanal dressing: a systematic review and meta-analysis," *International Endodontic Journal*, vol. 40, no. 1, pp. 2–10, 2007.

[12] L. S. Gonçalves, R. C. Rodrigues, C. V. Andrade Junior, R. G. Soares, and M. V. Vettore, "The effect of sodium hypochlorite and chlorhexidine as irrigant solutions for root canal disinfection: a systematic review of clinical trials," *Journal of Endodontia*, vol. 42, no. 4, pp. 527–532, 2016.

[13] S. Huumonen and D. Ørstavik, "Radiographic follow-up of periapical status after endodontic treatment of teeth with and without apical periodontitis," *Clinical Oral Investigations*, vol. 17, no. 9, pp. 2099–2104, 2013.

4

Novel Management for Severe Odontogenic Maxillary Sinusitis Based on Pathophysiology

Yoshio Ohyama,[1] **Masaru Ogawa**,[2] **and Satoshi Yokoo**[2]

[1]*Department of Oral and Maxillofacial Surgery, Shizuoka City Shizuoka Hospital, 10-93, Outemachi, Aoi-ku, Shizuoka-shi, Shizuoka 420-8690, Japan*
[2]*Department of Oral and Maxillofacial Surgery, and Plastic Surgery, Gunma University Graduate School of Medicine, 3-39-15, Showamachi, Maebashi-Shi, Gunma 371-8511, Japan*

Correspondence should be addressed to Yoshio Ohyama; yohyama1219@gmail.com

Academic Editor: Ozkan Ozgul

Endoscopic sinus surgery is commonly performed to treat odontogenic maxillary sinusitis. However, recurrence and natural ostium reclosure often occur due to the inadequate patency of the excretory route. Furthermore, classical maxillary sinus radical surgery is still performed for odontogenic maxillary sinusitis even though it can cause postoperative maxillary sinus deformation, loss of function, and a postoperative maxillary cyst. A management that addresses these issues has not yet been identified. This study reported a conservative maxillary sinus management, wherein a nasoantral window is prepared and the thickened maxillary sinus mucosa is preserved, using the Caldwell–Luc approach. This study presents a case of severe odontogenic maxillary sinusitis that spread to the frontal sinus. This novel management facilitated complete recovery from severe odontogenic maxillary sinusitis in this case.

1. Introduction

Odontogenic maxillary sinusitis (OMS) management initially involved classical maxillary sinus radical surgery (MSRS) [1, 2]. However, this surgery was found to cause postoperative maxillary cysts (POMCs) several decades after treatment [3].

The maxillary sinus mucosa (MSM) is essential for the elimination of foreign substances and bacteria from the maxillary sinus. Removing the MSM during MSRS changes the anatomy of the maxillary sinus. Moreover, the maxillary sinus loses its function following the procedure [4]. Minimally invasive endoscopic sinus surgery (ESS) with natural ostium winding, which treats the causative tooth, has been commonly performed to treat OMS [2, 5]. However, ESS provides an inadequate excretory tract for the OMS, which is a more serious condition than general nasal sinusitis [4, 6]. In addition, the causative site of OMS is located distally, below the natural ostium. This study described a conservative maxillary sinus management (CMSM) without MSM removal for severe OMS spreading to the frontal sinus.

1.1. Case Report. A 54-year-old man was referred to our oral and maxillofacial surgery department by the otolaryngology department for OMS treatment. The patient came in with the chief complaint of pain radiating from his right cheek to his forehead. Physical examination revealed left cheek tenderness without swelling. Teeth #25 and #26 (FDI World Dental Federation ISO-3950) were root-canal-treated; however, the roots were underfilled. Panoramic radiograph suggested that the root apex was exposed to the maxillary sinus (Figure 1(a)). Computed tomography revealed opacification extending from the left maxillary sinus to the left frontal sinus (Figure 1(b)). The patient was clinically diagnosed with OMS caused by teeth #25 and #26. As the patient was keen to preserve his teeth, he was referred for endodontic treatment. His symptoms did not improve despite endodontic treatment and long-term antibiotic administration. Thus,

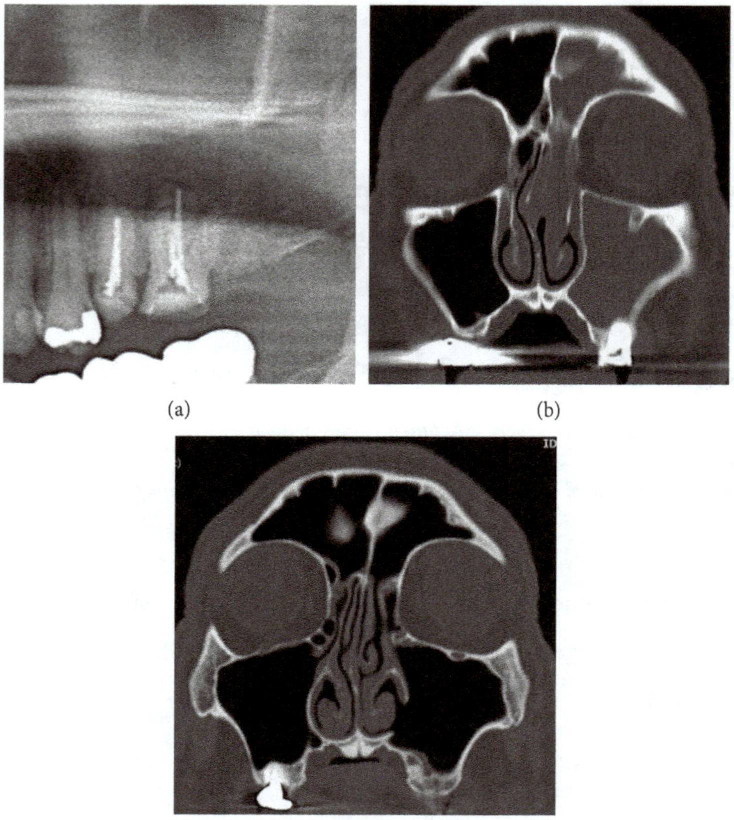

(a) (b) (c)

Figure 1: Radiographic findings. (a) Panoramic radiograph taken after the endodontic treatment of teeth #25 and #26 showing complete obturation of the roots except for the buccal distal root canal of #26. (b) Frontal plane of the preoperative computerized tomography (CT) scan revealed opacity extending from the left maxillary sinus to the left frontal sinus. (c) Frontal plane of the postoperative CT scan showed patency of the nasoantral window and the clearness of the left maxillary sinus and the left frontal sinus two years postoperatively.

CMSM was performed. Two years after the operation, recovery of OMS was observed. The anatomy and function of the maxillary sinus were completely restored. The nasoantral window was open, and the causative teeth were preserved (Figure 1(c)).

1.2. Surgical Procedure. Under general anesthesia, a 5- to 10-mm incision was made on the cervical side of the gingivobuccal fold of the left maxilla and the bone. The mucoperiosteal flap was raised, and the cortical bone around the canine fossa was removed to gain access to the left maxillary sinus. The root apices of teeth #25 and #26 protruded into the maxillary sinus, due to which the MSM corresponding to their root apices was removed through the left maxillary sinus followed by their apicoectomy (Figure 2). The root filling material of the buccal distal root canal of tooth #26 was not found (Figure 1(a)). Thus, retrograde filling was performed using 4-META/MMA-TBB resin. After irrigation with saline, the other thickened MSM was preserved (Figure 2). A large nasoantral window was prepared in the inferior nasal meatus. The vertical position of the nasoantral window was decided using the palatal wall as a guide. In addition, since the inferior nasal meatus was slightly raised on the inner wall of the maxillary sinus, the nasoantral window was created with a saw and hammer in this raised area atraumatically after removing the

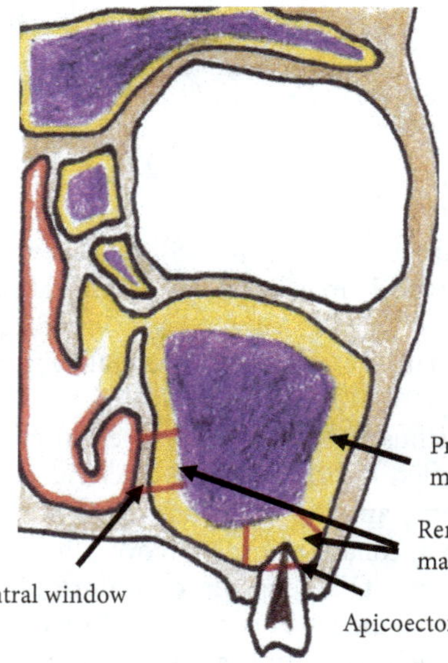

Figure 2: Schematic demonstration of CMSM. Apicoectomy was performed. A large nasoantral window in the inferior nasal meatus was prepared. The remainder of the thickened MSM was preserved.

surrounding MSM. Finally, the nasoantral window was enlarged with the bone forceps (Figure 2). Gauze, with acromycin, was inserted into the maxillary sinus from the nasal cavity through the nasoantral window. The gauze was removed one week postoperatively. Clarithromycin was administered for one month postoperatively.

2. Discussion

MSM derived from pseudostratified ciliated epithelium is essential for maxillary sinus ventilation and clearance [7]. MSM removal, associated with MSRS, disrupts the normal function and morphology of the maxillary sinus [6, 8], resulting in POMC and sclerosis of the maxillary sinus wall. CMSM, developed by Yokoo et al. [4], preserves the MSM, facilitating the healing of the thickened pseudostratified ciliated epithelium and the recovery of maxillary sinus function. ESS has been commonly performed to treat OMS; however, ESS provides an inadequate excretory passage and ventilation hole, and recloses easily. In OMS, pus accumulates from the inferior nasal meatus due to gravity [6]. Therefore, a large nasoantral window in the inferior nasal meatus should be created to prevent nasolacrimal duct damage and to secure an excretory passage and ventilation hole [4]. Furthermore, apicoectomy and retrograde root canal filling of the causative teeth, which cannot be performed with ESS, can be achieved with CMSM. In this case, the function of the maxillary sinus and the causative teeth were successfully preserved via CMSM with apicoectomy and retrograde root canal filling. Further investigations involving a larger group of patients are necessary to establish this procedure as a treatment option.

3. Conclusions

This study proposed a novel treatment method, CMSM, which preserved the function and morphology of the maxillary sinus while preventing POMC in an OMS patient.

References

[1] R. Aukštakalnis, R. Simonavičiūtė, and R. Simuntis, "Treatment options for odontogenic maxillary sinusitis: a review," *Stomatologija*, vol. 20, no. 1, pp. 22–26, 2018, (in eng).

[2] K. C. Lee and S. J. Lee, "Clinical features and treatments of odontogenic sinusitis," *Yonsei Medical Journal*, vol. 51, no. 6, pp. 932–937, 2010, (in eng).

[3] B. M. Niederquell, P. A. Brennan, M. Dau, M. Moergel, B. Frerich, and P. W. Kämmerer, "Bilateral postoperative cyst after maxillary sinus surgery: report of a case and systematic review of the literature," *Case Reports in Dentistry*, vol. 2016, Article ID 6263248, 8 pages, 2016, (in eng).

[4] Y. Satoshi, S. Takahiro, O. Masaru, and T. Yu, *Application of Endodontic Mircosurgery to the Causative Tooth of Maxillary Sinusitis*, Dental Diamond, Japan, 2015.

[5] F. Costa, E. Emanuelli, L. Franz, A. Tel, and M. Robiony, "Single-step surgical treatment of odontogenic maxillary sinusitis: a retrospective study of 98 cases," *Journal of Cranio-Maxillo-Facial Surgery*, vol. 47, no. 8, pp. 1249–1254, 2019, (in eng).

[6] S. S. B. James and A. Duncavage, Eds., *The Maxillary Sinus: Medical and Surgical Management*, Thieme, New York, 2011.

[7] W. T. Anselmo-Lima, M. D. Ferreira, F. C. Valera, M. Rossato, V. R. de Mello, and R. C. Demarco, "Histological evaluation of maxillary sinus mucosa after functional endoscopic sinus surgery," *American Journal of Rhinology*, vol. 21, no. 6, pp. 719–724, 2007, (in eng).

[8] S. Inanli, A. Tutkun, C. Batman, I. Okar, C. Uneri, and M. A. Sehitoğlu, "The effect of endoscopic sinus surgery on mucociliary activity and healing of maxillary sinus mucosa," *Rhinology*, vol. 38, no. 3, pp. 120–3, 2000, (in eng).

5

Long-Term Follow-up after Conservative Surgical Treatment of Odontogenic Myxoma: A Case Report and Literature Review

Hitoshi Sato, Yuji Kurihara, Sunao Shiogama, Kotaro Saka, Yuya Kurasawa, Masakatsu Itose, Atsutoshi Yaso, and Tatsuo Shirota

Department of Oral and Maxillofacial Surgery, School of Dentistry, Showa University, 2-1-1 Kitasenzoku, Ota-ku, Tokyo 145-8515, Japan

Correspondence should be addressed to Hitoshi Sato; h.sato@dent.showa-u.ac.jp

Academic Editor: Eugenio Maiorano

Odontogenic myxoma (OM) is a relatively rare, benign odontogenic tumor with locally aggressive behavior, but it is a nonmetastasizing neoplasm of the jaw bones. Although radical resection with an appropriate surgical margin is recommended, emerging evidence has suggested that a more conservative approach will result in acceptable recurrence rates with less morbidity if careful long-term follow-up is provided. A 56-year-old Japanese man with odontogenic myxoma of the left mandible was conservatively treated by surgical enucleation and curettage because he desired functional and cosmetic preservation. During a follow-up period of 100 months, the patient has remained clinically and radiologically free of recurrence. As far as we can ascertain, 20 reports published after 1990 described 37 patients with mandibular OM that had been treated by conservative surgery. Tumors recurred during a mean follow-up of 49.2 ± 42.8 months in 7 (18.9%) patients, and only one of five patients who were followed up for over 100 months developed recurrence. The rate of recurrence decreased from 24.0% to 8.3% when follow-up exceeded 60 months. Although enucleation and curettage have proven effective, the risk of recurrence remains considerable and long-term follow-up is indispensable. More evidence of long-term outcomes after conservative surgery for OM is needed.

1. Introduction

Odontogenic myxoma (OM) is a benign, locally invasive, aggressive, nonmetastasizing neoplasm of the jaw bones. It is the third most common odontogenic lesion with an annual incidence of ~0.07 new patients per million people [1, 2]. Although OM is a benign tumor, radical treatment is needed because the rate of local recurrence ranges from 10% - 33% [3-5]. Surgical resection with a minimum bone margin of 1 cm has been advocated [6-9], but emerging evidence suggests that a more conservative surgical approach will result in acceptable recurrence rates with less patient morbidity if follow-up can be over the long term [7, 10-12]. However, little has been reported about the actual long-term follow-up of patients with OM after conservative surgery. Here, we describe a mandibular odontogenic myxoma that was treated by conservative surgery and followed up for 100 months thereafter.

2. Case Report

2.1. Patient Information. A 56-year-old Japanese man was referred from a dental clinic for further examination of a radiolucent finding on the left side of his mandible in January 2010. The patient reported having no symptoms in his mouth including the left mandible area. His medical and dental history was noncontributory. An extraoral examination upon initial presentation revealed unremarkable findings and no complaints of paresthesia. An intraoral examination also confirmed the absence of redness and tender swelling of the left mandibular mucosa (Figure 1). Panoramic radiography revealed an extensive multilocular radiolucent area with imprecise borders and a "soap bubble appearance" (Figure 2). Computed tomography showed an approximately 39 × 19 × 11 mm tumor that extended to the roots of four teeth (#33 - 36; Figures 3(a) and 3(b)). We considered that the odontogenic tumor was benign and an incisional biopsy

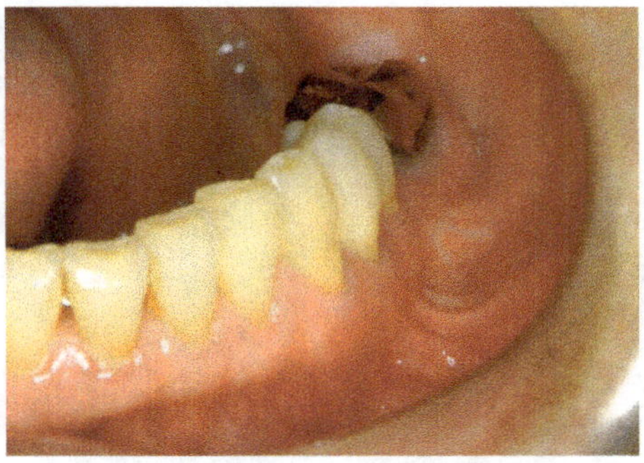

Figure 1: Intraoral photography before surgery. The image shows no symptoms such as redness or swelling of mucosa in the mandible.

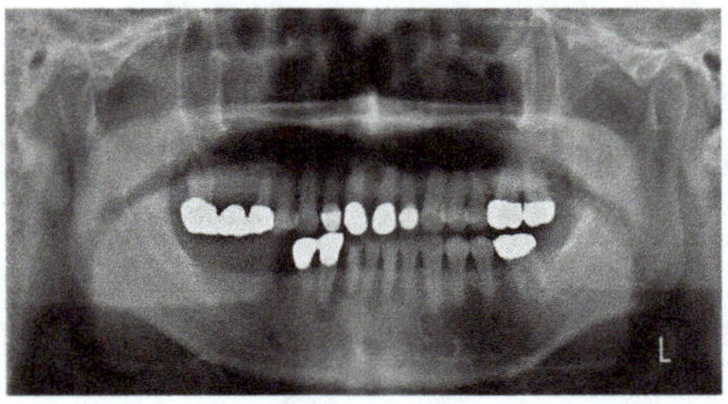

Figure 2: Panoramic dental radiography before surgery. The image shows extensive multilocular radiolucent area with imprecise borders and "soap bubble appearance".

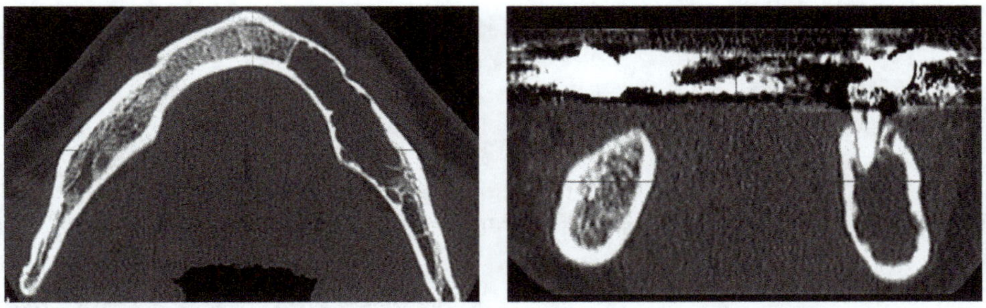

(a) (b)

Figure 3: Computed tomography (CT) image before surgery. The axial (a) and coronal (b) CT images show tumor infiltration of cortical bone extending to the inferior mandibular border.

was performed under local anesthesia. The histopathological findings revealed loosely arranged spindle-shaped cells in a myxoid fibrous stroma, indicating a clinical diagnosis of an odontogenic tumor. Segmental resection of the mandible was planned. The patient was given repeated and careful explanations about the high likelihood of recurrence, but he insisted upon a more conservative approach as he desired functional and cosmetic preservation. Conservative surgery then proceeded under general anesthesia after endodontic treatment of #33 - 36 was completed. The surgery consisted of extracting the second premolar from the left mandible, followed by total enucleation and vigorous curettage of the bone (Figure 4(a)). The surgical specimen (Figure 4(b)) revealed apparently benign, spindled-shaped cells in a loose and abundant mucoid stroma (Figures 5(a) and 5(b)). These findings confirmed the diagnosis of odontogenic myxoma. The immediate postoperative period and wound healing were uneventful. The patient underwent monthly clinical examinations for the first year thereafter, then every two months during the second year. Panoramic X-rays were obtained every three months for the first two years. Annual follow-up for eight years included panoramic X-rays and CT imaging (Figures 6(a) and 6(b), respectively), which showed no clinical or radiological signs of recurrence.

3. Discussion

Odontogenic myxomas are very rare (<10% all odontogenic tumors) benign tumors of the ectomesenchymal and/or mesenchymal origin [13, 14]. They are locally invasive and slow--growing, and their pathological characteristics in the tooth-bearing areas of the mandible and maxilla are well defined [13-17]. The radiographic features are described as those of a multilocular lesion with a "soap bubble" or "spider web" appearance [14-17]. Such lesions are often discovered incidentally during routine dental checkups, and about 60%

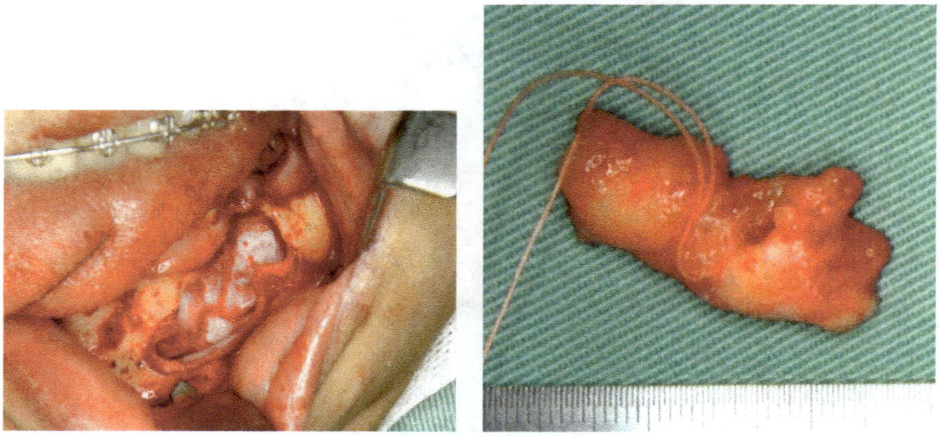

(a) (b)

FIGURE 4: Surgical procedures and resected specimen. The total enucleation and wide curettage of the surrounding bone (a) and resected specimen (b).

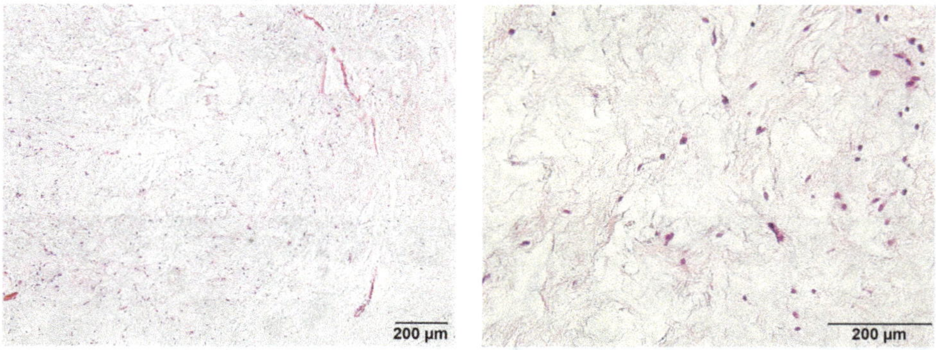

(a) (b)

FIGURE 5: Pathophysiological findings of stained specimen. Hematoxylin and eosin stain ×100 (a) and ×400 (b) magnification.

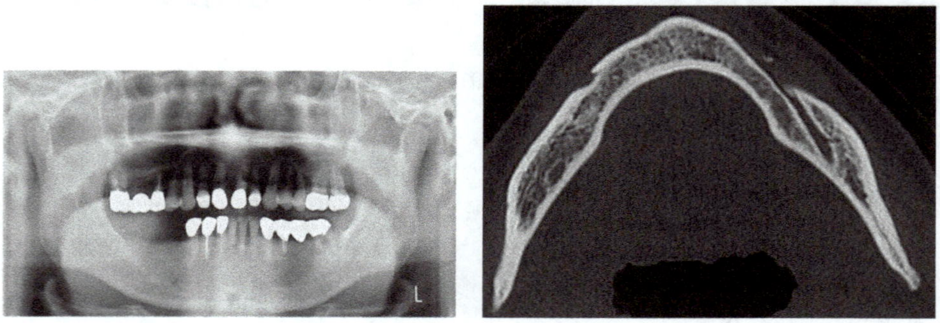

(a) (b)

FIGURE 6: Images of the jaw at 96 months after surgery. The panoramic dental radiograph (a) and computed tomography image (b) show no signs of recurrence.

of patients are in their second or third decade of life [4, 18]. Although the present patient was asymptomatic, panoramic radiography of the left mandible revealed an extensive radiolucent and multilocular area with imprecise borders that extended from the root of tooth #33 to that of tooth #36.

The treatment strategy for OM remains controversial. Because OM is locally aggressive and it can potentially cause extensive bony destruction, the treatment of choice seems to be radical surgery such as segmental resection. Indeed, complete surgical removal with curettage and peripheral ostectomy alone seems insufficient since OM is not encapsulated and myxomatous tissue infiltrates adjacent bone [3, 6-9]. Thus, the only initial treatment option for extended OM in principle is surgical resection because of the high risk of recurrence which reportedly ranges from 10% to 33% [4, 5]. In addition, recurrence rates can reach

TABLE 1: Clinical reports of mandibular odontogenic myxoma published after 1990.

No.	Author	Year	Age	Sex	Follow-up period (months)	Treatment	Recurrence	Size (mm)
1	Oliveira et al. [21]	2018	9	F	6	E/C	None	NA
2	Albanese et al. [22]	2012	25	F	6	E	None	21.2 × 47.6
3	Mauro et al. [23]	2012	6	M	6	E/C	None	NA
4	Subramaniam et al. [7]	2016	16	—	7	M	None	NA
5	Shivashankara et al. [24]	2017	13	M	12	E/N	None	40 × 20
6	Subramaniam et al. [7]	2016	18	—	12	E	None	NA
7	Miranda Rius et al. [25]	2013	55	M	12	E/C	None	33 × 28
8	Hammad et al. [26]	2016	45	F	13	M	None	50 × 30
9	Francisco et al. [27]	2017	9	F	14	E/C	Recurrence	NA
10	Francisco et al. [27]	2017	12	F	16	E/C	Recurrence	NA
11	Sumi et al. [28]	2000	48	M	22	E/C	None	70 × 25 × 15
12	Mittal et al. [29]	2016	48	F	24	E/C	Recurrence	25 × 20
13	Lin and Basile [30]	2010	25	F	24	E	None	NA
14	Lo Muzio et al. [4]	1996	21	M	24	E/C	None	NA
15	Lo Muzio et al. [4]	1996	28	M	24	E/C	Recurrence	NA
16	Bucci et al. [31]	1993	28	M	24	E/C	None	43 × 40
17	Francisco et al. [27]	2017	7	F	26	E/C	None	NA
18	Francisco et al. [27]	2017	15	F	27	E/C	Recurrence	NA
19	Lo Muzio et al. [4]	1996	16	F	31	E/C	None	NA
20	Francisco et al. [27]	2017	30	F	34	E/C	None	NA
21	Boffano et al. [11]	2011	38	M	38	E/C	None	25
22	Boffano et al. [11]	2011	42	F	40	E/C	None	30
23	Boffano et al. [11]	2011	20	M	42	E/C	None	20
24	Rajasekhar et al. [32]	2008	17	F	48	M	None	70 × 30
25	Lo Muzio et al. [4]	1996	22	F	48	E/C	Recurrence	NA
26	Takahashi et al. [6]	2018	37	F	73	E/C	None	40 × 19 × 12
27	Chaudhary et al. [33]	2015	25	F	84	E/C/M	None	NA
28	Li et al. [18]	2006	7	M	84	E/C	None	NA
29	Li et al. [18]	2006	32	M	84	E/C	None	NA
30	Lo Muzio et al. [4]	1996	65	F	84	E/C	None	NA
31	Francisco et al. [27]	2017	17	M	85	E/C	None	NA
32	Francisco et al. [27]	2017	11	F	98	E/C	None	NA
33	Present case		56	M	100	E/C	None	39 × 19 × 11
34	Francisco et al. [27]	2017	27	F	117	E/C	None	NA
35	Kawase-Koga et al. [10]	2014	40	M	120	E/C	None	40 × 30 × 15
36	Li et al. [18]	2006	37	M	132	C	None	NA
37	Kansy et al. [17]	2012	33	F	180	M	Recurrence	NA

Abbreviations: M: male, F: female, E: enucleation, C: curettage, M: marginal resection, and NA: not available.

25% after simple enucleation and curettage alone [19, 20]. On the other hand, some reports described that the choice of current recommended therapy depends on the size of the lesion and its nature and behavior between curettage and radical excision [3, 7]. In the present case, CT had shown that the tumor included the #33 - #36 apex and extended to the inferior border of the mandible. Therefore, radical resection such as block resection for mandible was strongly recommended. However, the patient rejected this strategy because he desired functional and cosmetic preservation, and in fact, conservative treatment with enucleation, curettage, and marginal resection would confer several advantages over the radical approach. It is substantially less invasive, it can be surgically implemented via an intraoral approach, and it offers the possibility of preserved nerve function and aesthetics and a shorter stay in the hospital. Recent evidence suggests that a more conservative approach will result in acceptable recurrence rates with less morbidity to patients if long-term follow-up is provided [7, 10-12]. Table 1 describes 20 reports of 37 patients with that was treated by conservative surgery [4, 6, 7, 10, 11, 17, 18, 21-33]. The mean age of the patients was 27.0 ± 15.2, and 20 (54%) were female. The tumors in almost all of them were managed by enucleation and curettage and recurred in 7 (18.9%). One and six of the procedures with recurrence had undergone marginal resection and enucleation with curettage, respectively. The patients were followed up for a mean of 49.2 ± 42.9 (range, 2 - 180) months. Including the present patient, only five have been followed up for over 100 months and the tumor recurred in one of them. The recurrence rate among all patients who were treated by conservative surgery was 19.0%. This rate is relatively lower than that previously described [19, 20]. Furthermore, our investigation of the literature indicated that the rate of recurrence decreases from 24.0% to 8.3% when the follow-up period exceeds 60 months.

The main reason for recurrence is thought to be incomplete removal rather than the intrinsic biological behavior of the OM [34]. Although the tendency is towards a more conservative surgical approach for children and a more radical approach for adults, Kansy et al. does not support this management strategy because the recurrence rates between enucleation and segmental resection are similar [17]. Tumor size has recently been considered to be a factor in the choice of a radical or more conservative surgical approach [4, 10, 11]. Conservative surgical procedures such as enucleation and curettage are recommended when the diameter of OM is <3 cm, whereas a radical approach such as segmental resection with immediate reconstruction is preferred when patients have larger tumors [11]. The conservative surgical recommendation is to enucleate a lesion with wide curettage of normal tissue or a generous amount of apparently intact tissue or even marginal resection of the mandible [12]. This approach has the advantage of preserving vital structures and maintaining oral function, and it could be applied to treat OM that recur after simple surgery [12]. However, one patient who developed recurrent OM 15 years after the initial procedure including tumor resection with the preservation of mandibular continuity has been described [17]. More radical surgery is inevitable for a large number of patients due to a tendency towards more extensive OM with significant destruction of key structures [17, 27]. Moreover, the rate of OM recurrence remains vague because few reports described long-term follow-up after conservative surgery. Thus, more evidence about long-term outcomes after conservative surgical treatment of OM is needed.

4. Conclusions

A conservative surgical approach comprising enucleation and curettage can be effective for OM management. Recurrence rates decreased from 24.0% to 8.3% among patients who were treated with conservative surgery and followed up for over 60 months. The risk of recurrence is likely to be considerable, and long-term follow-up is indispensable for the conservative management of OM.

References

[1] E. W. Odell and K. Adebiyi, "Odontogenic myxoma/myxofibroma," in *El-Naggar AK*, J. K. C. Chan, Ed., pp. 229-230, WHO Classification of Head and Neck Tumors. IARC Press, Lyon, 2017.

[2] E. N. M. Simon, M. A. W. Merkx, E. Vuhahula, D. Ngassapa, and P. J. W. Stoelinga, "Odontogenic myxoma: a clinicopathological study of 33 cases," *International Journal of Oral and Maxillofacial Surgery*, vol. 33, no. 4, pp. 333–337, 2004.

[3] Y. Leiser, I. Abu-El-Naaj, and M. Peled, "Odontogenic myxoma-a case series and review of the surgical management," *Journal of Cranio-Maxillo-Facial Surgery*, vol. 37, no. 4, pp. 206–209, 2009.

[4] L. L. Muzio, P. F. Nocini, G. Favia, M. Procaccini, and M. D. Mignogna, "Odontogenic myxoma of the jaws: a clinical, radiologic, immunohistochemical, and ultrastructural study," *Oral Surgery, Oral Medicine, Oral Pathology, Oral Radiology, and Endodontics*, vol. 82, no. 4, pp. 426–433, 1996.

[5] B. O. Abiose, H. A. Ajagbe, and O. Thomas, "Fibromyxomas of the jawbones–a study of ten cases," *British Journal of Oral & Maxillofacial Surgery*, vol. 25, no. 5, pp. 415–421, 1987.

[6] Y. Takahashi, K. Tanaka, H. Hirai, E. Marukawa, T. Izumo, and H. Harada, "Appropriate surgical margin for odontogenic myxoma: a review of 12 cases," *Oral Surgery, Oral Medicine, Oral Pathology, Oral Radiology*, vol. 126, no. 5, pp. 404–408, 2018.

[7] S. S. Subramaniam, A. A. Heggie, R. Kumar, and J. M. Shand, "Odontogenic myxoma in the paediatric patient: a review of eight cases," *International Journal of Oral and Maxillofacial Surgery*, vol. 45, no. 12, pp. 1614–1617, 2016.

[8] N. Kumar, M. Kohli, S. Pandey, and P. Agarwal, "Odontogenic myxoma," *Journal of Maxillofacial and Oral Surgery*, vol. 13, no. 2, pp. 222–226, 2014.

[9] T. J. King III, J. Lewis, L. Orvidas, and D. Kademani, "Pediatric maxillary odontogenic myxoma: a report of 2 cases and review of management," *Journal of Oral and Maxillofacial Surgery*, vol. 66, no. 5, pp. 1057–1062, 2008.

[10] Y. Kawase-Koga, H. Saijo, K. Hoshi, T. Takato, and Y. Mori, "Surgical management of odontogenic myxoma: a case report and review of the literature," *BMC Research Notes*, vol. 7, no. 1, p. 214, 2014.

[11] P. Boffano, C. Gallesio, A. Barreca, F. A. Bianchi, P. Garzino-Demo, and F. Roccia, "Surgical treatment of odontogenic myxoma," *Journal of Craniofacial Surgery*, vol. 22, no. 3, pp. 982–987, 2011.

[12] L. S. S. Zanetti, B. M. de Carvalho, I. R. Garcia, L. A. P. de Barros, P. L. dos Santos, and A. C. R. de Moraes Ferreira, "Conservative treatment of odontogenic myxoma," *The Journal of Craniofacial Surgery*, vol. 22, no. 5, pp. 1939–1941, 2011.

[13] P. J. Slootweg and A. R. M. Wittkampf, "Myxoma of the jaws. An analysis of 15 cases," *Journal of Maxillofacial Surgery*, vol. 14, no. 1, pp. 46–52, 1986.

[14] G. Martínez-Mata, A. Mosqueda-Taylor, R. Carlos-Bregni et al., "Odontogenic myxoma: clinico-pathological, immunohistochemical and ultrastructural findings of a multicentric series," *Oral Oncology*, vol. 44, no. 6, pp. 601–607, 2008.

[15] S. Singaraju, S. P. Wanjari, and R. N. Parwani, "Odontogenic myxoma of the maxilla: a report of a rare case and review of the literature," *Journal of Oral and Maxillofacial Pathology*, vol. 14, no. 1, pp. 19–23, 2010.

[16] C. E. E. Noffke, E. J. Raubenheimer, N. J. Chabikuli, and M. M. R. Bouckaert, "Odontogenic myxoma: review of the literature and report of 30 cases from South Africa," *Oral Surgery, Oral Medicine, Oral Pathology, Oral Radiology, and Endodontics*, vol. 104, no. 1, pp. 101–109, 2007.

[17] K. Kansy, P. Juergens, Z. Krol et al., "Odontogenic myxoma: diagnostic and therapeutic challenges in paediatric and adult patients–a case series and review of the literature," *Journal of Cranio-Maxillo-Facial Surgery*, vol. 40, no. 3, pp. 271–276, 2012.

[18] T. J. Li, L. S. Sun, and H. Y. Luo, "Odontogenic myxoma: a clinicopathologic study of 25 cases," *Archives of Pathology & Laboratory Medicine*, vol. 130, no. 12, pp. 1799–1806, 2006.

[19] D. C. Zimmerman and D. C. Dahlin, "Myxomatous tumors of the jaws," *Oral Surgery, Oral Medicine, and Oral Pathology*, vol. 11, no. 10, pp. 1069–1080, 1958.

[20] R. E. Barros, F. V. Dominguez, and R. L. Cabrini, "Myxoma of the jaws," *Oral Surgery, Oral Medicine, and Oral Pathology*, vol. 27, no. 2, pp. 225–236, 1969.

[21] S. V. Oliveira, A. C. Rocha, M. M. Ceccheti, C. de Barros Gallo, and F. A. Alves, "Odontogenic myxoma in a child treated with enucleation and curettage," *Autopsy & Case Reports*, vol. 8, no. 3, article e2018042, 2018.

[22] M. Albanese, P. F. Nocini, A. Fior et al., "Mandibular reconstruction using fresh frozen bone allograft after conservative enucleation of a mandibular odontogenic myxoma," *Journal of Craniofacial Surgery*, vol. 23, no. 3, pp. 831–835, 2012.

[23] A. Mauro, L. Lipari, S. Tortorici, A. Leone, A. Gerbino, and M. Buscemi, "Expression of MMP-2 and MMP-9 in odontogenic myxoma in a child: report of a clinical case," *Odontology*, vol. 101, no. 2, pp. 233–238, 2013.

[24] C. Shivashankara, M. Nidoni, S. Patil, and K. T. Shashikala, "Odontogenic myxoma: a review with report of an uncommon case with recurrence in the mandible of a teenage male," *The Saudi Dental Journal*, vol. 29, no. 3, pp. 93–101, 2017.

[25] J. Miranda Rius, A. Nadal, E. Lahor, B. Mtui, and L. Brunet, "Unusual presentation of localized gingival enlargement associated with a slow-growing odontogenic myxoma," *International Journal of Oral Science*, vol. 5, no. 3, pp. 172–175, 2013.

[26] H. M. Hammad, Y. M. Hasen, A.-A. M. Odat, A. M. Mikdadi, and R. A. Safadi, "Odontogenic myxoma with diffuse calcifications: a case report and review of a rare histologic feature," *Oral Surgery, Oral Medicine, Oral Pathology, Oral Radiology*, vol. 122, no. 4, pp. e116–e124, 2016.

[27] A. L. Francisco, T. C. Chulam, F. O. Silva et al., "Clinicopathologic analysis of 14 cases of odontogenic myxoma and review of the literature," *Journal of Clinical and Experimental Dentistry*, vol. 9, no. 4, pp. e560–e563, 2017.

[28] Y. Sumi, O. Miyaishi, K. Ito, and M. Ueda, "Magnetic resonance imaging of myxoma in the mandible: a case report," *Oral Surgery, Oral Medicine, Oral Pathology, Oral Radiology, and Endodontics*, vol. 90, no. 5, pp. 671–676, 2000.

[29] Y. Mittal, A. Chugh, K. G. Varghese, S. Dwivedi, and V. Goyal, "Management of recurrent odontogenic myxoma of mandible: a clinical case report," *Journal of Clinical and Diagnostic Research*, vol. 10, no. 10, pp. ZD30–ZD31, 2016.

[30] Y. L. Lin and J. R. Basile, "A case of odontogenic myxoma with unusual histological features mimicking a fibro-osseous process," *Head and Neck Pathology*, vol. 4, no. 3, pp. 253–256, 2010.

[31] E. Bucci, L. L. Muzio, M. D. Mignogna, and G. de Rosa, "Odontogenic myxoma: report of a case with peculiar features," *Journal of Oral and Maxillofacial Surgery*, vol. 49, no. 1, pp. 91–94, 1991.

[32] G. Rajasekhar, M. Mushtaq, N. G. Vura, R. Shekar, and S. Kumar, "Condyloma acuminatum associated with odontogenic myxoma: a case report," *Journal of Maxillofacial and Oral Surgery*, vol. 8, no. 4, pp. 384–387, 2009.

[33] Z. Chaudhary, P. Sharma, S. Gupta, S. Mohanty, M. Naithani, and A. Jain, "Odontogenic myxoma: report of three cases and retrospective review of literature in Indian population," *Contemporary Clinical Dentistry*, vol. 6, no. 4, pp. 522–528, 2015.

[34] J. G. Batsakis, "Myxomas of soft tissues and the facial skeleton," *Annals of Otology, Rhinology & Laryngology*, vol. 96, no. 5, pp. 618-619, 1987.

6

Acemannan Induced Bone Regeneration in Lateral Sinus Augmentation Based on Cone Beam Computed Tomographic and Histopathological Evaluation

Hai Anh Trinh,[1] Van Viet Dam,[2] Wijit Banlunara,[3] Polkit Sangvanich,[4] and Pasutha Thunyakitpisal[5]

[1]Multidisciplinary Dental Biomaterials Science Program, Graduate School, Chulalongkorn University, Bangkok 10330, Thailand
[2]Department of Implantology, Hanoi National Hospital of Odonto-Stomatology, Hanoi 100000, Vietnam
[3]Department of Pathology, Faculty of Veterinary Science, Chulalongkorn University, Bangkok 10330, Thailand
[4]Department of Chemistry, Faculty of Science, Chulalongkorn University, Bangkok 10330, Thailand
[5]Department of Anatomy, Multidisciplinary Dental Biomaterials Science Program, Research Unit of Herbal Medicine, Biomaterial and Material for Dental Treatment, Faculty of Dentistry, Chulalongkorn University, Bangkok 10330, Thailand

Correspondence should be addressed to Pasutha Thunyakitpisal; pthunyak@yahoo.com

Academic Editor: Jose López-López

Acemannan, the major polysaccharide extracted from Aloe vera, is biomaterial that has demonstrated osteoinductive effects *in vitro* and *in vivo*. However, the effect of acemannan sponges on bone formation in open-type sinus augmentation has not evaluated. Here, we report a case study using radiographic and histological analyses to investigate the effect of acemannan on bone formation after lateral sinus lift surgery. The case was a 57-year-old female patient with an atrophic left posterior maxilla who underwent lateral sinus lift using an acemannan sponge using the two-stage procedure. In the first stage, an acemannan sponge was inserted through the bony window and placed between the antral floor and the elevated sinus membrane. Cone beam computed tomography (CBCT) images were taken immediately as baseline and 6-month postoperation for evaluation. A bone core specimen was also obtained for histological examination at the time of implant placement. The histological results revealed new bone formation, and the CBCT images demonstrated increased alveolar bone height at 6-month postoperation. Our findings suggest that an acemannan sponge could be a biomaterial for inducing bone formation in sinus lift surgery.

1. Introduction

Limited residual alveolar bone height is frequently encountered in the edentulous posterior maxilla due to its anatomy and physiology, sinus enlargement, and postextraction alveolar bone resorption [1]. These circumstances result in thin antral floor bone, which is unfavorable for dental implant placement. Thus, various bone augmentation techniques have been introduced to overcome this problem. A lateral sinus lift is the recommended technique when the residual bone height is less than 5 mm, which is performed by creating a bony window in the lateral wall of the maxillary sinus, followed by lifting the sinus membrane and placing a grafting material to enhance bone formation [2, 3]. This procedure can be performed as a one- or two-stage procedure. In cases of extremely minimal residual bone (1–3 mm), it may be difficult to achieve implant stability; in these cases, a two-stage procedure is performed [4]. The sinus bone is augmented at the first operation. The implant is then placed at the second operation at 6-month postoperation after the bone healing period.

Many bone substitute materials have been used for sinus bone augmentation including autografts, allografts, xenografts, and alloplasts [5]. Although an autograft is considered the optimum material for a bone graft due to its osteoconductive, osteoinductive, and osteogenic properties, donor site morbidity and limited quantities are disadvantages of this material [6]. In addition, allografts and xenografts have a risk

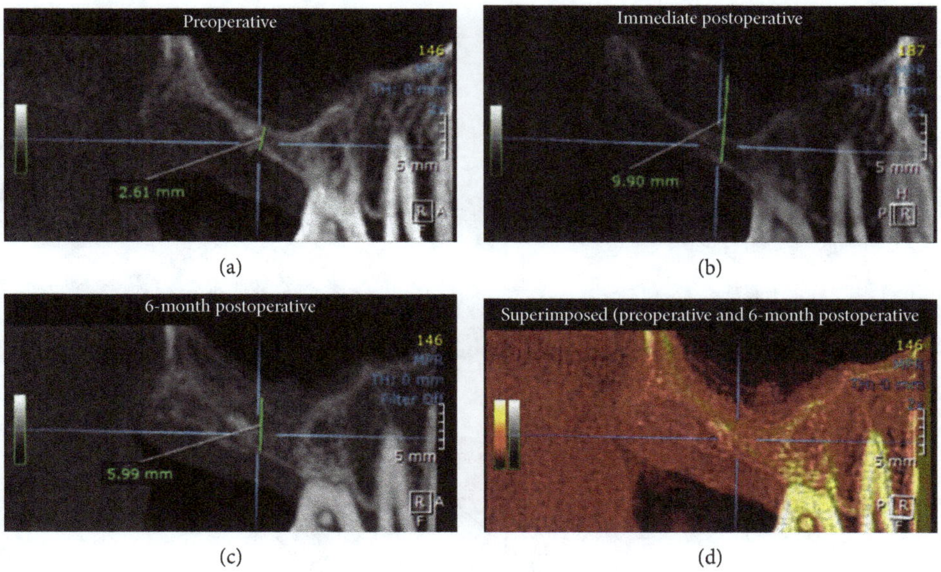

FIGURE 1: The sagittal view CBCT images show the left posterior edentulous maxillary region of the patient at preoperation (a), immediate postoperation (b), 6-month postoperation (c), and superimposed CBCT image between preoperation and 6-month postoperation of the lateral sinus augmentation (d).

of disease transmission and religious concerns [7]. Many researchers have been searching for alternative biomaterials to overcome these drawbacks.

Aloe vera is known for its wound healing effect. Acemannan, the major polysaccharide fraction from Aloe vera, has been reported as a promising biomaterial for bone regeneration [8]. Acemannan has shown osteoinductive effects, enhancing the alveolar bone and bone density in tooth extraction sockets [9, 10]. However, the radiographic and histological evaluation of acemannan on bone formation in direct sinus lift surgery has not been investigated. In this study, acemannan was extracted from fresh Aloe vera pulp gel and characterized with ^{13}C- and ^{1}H-nuclear magnetic resonance spectroscopy and Fourier transform infrared spectroscopy as previously described [11, 12]. The acemannan sponge was prepared by dissolved 150 mg acemannan in 3 ml sterile distilled water, frozen at -80°C overnight, and then lyophilized for 24 h [10]. The sponge was sterilized by gamma irradiation (Thailand Institute of Nuclear Technology, Bangkok, Thailand) and stored in a desiccator until used. In this case, the patient underwent lateral sinus augmentation with an acemannan sponge at the first stage without immediate implant placement. The outcome was evaluated radiographically and histologically.

2. Case Presentation

A 57-year-old, nonsmoking female patient with good general health was referred to the Department of Implantology, National Hospital of Odonto-Stomatology, Hanoi, Vietnam, with a complaint of loss of chewing ability on the upper left side. Her clinical examination found that the upper left second and third molars were missing. The patient's dental history revealed that the upper left second and third molars were extracted due to severe aggressive periodontal disease many years ago, and the patient refused to use a removable denture. The initial CBCT evaluation demonstrated left maxillary sinus pneumatization and a 2.61 mm residual bone height in the edentulous region underneath the sinus (Figure 1(a)). Based on these findings, a two-stage lateral sinus lift procedure was planned. Bleeding time, coagulation time, and clot retraction time assays were performed. The patient was informed about the study and procedure protocol and agreed to participate in this study.

The patient was prescribed 600 mg clindamycin 1 h before surgery [13] and rinsed with 0.12% chlorhexidine solution (Peridex 3M ESPE, 3M Dental Products, St. Paul, MN, USA) for 1 min prior to the operation. Local anesthesia (2% lidocaine with epinephrine 1 : 80,000, Lignospan Special, Septodont, Saint-Maur-des-Fosses, France) was administered. Subsequently, a midcrestal incision and releasing incisions were performed, and a full-thickness mucoperiosteal buccal flap was raised to expose the alveolar bone. A bony window in the lateral wall of the sinus was created using an SLA KIT (Neobiotech, Seoul, South Korea). The lateral bony window wall was removed with a periosteal elevator, and the sinus membrane was lifted. A 150 mg acemannan sponge was placed on the antral floor under the elevated sinus membrane. The bony window wall was repositioned, and the incisions were sutured using a 4.0 nonabsorbable suture (Ethicon, Inc., Somerville, NJ, USA). A CBCT scan was immediately performed as baseline.

Postoperatively, the patient was prescribed 300 mg clindamycin 3 times daily for 7 days, 0.12% chlorhexidine solution for mouthwash (10 ml for 1 min, 3 times/day for 10 days), and a nonsteroidal analgesic (ibuprofen 400 mg, 3 times/day for 3 days; as needed) [14]. The patient was called to ask about any postoperative complications at days 1 and 3. The patient was seen 7 days postoperatively for suture removal and clinical evaluation. The patient was then recalled at 6-month postoperation to assess bone formation using CBCT. Implant placement was performed at the

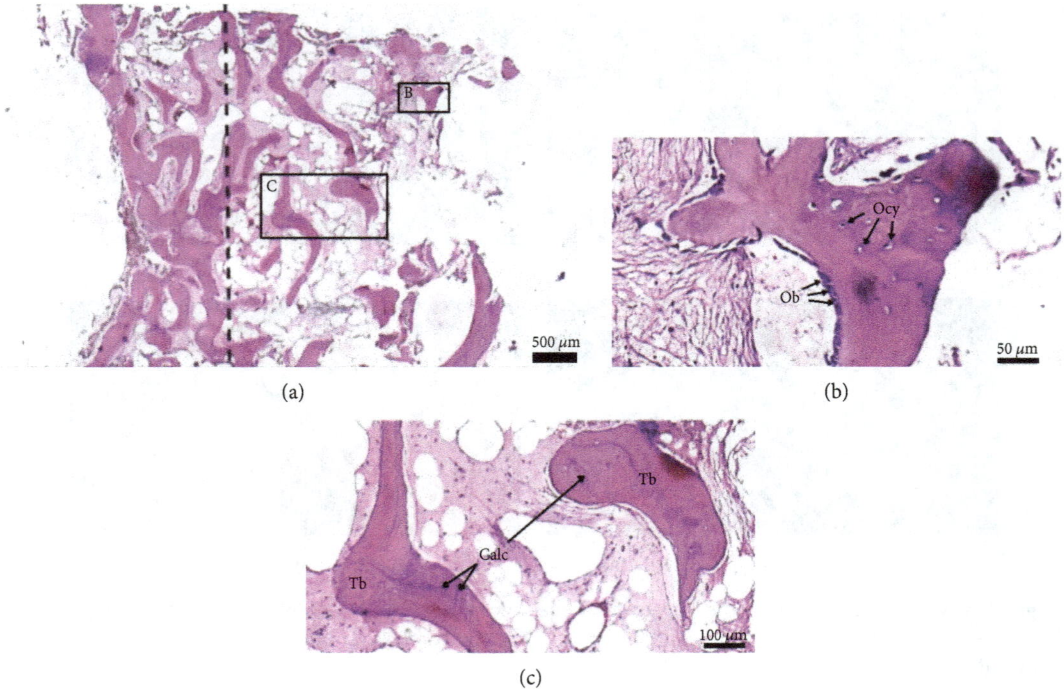

Figure 2: (a) Low-magnification image of the histopathological evaluation using H&E staining of the 6-month postoperation bone core specimen. The dashed line represents the border between the pre- and postoperation residual bone. (b) High-magnification image demonstrates active cuboidal osteoblasts (Ob) and osteocytes (Ocy) in lacunae. (c) High-magnification image shows thick trabeculae (Tb), bone lacunae, and calcification zone (Calc).

second stage. A sinus core biopsy specimen was obtained at the implant site prior to implant placement using a 3 mm trephine bur and stored in Bouin's fixative. The bone core sample was submitted for histopathological examination. During the study, the patient was instructed not to wear any denture to prevent interference with wound healing.

2.1. Radiographic Image Acquisition. The CBCT radiograph was performed immediately and 6-month postoperation using a Planmeca ProMax 3D (Planmeca, Helsinki, Finland) with fixed exposure parameters of 96 kV, 7 mA, 50 × 55 mm FOV, 75 μm slice thickness, and 15.152 seconds. The images were obtained to evaluate the residual bone quality and quantity and any possible maxillary sinus pathology. To minimize the error from radiographic image alignment, the OnDemand3D™ fusion module software (Cybermed Inc., Seoul, South Korea) was used to generate a superimposed image in the sagittal plane. With the advancement of this technology, the difference between pre- and postoperative images could be accurately and reliably observed in the superimposed image to evaluate the treatment results [15]. The method uses a basic concept from information theory and mutual information (MI) as a matching criterion [16]. To perform the image fusion process, the manual registration was used first to roughly align the image datasets. Next, an automated registration tool was used to automatically fuse the image datasets. The residual bone heights between baseline and 6-month postoperation were determined and compared. The residual bone heights were measured at the site where the implant would be placed.

2.2. Histopathological Processing. The bone core specimen was demineralized in 10% formic acid, dehydrated in ethanol–acetone, and embedded in paraffin. 6 μm thickness sections were prepared in the longitudinal midline direction and stained with hematoxylin-eosin (H&E). The sections were scanned, recorded by slide digitalization (Pannoramic Scan, 3DHistech Ltd., Budapest, Hungary), and analyzed using the CaseViewer 2.0 (3DHistech Ltd., Budapest, Hungary) program. The sections were examined by a blinded pathologist. The results are presented descriptively.

2.3. Clinical and CBCT Evaluation. There were no adverse events during the surgical procedure or healing period. The patient did not experience any postsurgical complications. The immediate postoperative CBCT images showed that the sinus wall membrane was elevated and the space was filled by the acemannan sponge (Figure 1(b)). The 6-month postoperative CBCT images revealed that the radiographic bone height had increased from 2.61 to 5.99 mm (Figures 1(c) and 1(d)).

2.4. Histopathological Evaluation. The sections did not demonstrate any signs of inflammation. New bone formation was observed. Active osteoblasts were present on the periphery of the newly formed bone. Numerous osteocytes in lacunae illustrated the vitality of the bone specimen (Figures 2(a) and 2(b)). A zone of calcification confirmed the mineralization process. Thick bone trabeculae with lamellae were noted (Figure 2(c)).

3. Discussion

The use of allografts, xenografts, and alloplasts has been recommended to increase bone height in sinus augmentation procedures, rather than using an autograft. Because the radiodensity of a bone graft is similar to that of a native bone, the quality of the increased bone height as a living hard tissue for a sustainable outcome has been questioned.

In the present study, the CBCT images showed alveolar bone height increased approximately 2-fold from the baseline height at 6-month postoperation. The histological images confirmed the new bone formation with many osteoblasts and osteocytes present. Bone trabeculae with lamella and calcification zones were also observed. In addition, no inflammatory response or tissue reaction was observed. The sponge was resorbed and replaced with new bone. This finding indicated that the acemannan sponge was biocompatible with the maxillary sinus. Taken together, our results demonstrated the osteoinductive property of the acemannan sponge. These results correspond with our report that demonstrated using acemannan in indirect sinus augmentation and simultaneous implant placement increased bone formation [17].

Based on the study's limitations, a precise explanation of the underlying mechanism of acemannan on osseous regeneration could not be determined. A possible explanation is that, as a 3-dimensional interconnected porous scaffold, the acemannan sponge absorbs blood and/or serum from the surrounding tissue to stabilize the blood clot to maintain its volume for bone growth [9]. Acemannan may increase bone formation by increasing cell proliferation, osteoblast differentiation, growth factor and extracellular matrix secretion, and mineralization [8, 9]. Moreover, the anti-inflammatory and immunomodulatory effects of acemannan have been reported [18].

This polysaccharide will facilitate the inflammatory reaction through macrophage activation and the release of cytokines and growth factors. Interleukins (ILs), tumor necrosis factor alpha (TNF-α), transforming growth factor beta (TGF-β), platelet-derived growth factor (PDGF), endothelial growth factor (EGF), bone morphogenetic proteins (BMPs), and vascular endothelial growth factor (VEGF) have been associated with bone repair and regeneration [19, 20].

It should be noted that the increased bone height in this study is limited. The postoperative bone height gain was approximately 6 mm from the 3 mm initial bone height; however, the minimum implant length for predictable success is 10 mm [21]. Therefore, adding acemannan as a biomolecule in an osteoconductive scaffold (such as xenograft, allograft, or synthetic calcium phosphate) in sinus augmentation and in implant placement in the esthetic zone should be investigated.

4. Conclusion

The safety and biocompatibility of the acemannan sponge with the maxillary sinus were investigated. The osteoinductive property of acemannan in a sinus lift procedure was demonstrated using CBCT and histological analysis. Further studies with a larger sample size should be performed.

Acknowledgments

We thank Prof. Dr. Visaka Limwong, Assoc. Prof. Dr. Dolly Methatharathip, and Dr. Kevin A. Tompkins for their valuable suggestions. This study was supported by the Research Unit of Herbal Medicine, Biomaterial and Material for Dental Treatment, Chulalongkorn University (Government Budget) and the 90th Anniversary of Chulalongkorn University Scholarship, Ratchapisek Sompote Fund, Bangkok, Thailand.

References

[1] I. Woo and B. Le, "Maxillary sinus floor elevation: review of anatomy and two techniques," *Implant Dentistry*, vol. 13, no. 1, pp. 28–32, 2004.

[2] T. Starch-Jensen and J. D. Jensen, "Maxillary sinus floor augmentation: a review of selected treatment modalities," *Journal of Oral and Maxillofacial Research*, vol. 8, no. 3, article e3, 2017.

[3] S. Balaji, "Direct v/s indirect sinus lift in maxillary dental implants," *Annals of Maxillofacial Surgery*, vol. 3, no. 2, pp. 148–153, 2013.

[4] P. Felice, R. Pistilli, M. Piattelli, E. Soardi, C. Barausse, and M. Esposito, "1-stage versus 2-stage lateral sinus lift procedures: 1-year post-loading results of a multicentre randomised controlled trial," *European Journal of Oral Implantology*, vol. 7, no. 1, pp. 65–75, 2014.

[5] H. Ghanbari, A. Moeintaghavi, N. Sargolzaei, A. Foroozanfar, and Y. Dadpoor, "Comparative study of algipore and decalcified freeze-dried bone allograft in open maxillary sinus elevation using piezoelectric surgery," *Journal of Periodontology*, vol. 5, no. 1, pp. 1–6, 2013.

[6] L. F. Rodella, G. Favero, and M. Labanca, "Biomaterials in maxillofacial surgery: membranes and grafts," *International Journal of Biomedical Sciences*, vol. 7, no. 2, pp. 81–88, 2011.

[7] N. Tajima, S. Ohba, T. Sawase, and I. Asahina, "Evaluation of sinus floor augmentation with simultaneous implant placement using platelet-rich fibrin as sole grafting material," *The International Journal of Oral & Maxillofacial Implants*, vol. 28, no. 1, pp. 77–83, 2013.

[8] S. Boonyagul, W. Banlunara, P. Sangvanich, and P. Thunyakitpisal, "Effect of acemannan, an extracted polysaccharide from *Aloe vera*, on BMSCs proliferation, differentiation, extracellular matrix synthesis, mineralization, and bone formation in a tooth extraction model," *Odontology*, vol. 102, no. 2, pp. 310–317, 2014.

[9] P. Chantarawaratit, P. Sangvanich, W. Banlunara, K. Soontornvipart, and P. Thunyakitpisal, "Acemannan sponges stimulate alveolar bone, cementum and periodontal ligament regeneration in a canine class II furcation defect model," *Journal of Periodontal Research*, vol. 49, no. 2, pp. 164–178, 2014.

[10] P. Jansisyanont, S. Tiyapongprapan, V. Chuenchompoonut, P. Sangvanich, and P. Thunyakitpisal, "The effect of aceman-

nan sponges in post-extraction socket healing: a randomized trial," *Journal of Oral and Maxillofacial Surgery, Medicine, and Pathology*, vol. 28, no. 2, pp. 105–110, 2016.

[11] Y. Ni, D. Turner, K. M. Yates, and I. Tizard, "Isolation and characterization of structural components of *Aloe vera* L. leaf pulp," *International Immunopharmacology*, vol. 4, no. 14, pp. 1745–1755, 2004.

[12] N. Jittapiromsak, S. Jettanacheawchankit, P. Lardungdee, P. Sangvanich, and P. Thunyakitpisal, "Effect of acemannan on BMP-2 expression in primary pulpal fibroblasts and periodontal fibroblasts, in vitro study," *Journal of Tissue Engineering and Regenerative Medicine*, vol. 4, no. 3, pp. 149–154, 2007.

[13] A. Pozzi and P. K. Moy, "Minimally invasive transcrestal guided sinus lift (TGSL): a clinical prospective proof-of-concept cohort study up to 52 months," *Clinical Implant Dentistry and Related Research*, vol. 16, no. 4, pp. 582–593, 2014.

[14] M. Falah, D. S. Sohn, and S. Srouji, "Graftless sinus augmentation with simultaneous dental implant placement: clinical results and biological perspectives," *International Journal of Oral and Maxillofacial Surgery*, vol. 45, no. 9, pp. 1147–1153, 2016.

[15] J. H. Lee, M. J. Kim, S. M. Kim, O. H. Kwon, and Y. K. Kim, "The 3D CT superimposition method using image fusion based on the maximum mutual information algorithm for the assessment of oral and maxillofacial surgery treatment results," *Oral Surgery, Oral Medicine, Oral Pathology and Oral Radiology*, vol. 114, no. 2, pp. 167–174, 2012.

[16] F. Maes, A. Collignon, D. Vandermeulen, G. Marchal, and P. Suetens, "Multimodality image registration by maximization of mutual information," *IEEE Transactions on Medical Imaging*, vol. 16, no. 2, pp. 187–198, 1997.

[17] H. A. Trinh, V. V. Dam, B. Le, P. Pittayapat, and P. Thunyakitpisal, "Indirect sinus augmentation with and without the addition of a biomaterial: a randomized controlled clinical trial," *Implant Dentistry*, vol. 28, no. 6, pp. 571–577, 2019.

[18] K. Bhalang, P. Thunyakitpisal, and N. Rungsirisatean, "Acemannan, a polysaccharide extracted from *Aloe vera*, is effective in the treatment of oral aphthous ulceration," *The Journal of Alternative and Complementary Medicine*, vol. 19, no. 5, pp. 429–434, 2013.

[19] A. Bhat, R. M. Wooten, and A. C. Jayasuriya, "Secretion of growth factors from macrophages when cultured with microparticles," *Journal of Biomedical Materials Research Part A*, vol. 101, no. 11, pp. 3170–3180, 2013.

[20] N. Fujiwara and K. Kobayashi, "Macrophages in inflammation," *Current Drug Target -Inflammation & Allergy*, vol. 4, no. 3, pp. 281–286, 2005.

[21] T. J. Griffin and W. S. Cheung, "The use of short, wide implants in posterior areas with reduced bone height: a retrospective investigation," *The Journal of Prosthetic Dentistry*, vol. 92, no. 2, pp. 139–144, 2004.

7

Prelacrimal Window Approach in the Management of Odontogenic Maxillary Sinusitis from Dental Foreign Body

Saikrishna Ananthapadmanabhan,[1] Anthony Noor,[1] and Niranjan Sritharan[1,2]

[1]*Department of Otolaryngology, Nepean Hospital, Kingswood, NSW 2747, Australia*
[2]*Department of Otolaryngology, Westmead Hospital, Westmead, NSW 2145, Australia*

Correspondence should be addressed to Saikrishna Ananthapadmanabhan; saikrishnaanantha96@gmail.com

Academic Editor: Giovanni Mergoni

The floor of the maxillary sinus is partly formed by the alveolar process of the maxilla, and this anatomical relationship forms an interface for collaboration between rhinologists, maxillofacial and dental surgeons, and dentists. Odontogenic maxillary sinusitis (ODMS) occurs secondary to infectious processes of the maxillary molar and premolar teeth or following complications from dental procedures. Extruded dental foreign bodies within the sinus can cause chronic mucosal irritation leading to mucociliary dysfunction and sinogenic symptoms. Anteriorly placed foreign bodies are difficult to access via the conventional endoscopic maxillary antrostomy. Endoscopic approaches to access the anterior maxillary sinus involve extended resection of the medial maxillary wall, potentially with the removal of the inferior turbinate and nasolacrimal duct mobilisation. The prelacrimal window approach (PLWA) is a favourable modification that provides excellent visualisation of the maxillary sinus with minimal tissue resection and displacement. We describe the case of an extruded distobuccal 27 tooth root into the anterior maxillary sinus, presenting with acute sinusitis. The patient was successfully managed via a PLWA. This case represents the importance of recognition of ODMS with early referral to otorhinolaryngologists.

1. Introduction

Odontogenic maxillary sinusitis (ODMS) is a common form of paranasal sinus disease and can be secondary to endodontic or periodontal pathology or as a complication of dental procedures, which includes extraction-related oroantral communication or extrusion of dental foreign bodies [1–4]. In the former, there is inflammatory spread through the alveolar process of the maxilla with subsequent infection of the Schneiderian membrane that lines the maxillary sinus. In the latter, the sinus mucosa is vulnerable to an altered microbiome, with oral pathogens and extruded foreign bodies acting as vectors for infection. Ultimately, there is mucosal inflammation, impaired mucociliary clearance and host defences, obstruction of natural sinus drainage pathways, and superimposed bacterial infection.

Foreign bodies in the maxillary sinus are often an iatrogenic complication of dental surgery [5], and may include tooth roots [6], burs [7], implants [8], needles [9], endodontic obturation materials [10, 11], and amalgam [12]. Inadvertent formation of an oroantral communication is the primary route of access for an extruded material, with less common pathways including the tooth socket, the pulp chamber, or operations involving the maxillary antrum. In the case of ODMS from a retained foreign body, the mainstay of surgical treatment is the removal of the offending agent [4]. We describe a case of accidental extrusion of a tooth root into the anterior maxillary sinus, which was removed using an innovative endoscopic technique termed prelacrimal window approach (PLWA).

The anterior wall of the maxillary sinus has proved to be challenging for surgical access, with difficulty in visualizing and instrumenting this region via the natural ostium [13]. Historical external approaches have included Caldwell-Luc, canine fossa puncture, and midfacial gloving, which have unfavourable morbidity. Subsequent endoscopic endonasal techniques have included Denker's approach and the endoscopic medial maxillectomy (EMM), which usually involve resection of the inferior turbinate (IT) and potentially the nasolacrimal duct (NLD). This may create issues with epiphora and inefficient nasal airflow and humidification causing crusting [14]. The PLWA is a favourable minimal access approach, with preservation of the IT and NLD. The prelacrimal recess, shown in Figure 1, is the area bounded by the medial wall of the maxillary sinus medially, the anterior wall of the maxillary sinus anteriorly, the infraorbital laterally, and the level of the nasolacrimal duct posteriorly. It extends in a craniocaudal direction from the orbital floor to the floor of the nasal cavity. The medial boundary of the prelacrimal recess on the medial wall of the maxillary sinus is defined between the nasolacrimal duct posteriorly and the pyriform aperture anteriorly. The prelacrimal window provides wide surgical access to the maxillary sinus with preservation of normal structures. The technique was first reported by Zhou et al. [15] and has been extrapolated in approaches to the pterygopalatine and infratemporal fossa [16]. Studies have reported the efficacy of the PLWA in addressing multiple maxillary sinus pathologies including inflammatory and neoplastic diseases [17–19]. The dimensions of the prelacrimal window have been described by Simmen et al. [20] and Kashlan and Craig [21].

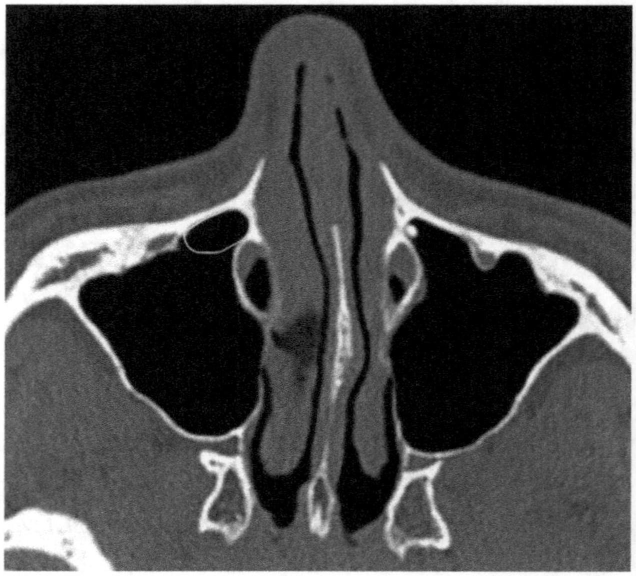

FIGURE 1: CT representation of the prelacrimal recess shown bounded by the anterior and medial walls of the maxillary sinus, nasolacrimal duct, and infraorbital nerve. The medial boundary defined as the bone between the pyriform aperture and nasolacrimal duct can be instrumented to provide surgical access to the anterior and inferior walls of the maxillary sinus.

2. Case Description

A 30-year-old female was referred to our otolaryngology outpatient clinic by the dental surgeons with distobuccal 27 tooth root extrusion into the left maxillary sinus following an extraction 2 weeks previously. This is on a background of known dental caries with previous extractions of teeth 18, 28, 38, and 48. She presented with a 10-day history of left-sided sinofacial pain and progressively worsening headache, with 3 days of anterior and posterior purulent rhinorrhoea. Initial nasal endoscopy at 2 weeks showed pus in the middle meatus. The postnasal space was normal and oral examination revealed a healed 27 socket without evidence of oroantral communication. CT paranasal sinuses with fine slices, arranged by the dental team on day 5 postdental extraction, once headache started to develop, demonstrated a $4 \times 2 \times 5$ m sclerotic density placed anteromedially in the left maxillary sinus with mucosal thickening obstructing the ostiomeatal unit (Figure 2). Her acute infective symptoms were managed with oral antibiotics, nasal irrigation washes, and nasal sprays. The patient reported persistent sinofacial pain and headaches that interfered with her quality of life over the next 2 months, and to provide symptomatic relief and to prevent recurrent exacerbations of acute infective sinusitis, definitive surgical management was pursued. Using the technique described by Simmen et al. [20], a Type II bony prelacrimal recess of 5.6 mm was measured representing suitability for the PLWA.

She underwent the prelacrimal maxillary window approach with removal of the dental foreign body and preservation of the IT and NLD (Figures 3–5). The nasal cavity was prepared with cophenylcaine, 1 : 10,000 adrenaline, and topical vasoconstrictors applied onto neuropatties. A mucosal incision was made on the lateral nasal wall anterior to the IT using monopolar diathermy and the mucoperiosteal flap was raised. A burr was used to skeletonise the nasolacrimal apparatus, which was preserved. An endoscopic prelacrimal medial maxillotomy was created to access the anterior part of the maxillary sinus. Excellent visualisation was achieved with the 0° endoscope, and the tooth fragment was identified and removed intact. The flap was replaced and closed with Monocryl sutures. The patient had a good recovery with full resolution of sinus symptoms.

3. Discussion

The maxillary sinus is the most common site of paranasal sinus disease. Certain factors that may contribute to this observation include its large volume, the anatomic relationship to the maxillary teeth, and the upward mucociliary drainage pattern towards the superiorly placed natural sinus ostium [22, 23]. Studies have reported that 25–40% of chronic maxillary sinusitis is odontogenic [24] and a 2010 meta-analysis of ODMS suggested that 55% of cases are iatrogenic [25]. Dental instrumentation of the maxillary molars presents the greatest risk to iatrogenic ODMS due to the challenging root canal anatomy and location [4]. Thin or dehiscent bone in the maxillary sinus floor can cause premolar and molar teeth roots to project into the sinus, in close contact with the respiratory epithelium [26]. Previous case reports have documented extrusion of various dental foreign bodies including displaced teeth fragments, endodontic obturation materials, dental burs, drill bits, and amalgam, whereas our case developed symptoms within 2 months of dental surgery, and a latency period between initial insult and sinogenic symptoms of up to 4 years has been described [27]. The management of ODMS includes dental and/or sinus surgery, depending on the underlying aetiology [28, 29]. In

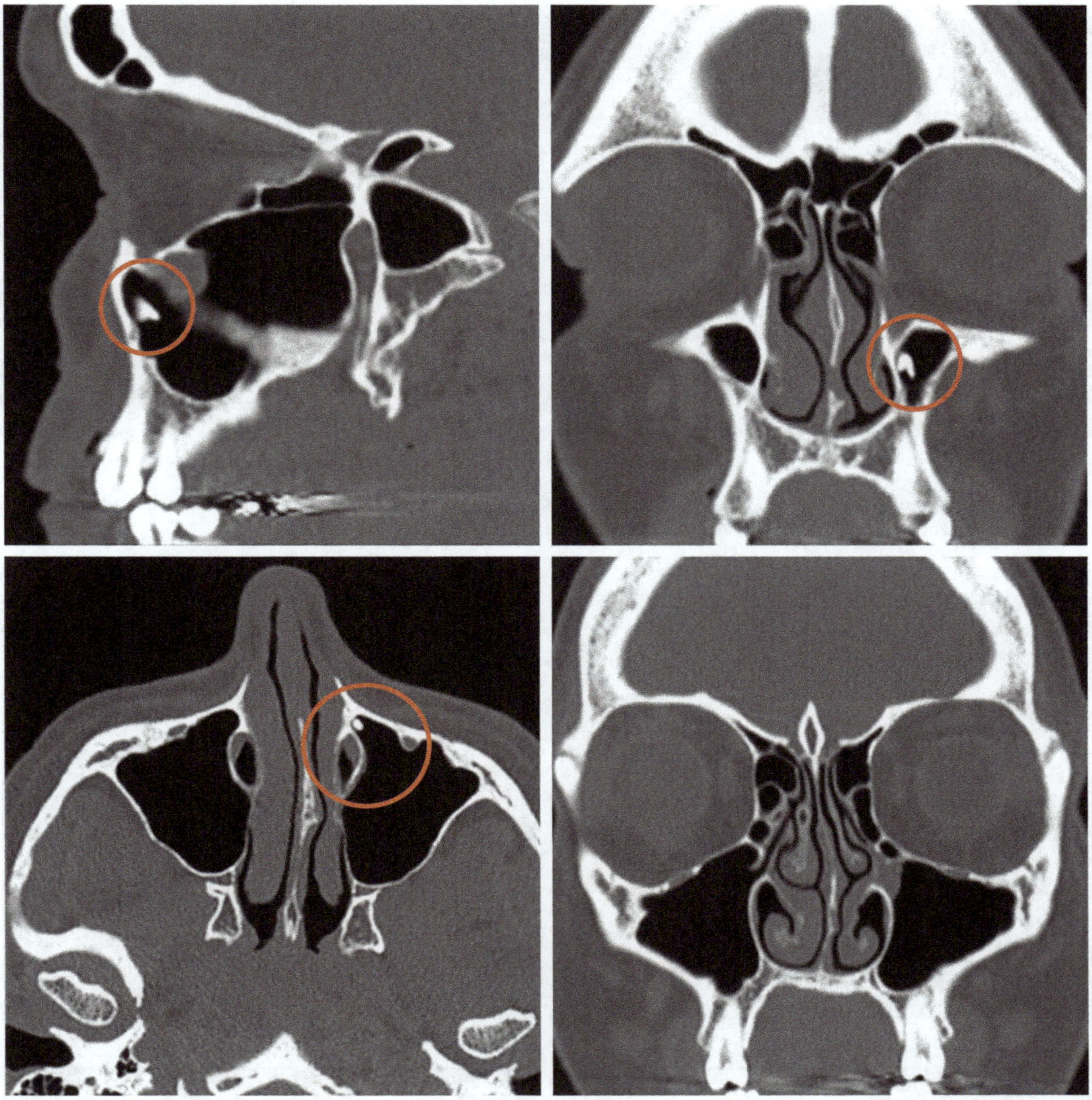

FIGURE 2: Non-contrast CT paranasal sinuses, bony windows: Top left (sagittal), Top right (coronal), Bottom left (axial) demonstrating 4 × 2 × 5 mm sclerotic, radio-opaque density anteriorly in the left maxillary sinus. The NLD and infraorbital foramen are noted within the red circle. The bottom right (coronal) figure shows lobulated mucosal thickening surrounding the left ostiomeatal unit with occlusion. No periapical lucencies or other radiologic stigmata of endodontic or periodontal disease were present. No osteitis or significant maxillary sinus opacification was observed as the CT was performed within 5 days of the initial dental procedure, and it was organised by the dental team to confirm the existence of the foreign body when the patient had begun to develop headaches but before reporting nasal discharge and infective symptoms. As there was no concern for complicated sinusitis and operative anatomy was already detailed in the initial CT, a repeat CT was not indicated when the patient's nasal obstruction and sinofacial pain were worsening.

cases of foreign body ODMS, removal of the agent is needed to prevent chronic irritation of the Schneiderian membrane and mucociliary dysfunction. The caveat is in the case of implant-related ODMS where removal may introduce the risk of oroantral communication, difficult reimplantation, and cost to the patient [4]. In this cohort, consideration of functional endoscopic sinus surgery (ESS) alone can be entertained to enlarge drainage pathways. The presence of obstruction at the maxillary sinus ostium or ostiomeatal complex and retained dental foreign bodies are strong predictors of the eventual need for ESS [2]. A pressing concern depending on the immune status of the patient and type of foreign body is fungal maxillary sinusitis.

Studies have shown that despite the use of a combination of angled microdebrider blades and antrostomy sites, the anterior and inferior walls of the maxillary sinus remain difficult to access and necessitate extended approaches beyond a standard middle meatal antrostomy [13]. Endoscopic sinus

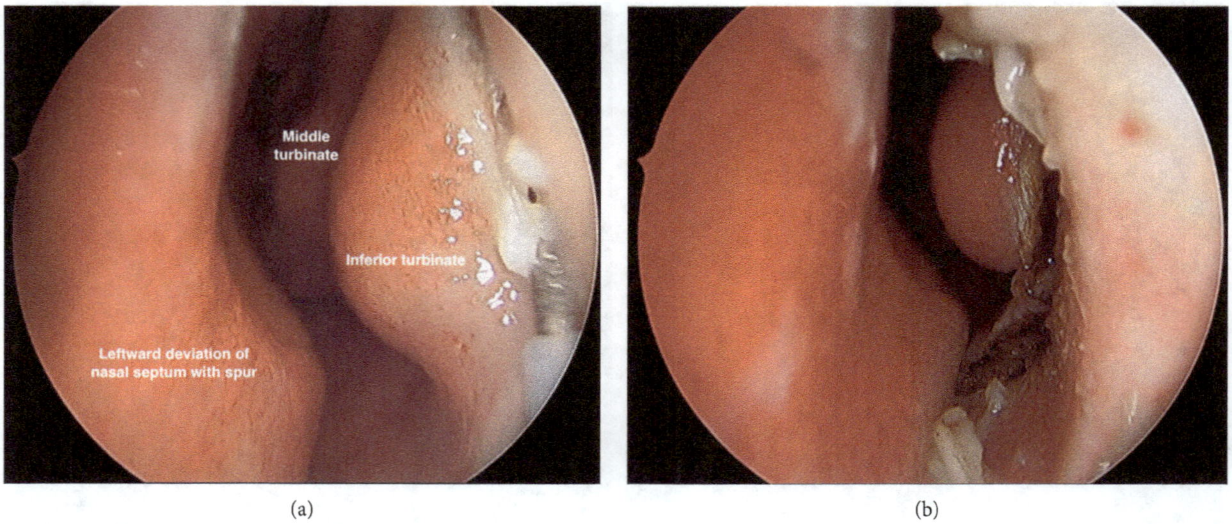

FIGURE 3: Endoscopic view of nasal cavity. (a) Monopolar diathermy is used to create mucosal incision anterior to the head of the IT; and (b) mucosal incision is extended to the floor of the nasal cavity, allowing a mucoperiosteal flap to be raised.

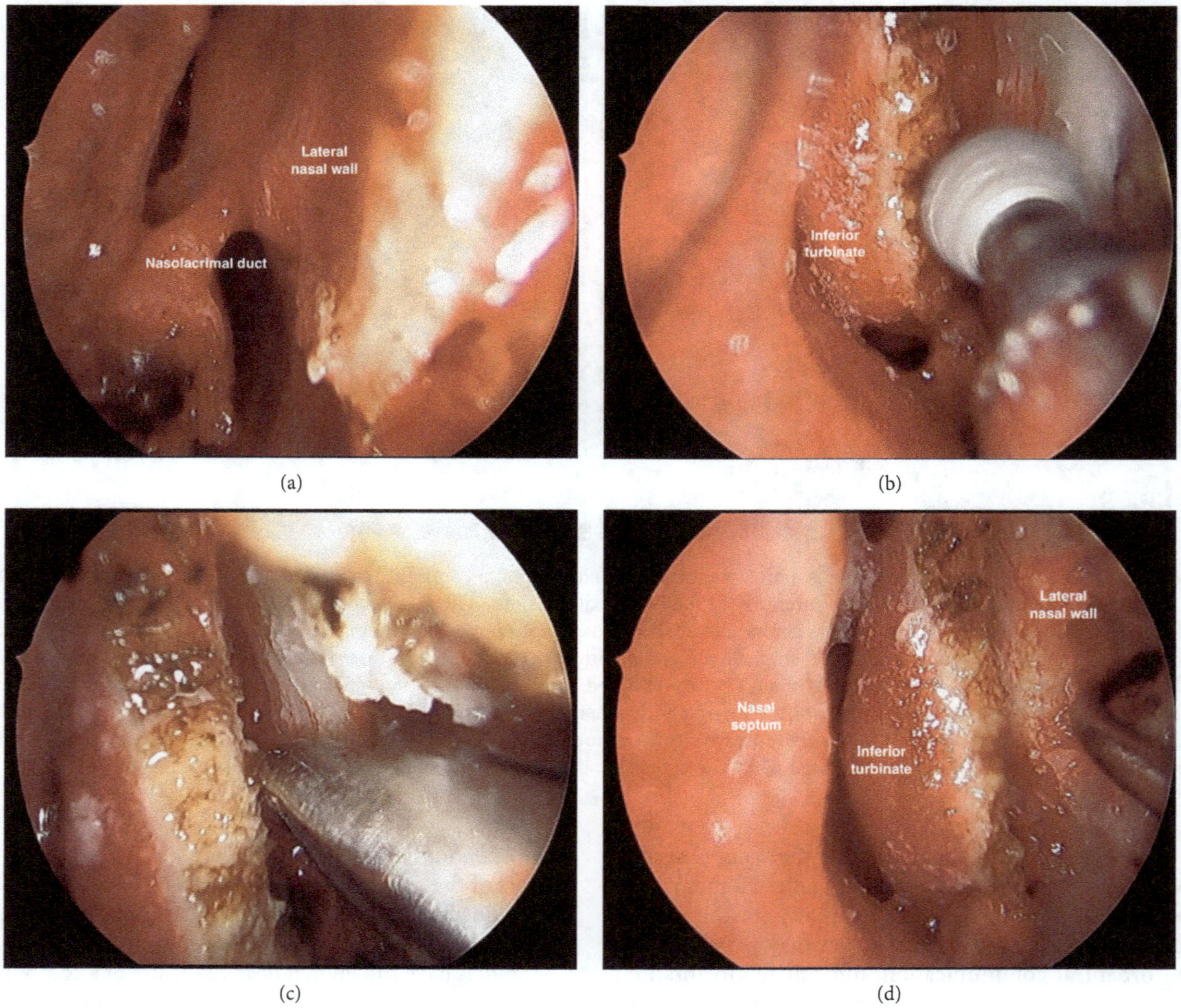

FIGURE 4: (a) Skeletonization of the NLD. (b) Burr used to commence the prelacrimal medial maxillectomy anterior to the NLD and IT. (c) Bony removal of the lateral nasal wall to access the maxillary sinus. (d) Instrumentation through the prelacrimal window into the maxillary sinus.

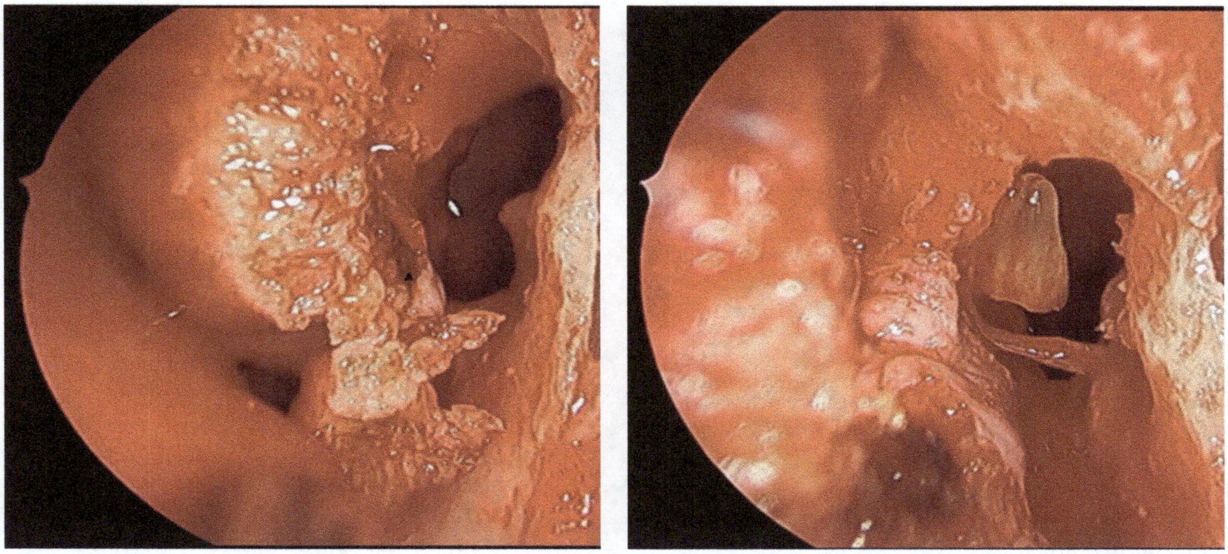

(a) (b)

FIGURE 5: (a) Endoscopic view of the prelacrimal maxillary window accessing the anterior maxillary sinus. (b) Identification and retrieval of the displaced tooth root through the PLWA.

surgery has largely replaced historical nonendoscopic approaches in addressing maxillary sinus disease due to concerns about high rates of permanent facial paraesthesia and neuralgia. With more extensive endonasal approaches, the risk of epiphora, nasal crusting, and ineffective nasal humidification arises. Some authors have raised concerns about the empty nose syndrome with IT resection [30], though this remains controversial. In our patient with ODMS from a dental foreign body, the goal of surgery is straightforward, as the removal of the offending agent should halt sinogenic symptoms. Hence, a minimal access approach is ideal. The IT and medial maxillary wall were replaced to their original anatomical status at the end of the surgery, reducing any potential functional morbidity. A maxillary antrostomy for long-term ventilation and topical medical delivery of the sinus may be considered by some surgeons but was not indicated since the mucosal inflammation causing ostiomeatal complex obstruction will resolve with the removal of the tooth root.

Preoperative CT evaluation of the distance between the anterior maxillary wall and the anterior margin of the NLD is important before PLWA [20]. A radiologic study by Kashlan and Craig [21] provided a comprehensive description of the anteroposterior and superoinferior distances of the prelacrimal recess, with the former distance on the medial wall requiring instrumentation to access the maxillary sinus [21]. The anteroposterior dimension increases in a craniocaudal direction moving from the orbital floor to the opening of the NLD orifice towards the nasal floor, which is consistent with known observations that the nasolacrimal duct has a slight posterior course as it descends down the lateral nasal wall. Distances of the prelacrimal window ≤3 mm can represent high complexity with the need for bone removal and mobilisation of the NLD. Distances ≥7 mm permit the easiest access to the anterior maxillary sinus, and distances between 3 and 7 mm represent intermediate complexity. Even with short distances, modifications to the technique involving the removal of the bony nasolacrimal canal and mobilisation of the NLD to create an adequate working channel have been described in the literature [20, 21, 31]. There is variability among the population in the length of this bony window, with gender differences reported in some studies, with females having shorter distances and greater surgical complexity in accessing the anterior maxillary sinus [32].

4. Conclusion

Odontogenic maxillary sinusitis from tooth root extrusion is an iatrogenic complication that should be recognised and referred early. The PLWA is an innovative rhinologic technique that provided excellent surgical access to the anterior maxillary sinus and demonstrated advantages over conventional external and endoscopic techniques.

Abbreviations

EMM: Endoscopic medial maxillectomy
IT: Inferior turbinate
NLD: Nasolacrimal duct
ODMS: Odontogenic maxillary sinusitis
PLWA: Prelacrimal window approach.

References

[1] B. Nandakumar, N. Niles, and L. Kalish, "Odontogenic maxillary sinusitis: the interface and collaboration between rhinologists and dentists," *Journal of Otorhinolaryngology, Hearing and Balance Medicine*, vol. 2, no. 4, p. 8, 2021.

[2] R. Little, C. Long, T. Loehrl, and D. M. Poetker, "Odontogenic sinusitis: a review of the current literature," *Laryngoscope Investigative Otolaryngology*, vol. 3, no. 2, pp. 110–114, 2018.

[3] J. Craig, D. Poetker, U. Aksoy et al., "Diagnosing odontogenic sinusitis: an international multidisciplinary consensus statement," *International Forum of Allergy & Rhinology*, vol. 11, no. 8, pp. 1235–1248, 2021.

[4] J. Craig, R. Tataryn, T. Aghaloo et al., "Management of odontogenic sinusitis: multidisciplinary consensus statement," *International Forum of Allergy & Rhinology*, vol. 10, no. 7, pp. 901–912, 2020.

[5] M. Tanasiewicz, A. Bubilek-Bogacz, H. Twardawa, M. Skucha-Nowak, and T. Szklarski, "Foreign body of endodontic origin in the maxillary sinus," *Journal of Dental Sciences*, vol. 12, no. 3, pp. 296–300, 2017.

[6] M. Seigneur, A. Cloitre, O. Malard, and P. Lesclous, "Teeth roots displacement in the maxillary sinus: characteristics and management," *Journal of Oral Medicine and Oral Surgery*, vol. 26, no. 3, p. 34, 2020.

[7] J. Smith and P. Emko, "Management of a maxillary sinus foreign body (dental bur)," *Ear, Nose, & Throat Journal*, vol. 86, no. 11, pp. 677–678, 2007.

[8] S. Iida, N. Tanaka, M. Kogo, and T. Matsuya, "Migration of a dental implant into the maxillary sinus: a case report," *International Journal of Oral and Maxillofacial Surgery*, vol. 29, no. 5, pp. 358–359, 2000.

[9] V. Fan and S. Korvi, "Sewing needle in the maxillary antrum," *Journal of Oral and Maxillofacial Surgery*, vol. 60, no. 3, pp. 334–336, 2002.

[10] K. Yamaguchi, T. Matsunaga, and Y. Hayashi, "Gross extrusion of endodontic obturation materials into the maxillary sinus: a case report," *Oral Surgery, Oral Medicine, Oral Pathology, Oral Radiology, and Endodontics*, vol. 104, no. 1, pp. 131–134, 2007.

[11] P. Khongkhunthian and P. Reichart, "Aspergillosis of the maxillary sinus as a complication of overfilling root canal material into the sinus: report of two cases," *Journal of Endodontia*, vol. 27, no. 7, pp. 476–478, 2001.

[12] D. Macan, T. Ćabov, P. Kobler, and Z. Bumber, "Inflammatory reaction to foreign body (amalgam) in the maxillary sinus misdiagnosed as an ethmoid tumour," *Dento Maxillo Facial Radiology*, vol. 35, pp. 303–306, 2014.

[13] A. Robey, E. O'Brien, and D. Leopold, "Assessing current technical limitations in the small-hole endoscopic approach to the maxillary sinus," *American Journal of Rhinology & Allergy*, vol. 24, no. 5, pp. 396–401, 2010.

[14] F. Pagella, A. Pusateri, E. Matti et al., "TuNa-saving endoscopic medial maxillectomy: a surgical technique for maxillary inverted papilloma," *European Archives of Oto-Rhino-Laryngology*, vol. 274, no. 7, pp. 2785–2791, 2017.

[15] B. Zhou, D. Han, and S. Cui, "Endoscopic nasal lateral wall dissection approach to maxillary sinus," *Zhonghua Er Bi Yan Hou Tou Jing Wai Ke Za Zhi*, vol. 42, pp. 743–748, 2007.

[16] B. Zhou, Q. Huang, P. Shen et al., "The intranasal endoscopic removal of schwannoma of the pterygopalatine and infratemporal fossae via the prelacrimal recess approach," *Journal of Neurosurgery*, vol. 124, no. 4, pp. 1068–1073, 2016.

[17] Y. Lin, C. Lin, and T. Yeh, "Application of the endoscopic prelacrimal recess approach to the maxillary sinus in unilateral maxillary diseases," *International Forum of Allergy & Rhinology*, vol. 8, no. 4, pp. 530–536, 2018.

[18] L. Koh and R. Dhepnorrarat, "The modified endoscopic prelacrimal approach: how I do it," *The Journal of Otolaryngology*, vol. 1, no. 30, 2018.

[19] Q. Yu, G. Guan, N. Zhang et al., "Intranasal endoscopic prelacrimal recess approach for maxillary sinus inverted papilloma," *European Archives of Oto-Rhino-Laryngology*, vol. 275, no. 9, pp. 2297–2302, 2018.

[20] D. Simmen, N. Veerasigamani, H. Briner, N. Jones, and B. Schuknecht, "Anterior maxillary wall and lacrimal duct relationship – CT analysis for prelacrimal access to the maxillary sinus," *Rhinology*, vol. 55, no. 2, pp. 170–174, 2017.

[21] K. Kashlan and J. Craig, "Dimensions of the medial wall of the prelacrimal recess," *International Forum of Allergy & Rhinology*, vol. XX, pp. 1–5, 2018.

[22] G. Bell, B. Joshi, and R. Macleod, "Maxillary sinus disease: diagnosis and treatment," *British Dental Journal*, vol. 210, no. 3, pp. 113–118, 2011.

[23] K. Ganesan and N. Rathod, "Maxillary sinusitis," in *Oral and Maxillofacial Surgery for the Clinician*, K. Bonanthaya, E. Panneerselvam, S. Manuel, V. Kumar, and A. Rai, Eds., pp. 475–489, Springer, Singapore, 2021.

[24] S. Albu and M. Baciut, "Failures in endoscopic surgery of the maxillary sinus," *Otolaryngology and Head and Neck Surgery*, vol. 142, no. 2, pp. 196–201, 2010.

[25] O. Arias-Irimia, C. Barona-Dorado, J. Santos-Marino, N. Martínez-Rodriguez, and J. M. Martínez-González, "Meta-analysis of the etiology of odontogenic maxillary sinusitis," *Medicina Oral, Patologia Oral y Cirugia Bucal*, vol. 15, no. 1, pp. e70–e73, 2009.

[26] R. Fry, D. Patidar, S. Goyal, and A. Malhotra, "Proximity of maxillary posterior teeth roots to maxillary sinus and adjacent structures using Denta scan®," *Indian Journal of Dental*, vol. 7, no. 3, pp. 126–130, 2016.

[27] M. Troeltzsch, C. Pache, M. Troeltzsch et al., "Etiology and clinical characteristics of symptomatic unilateral maxillary sinusitis: a review of 174 cases," *Journal of Cranio-Maxillo-Facial Surgery*, vol. 43, no. 8, pp. 1522–1529, 2015.

[28] J. Craig, C. McHugh, Z. Griggs, and E. I. Peterson, "Optimal timing of endoscopic sinus surgery for odontogenic sinusitis," *The Laryngoscope*, vol. 129, no. 9, pp. 1976–1983, 2019.

[29] S. Kim, J. Park, H. Tim, C. Lee, Y. Park, and J. Bae, "Clinical features and treatment outcomes of dental implant-related paranasal sinusitis: a 2-year prospective observational study," *Clinical Oral Implants Research*, vol. 27, no. 11, pp. e100–e104, 2016.

[30] T. Nakayama, Y. Tsunemi, A. Kuboki et al., "Prelacrimal approach vs conventional surgery for inverted papilloma in the maxillary sinus," *Head & Neck*, vol. 42, no. 11, pp. 3218–3225, 2020.

[31] D. Morrissey, P. Wormald, and A. Psaltis, "Prelacrimal approach to the maxillary sinus," *International Forum of Allergy & Rhinology*, vol. 6, pp. 214–218, 2016.

[32] A. Andrianakis, U. Moser, A. Wolf et al., "Gender-specific differences in feasibility of pre-lacrimal window approach," *Scientific Reports*, vol. 11, no. 1, p. 7791, 2021.

8

Mental Nerve Paraesthesia: A Report of Two Cases Associated with Endodontic Etiology

Neeta Patel,[1] Akshayraj Langaliya,[1] Shikha Kanodia,[2] Aravind Kumbhar,[1] Aastha Buch,[3] Aarshvi Shah,[1] Himani Bhatt,[1] Drashti Panchal,[1] Sharan Shah,[1] and Jinali Shah[1]

[1]*AMC Dental College and Hosptial, Bhalakhiya Mill Compound, Opp. Anupam Cinema, Ahmedabad 380008, India*
[2]*Government Dental College and Hospital, Civil Hospital Campus, Asarwa, Ahmedabad 380016, India*
[3]*Faculty of Dental Sciences, Dharmsinh Desai University, Nadiad 387001, India*

Correspondence should be addressed to Akshayraj Langaliya; akshaylangalia@gmail.com

Academic Editor: Darko Macan

Paraesthesia of the mental nerve can occur due to various etiological factors. Rarely, dental infections can cause paraesthesia. However, this article discusses two cases of endodontic etiology in the mental nerve region as a causative factor for paraesthesia. In the first case, the patient had severe pain localized to his right mandible, with numbness of his lower lip. Endodontic treatment led to quick regression and resolution of paraesthesia. In the second case, a patient who was referred for retreatment of a mandibular second premolar infection developed profound paraesthesia in the region of the mental nerve distribution following prior therapy. Possible mechanisms responsible for periapical infection-related paraesthesia are discussed here. CBCT imaging may be useful in the diagnosis and management of such conditions.

1. Introduction

Paraesthesia is a feeling that is rare, provocative, or spontaneous and is commonly described by patients as a burning, tickling, or tingling sensation [1]. According to the taxonomy of the International Association of Study of Pain (IASP), paraesthesia, although abnormal, is not unpleasant [2]. Patients have often described it as warmth, cold, burning, aching, prickling, tingling, pin and needle sensation, or numbness.

The mental foramen in dentistry is an essential anatomical feature on the lateral surface of the mandible. This marks the culmination of the mandibular canal that opens in an oblique direction to the surface. The mental nerve bundle passes through the mental foramen and supplies the soft tissues of the chin, lower lip, and gingiva on the ipsilateral side of the mandible with sensory innervation and nutrition [3].

Radiographically, the mental foramen may result in misdiagnosis of a radiolucent lesion in the apical area of the mandibular premolar teeth. For diagnostic and clinical procedures, accurately locating the mental foramen is important [4]. The intimate anatomical proximity between the root apices of the mandibular premolars and the mental nervous bundle should also be meticulously examined. Periapical infection before and after endodontic therapy leading to mental and inferior alveolar nerve paraesthesia is also well documented [5]. The mechanism of induction of paraesthesia due to periapical infection may be threefold.

(1) The inflammatory process causes purulent exudate to accumulate in the mandibular bone, causing local mechanical pressure on the mental nerve [6, 7]

(2) Toxic or inflammatory bacterial products [6–8]

(3) Adequate subsequent hematoma pressure [6, 7]

(4) Direct invasion of nerve structures by bacteria themselves [9]

2. Case Reports

2.1. Case 1. A 21-year-old healthy male patient reported to our institute with severe pain localized to his right mandible and numbness on the right side of the lower lip. On examination, the patient was apyrexic with normal vital signs, no apparent facial asymmetry, and a 42 mm incisal mouth opening without pain. The patient had a trauma history on the same side 1 month prior. No carious lesion was evident on clinical assessment. The lower right second premolar was tender on percussion. Electric pulp testing revealed an intact sensation in the mandibular right first molar and right first premolar but no response in the mandibular right second premolar. Two-point discrimination light-touch and pin-prick tests were performed on the right mentum region encompassing the area of the skin below the right half of the lower lip and anterior part of the cheek on the same side, which confirmed persistent paraesthesia (Figure 1(a)). A RadioVisio Graphic (RVG) image revealed radiolucency in the apical region involving the mental foramen (Figure 1(b)). To further confirm the diagnosis, a cone-beam computed tomography (CBCT) scan (Vatech PaX I 3D Smart, 74 kV, 10 mA, 10.8 sec) of the same region revealed a large periapical radiolucency involving the second premolar extending into the mental foramen (Figure 1(c)). Nonsurgical endodontic treatment was planned. Informed consent was obtained before initiation of treatment.

Root canal treatment was initiated under isolation with a dental dam (Figure 1(d)). Patency filing was performed with a stainless steel 10# K file (Dentsply-Maillefer, Switzerland). The working length was determined using an electronic apex locator (Root ZX mini, Morita, Osaka, Japan), which was later confirmed by the RVG image (Figure 2(a)). Cleaning and shaping were performed by Protaper Gold files (Dentsply-Maillefer, Switzerland) until F2 size with careful intermittent copious irrigation with 3% sodium hypochlorite (Vishal Dentcare, Ahmedabad, India) solution followed by normal saline and a final rinse of 17% EDTA (Prime Dental Products, Thane, India). The canal was carefully dried with paper points, and an intracanal medicament of calcium hydroxide with a mixture of 2% CHX (Vishal Dentcare, Ahmedabad India) was placed (Figure 2(b)). The tooth was restored with an interim restoration (Cavit 3M, USA), and the patient was discharged with oral antibiotics Tab. Amoxycillin-Clavulanic acid–625 mg twice daily for seven days and vitamin B oral supplements.

The patient was recalled after 7 days and evaluated for symptoms of paraesthesia. There seemed to be a mild recovery from numbness in the chin region and complete recovery from pain and tenderness. Two weeks later, the paraesthesia had almost disappeared except for a small patch on the right side of the lower lip. The tooth was completely asymptomatic; therefore, obturation was performed at this visit with laterally compacted gutta-percha with MTA-based sealer (MTA Plus, Prevest Denpro, India) (Figure 2(d)). At three- and six-month subsequent follow-ups, examination showed reconstitution of the apical region, cortical lining of the inferior alveolar canal, and paraesthesia was completely resolved (Figures 2(e) and 2(f)).

2.2. Case 2. A 45-year-old male reported to our institute with pain, swelling, and tingling sensations in the lower right second premolar region. On examination, the patient was apyrexic with normal vital signs and had adequate mouth opening. The patient had previously undergone root canal treatment in tooth #45 before one year by a general dentist. The patient described that almost after 6 months of the initial treatment, he had an episode of sudden pain in relation to the same tooth but he took over-the-counter medications and the pain soon subsided. The next episode was a drastic one as described above which urged him to visit our department. On palpation, the right second premolar was tender, and two-point discrimination, light-touch, and pin-prick tests were performed as the above-mentioned case, which confirmed persistent paraesthesia (Figure 3(a)). To confirm the diagnosis of mental nerve involvement, CBCT was directly performed at the insistence of the patient. A small field of view (FOV) CBCT (Vatech PaX I 3D Smart, 74 kV, 10 mA, 10.8 sec) was obtained, which apparently depicted mental foramen involvement and improper root canal filling, necessitating retreatment in relation to the right second premolar (Figures 3(b) and 3(c)). Informed consent was obtained before beginning the treatment, and all possible outcomes were explained.

Under dental dam isolation, the previous restoration was removed, and gutta-percha was removed using a combination of H files (Dentsply Maillefer, Switzerland), ProTaper retreatment files D1 and D2 (Dentsply Maillefer, Switzerland), and gutta-percha solvent (Carvene Prevest Denpro, India) (Figure 3(d)). Intermittent copious irrigation was performed with 3% NaOCl followed by a final rinse with generically prepared 7% maleic acid and 2% CHX (Vishal Dentcare, Ahmedabad, India). An intracanal medicament of injectable calcium hydroxide (RC cal, Prime Dental Products, Thane, India) dressing was given in interim appointments (twice for three weeks), allowing the patient to be discharged with Tab. Amoxycillin-Clavulanic acid–625 mg twice daily for seven days and vitamin B oral supplements.

The pain completely resolved within a span of three days, and a gradual reduction in paraesthesia occurred over a period of one and a half months. Subsequently, obturation was performed using the lateral condensation technique with an Endosequence Bioceramic sealer (Brasseler, Endo, USA). Three- and twelve-month follow-up examinations showed reconstitution of the apical region, labial cortex, and cortical lining of the mental foramen, and paraesthesia was completely resolved (Figures 4(c)–4(e)).

3. Discussion

Paraesthesia due to endodontic etiology can be attributed to various factors such as periapical infection in relation to an affected premolar. Localized pressure on the mental nerve due to an acute inflammatory response can cause Mental Nerve Paraesthesia (MNP). Gilbert and Dickerson reported

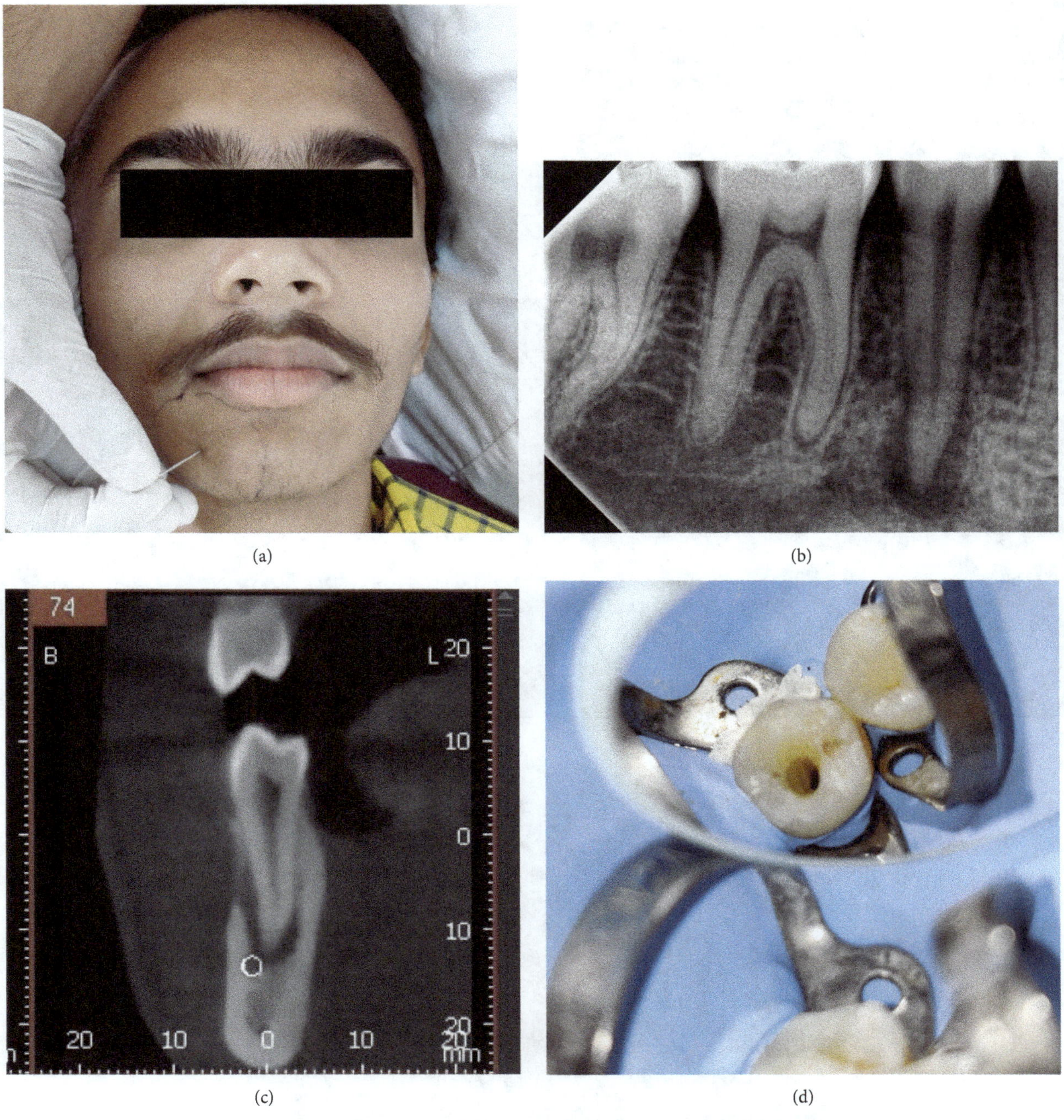

FIGURE 1: (a) Paraesthesia testing, (b) preoperative RVG, (c) preoperative CBCT, and (d) access cavity under dental dam.

a case of asymptomatic apical periodontitis that had undergone acute exacerbation leading to paraesthesia of the area supplied by the mental nerve [8]. It was found that the patient's use of home remedies and local aspirin tablets caused burns in the mental region and may have exacerbated the problem.

In the cases enumerated here, the causes of paraesthesia prior to and after previous endodontic treatment were carefully evaluated and individually considered in an attempt to establish the exact etiology. The patient was asked additional questions regarding the presence of other symptoms of neuropathy, such as numbness or altered sensation, and chairside examination was performed [10]. Flare-up-related paraesthesia was ruled out due to a lack of other characteristic signs of infection [11].

CBCT offers a small field of view with relatively less radiation and is recommended as a diagnostic aid in examining causes, suggesting a safety zone for any procedure, and delineating important structures missed with conventional periapical radiography. There were no extra canals visible in CBCT imaging [12].

Paraesthesia due to direct injection of local anaesthetic solutions into the nerve or needle injury is common. Trauma caused by the contact of the needle with the nerve is probably related to an improper or misguided anaesthetic technique, causing haemorrhage that may lead to compression

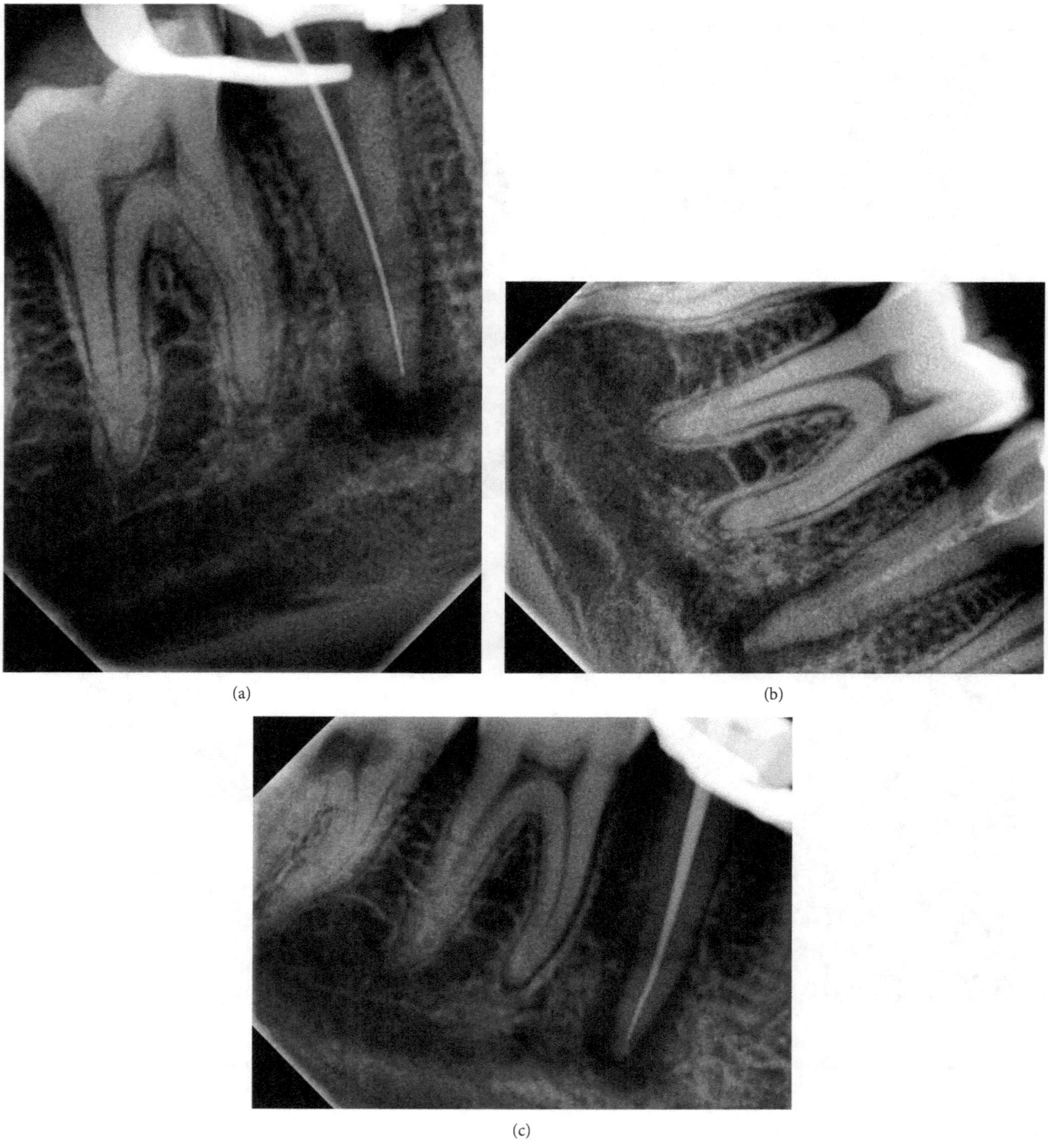

(a) (b) (c)

FIGURE 2: Continued.

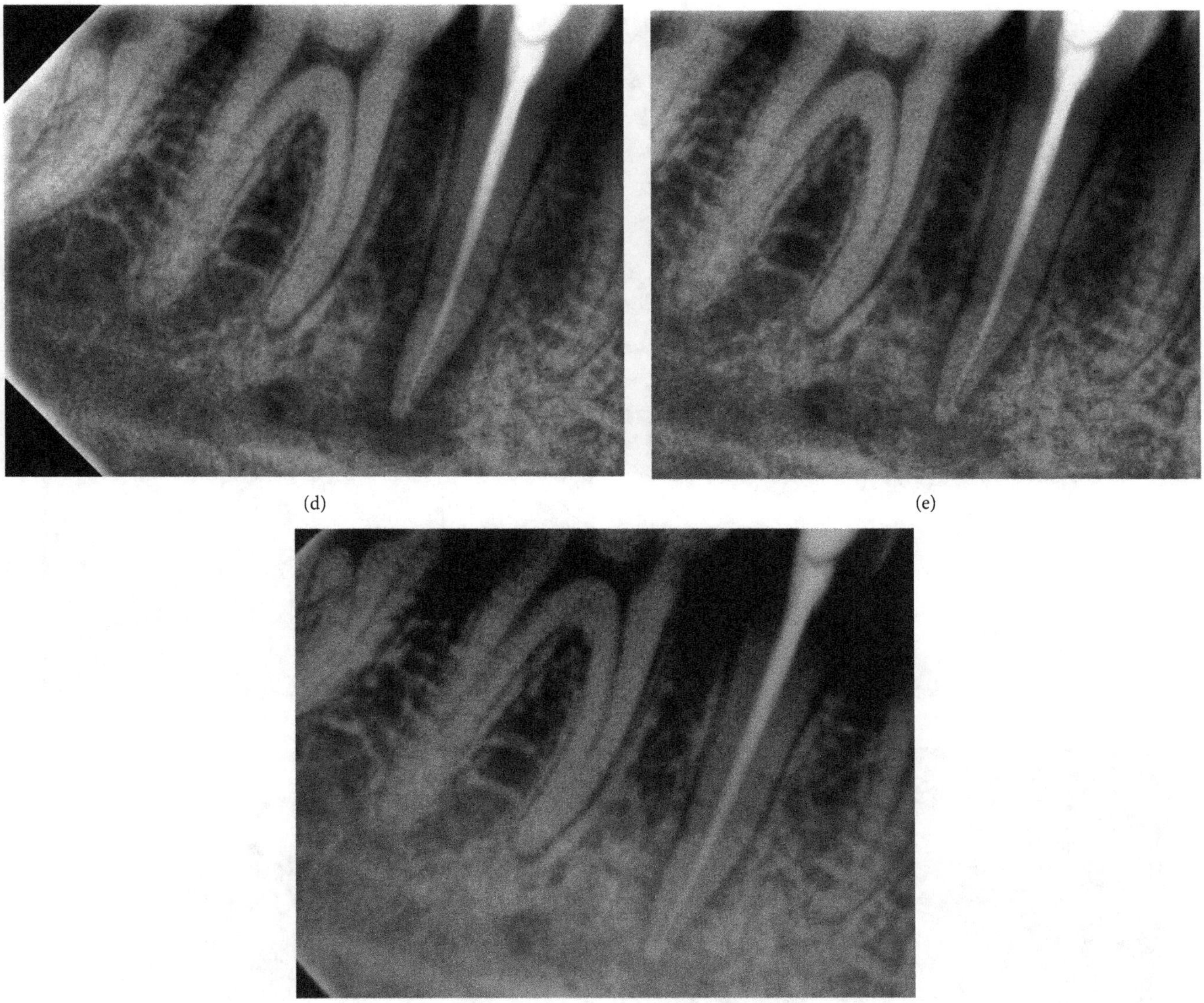

(d) (e) (f)

FIGURE 2: (a) Working length determination, (b) calcium hydroxide placement, (c) master cone selection, (d) obturation, (e) 3-month follow-up, and (f) 6-month follow-up.

of the nerve and then paraesthesia. The hydrostatic pressure of the injection and mechanical nerve compression cause a reduction in blood flow to the nerve and its deformation, subsequently causing paraesthesia [13]. Inferior alveolar nerve paraesthesia is common due to local anaesthesia, but MNP rarely occurs due to the anaesthetic technique. Flanagan reported a case in which needle injury caused a hematoma in the mental region and compression of the mental nerve occurred, resulting in MNP [14]. Our cases did not warrant administration of local anaesthetic; hence, the possibility of this etiology was eliminated.

Extrusion of sodium hypochlorite is another factor to be considered. It is known that sodium hypochlorite when comes in contact with vital tissue causes haemolysis, ulceration, preventing neutrophil migration leading to injury to endothelial and fibroblast cells. The immediate sequel of such accidents includes acute sudden excruciating pain and an immediate swelling in the affected area. In severe cases, a necrotic ulceration of the tissue adjacent to the tooth usually follows which may appear immediately or a few days to weeks later. However, no such symptoms were observed in either of the cases and hence extrusion of the irrigant cannot consider a likely cause [15]. Consideration and careful attention were given to maintain the working length within the confines of the root. Overinstrumentation, causing trauma to the neurovascular bundle is unlikely in this case [16].

Several cases have been documented suggesting paraesthesia can be induced by extrusion of different sealers. Although sealers are biocompatible and nontoxic, some studies also indicate that endodontic materials can be neurotoxic at some level, initiating a host-dependent inflammatory process, which causes cellular damage, ulceration, and haemolysis when in contact with vital tissue. Some cases of MNP are reported due to the overfilling of sealer paste in the vicinity of the mental nerve.

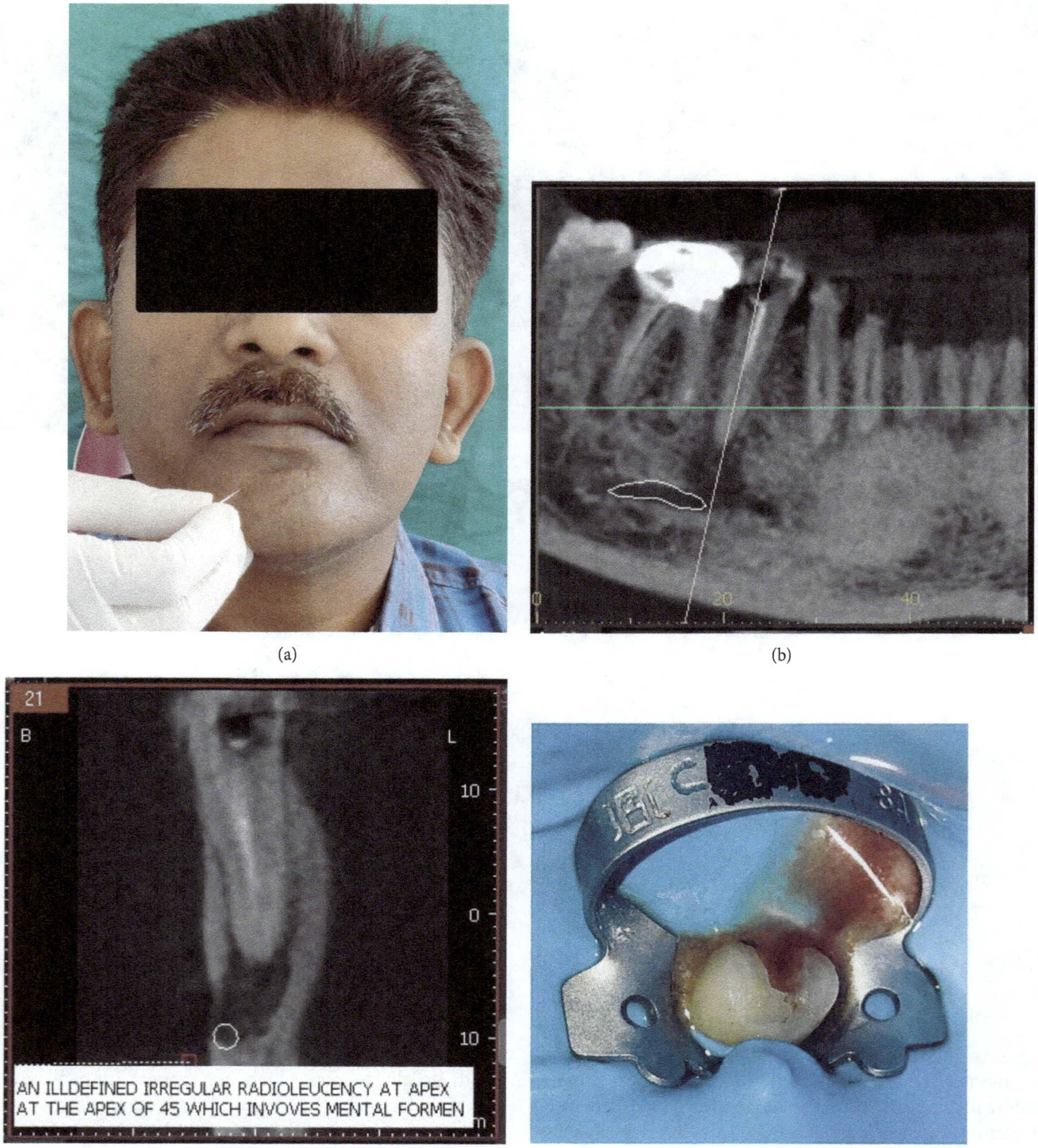

Figure 3: (a) Paraesthesia testing, (b, c) preoperative CBCT, and (d) access cavity under rubber dam isolation.

Gutta-percha is considered a biologically inert material. The collective effect of overinstrumentation and excessive vertical pressure during compaction of the filling material cause extrusion of the filling material, and paraesthesia usually results from the overfilling of gutta-percha [17, 18].

Additionally, continuous wave of the condensation technique could possibly produce higher temperatures; hence, in these cases, we performed the cold lateral condensation technique, which was associated with a lack of bone necrosis or symptoms due to overheating. Meticulous attention to detail was exercised with regard to sealer placement and apical tug back of gutta-percha to avoid any overextension into the periapical area [19].

Vitamin B complex is the key pharmacological choice. The B complex used in this case was based on its safety profile and its potential to support recovery from nerve damage. Early treatment and prevention of periapical lesions by regular dental care is the most important and effective way to prevent MNP.

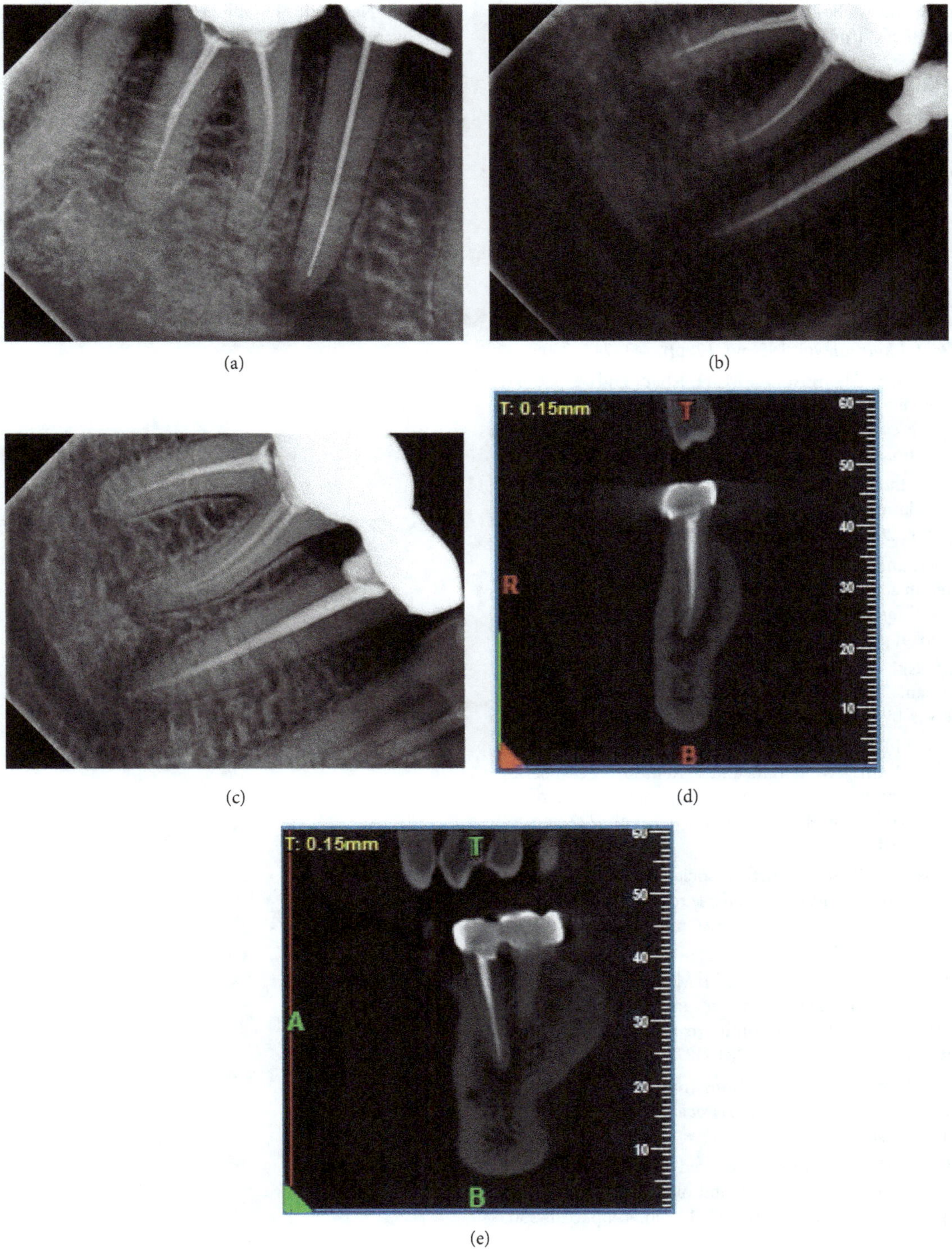

FIGURE 4: (a) Working length determination, (b) obturation, (c) 3-month follow-up RVG, and (d, e) 12-month follow-up CBCT.

4. Conclusion

Two cases presented with periapical infection in the second premolar, which led to MNP. The most important part of managing such a condition associated with endodontic involvement is accurate diagnosis and/or prevention of iatrogenic errors. CBCT imagery strengthens our understanding of anatomy in this respect and may offer additional support. Elimination of endodontic etiology through conventional nonsurgical endodontic therapy in conjunction with vitamin B supplements led to successful and complete elimination of paraesthesia in due course of time.

References

[1] American Association of Endodontics, *Glossary*, AAE, Chicago, Ill, USA, 1994.

[2] H. Merskey and N. Bogduk, *IASP Task Force on Taxonomy. Classification of Chronic Pain*, IASP Press, Seattle, 2nd edition, 1994.

[3] D. R. Morse, "Infection-related mental and inferior alveolar nerve paresthesia: literature review and presentation of two cases," *Journal of Endodontia*, vol. 23, no. 7, pp. 457–460, 1997.

[4] R. Di Lenarda, M. Cadenaro, and C. Stacchi, "Paresthesia of the mental nerve induced by periapical infection: a case report," *Oral Surgery, Oral Medicine, Oral Pathology, Oral Radiology, and Endodontics*, vol. 90, no. 6, pp. 746–749, 2000.

[5] W. Jerjes, B. Swinson, B. Banu, M. Al Khawalde, and C. Hopper, "Paraesthesia of the lip and chin area resolved by endodontic treatment: a case report and review of literature," *British Dental Journal*, vol. 198, no. 12, pp. 743–745, 2005.

[6] S. M. Andrabi, S. Alam, A. Zia, M. H. Khan, and A. Kumar, "Mental nerve paresthesia secondary to initiation of endodontic therapy: a case report," *Restorative Dentistry & Endodontics*, vol. 39, no. 3, pp. 215–219, 2014.

[7] O. Genc Sen and V. Kaplan, "Temporary Mental Nerve Paresthesia Originating from Periapical Infection," *Case Reports in Dentistry*, vol. 2015, Article ID 457645, 4 pages, 2015.

[8] B. O. Gilbert and A. W. Dickerson, "Paresthesia of the mental nerve after an acute exacerbation of chronic apical periodontitis," *Journal of the American Dental Association (1939)*, vol. 103, no. 4, pp. 588–590, 1981.

[9] S. Szmigielski, M. Blankenship, J. P. Robinson, and S. Harshman, "Injury of myelin sheaths in isolated rabbit vagus nerves by α-toxin of *Staphylococcus aureus*," *Toxicon*, vol. 17, no. 4, pp. 363–371, 1979.

[10] M. Devine, Z. Yilmaz, M. Hirani, and T. Renton, "A case series of trigeminal nerve injuries caused by periapical lesions of mandibular teeth," *British Dental Journal*, vol. 222, no. 6, pp. 447–455, 2017.

[11] G. D. Glassman, "Flare-up with associated paresthesia of a mandibular second premolar with three root canals," *Oral Surgery, Oral Medicine, Oral Pathology, Oral Radiology*, vol. 64, no. 1, pp. 110–113, 1987.

[12] B. S. Chong, K. Gohil, R. Pawar, and J. Makdissi, "Anatomical relationship between mental foramen, mandibular teeth and risk of nerve injury with endodontic treatment," *Clinical Oral Investigations*, vol. 21, no. 1, pp. 381–387, 2017.

[13] D. A. Haas, "Localized complications from local anesthesia," *Journal of the California Dental Association*, vol. 26, no. 9, pp. 677–682, 1998.

[14] D. Flanagan, "Delayed onset of altered sensation following dental implant placement and mental block local anesthesia: a case report," *Implant Dentistry*, vol. 11, no. 4, pp. 324–330, 2002.

[15] S. Perotti, P. Bin, and R. Cecchi, "Hypochlorite accident during wndodontic therapy with nerve damage - a case report," *Acta Bio-Medica*, vol. 89, no. 1, pp. 104–108, 2018.

[16] E. Shadmehr and N. Shekarchizade, "Endodontic periapical lesion-induced mental nerve paresthesia," *Dental Research Journal*, vol. 12, no. 2, pp. 192–196, 2015.

[17] R. A. Barkhordar and N. T. Nguyen, "Paresthesia of the mental nerve after overextension with AH26 and gutta- percha: report of case," *Journal of the American Dental Association (1939)*, vol. 110, no. 2, pp. 202-203, 1985.

[18] E. J. Neaverth, "Disabling complications following inadvertent overextension of a root canal filling material," *Journal of Endodontia*, vol. 15, no. 3, pp. 135–139, 1989.

[19] B. T. Ozkan, S. Celik, and E. Durmus, "Paresthesia of the mental nerve stem from periapical infection of mandibular canine tooth: a case report," *Oral Surgery, Oral Medicine, Oral Pathology, Oral Radiology, and Endodontics*, vol. 105, no. 5, pp. e28–e31, 2008.

9

A Case Series of Psychological Stress Evaluation as a Risk Factor for Oral Lichen Planus

Irna Sufiawati,[1] **Ani Megawati**,[2] **Muhammad Al Farisyi**,[3] **and I. Nyoman Gede Juwita Putra**[4]

[1]*Department of Oral Medicine, Faculty of Dentistry, Padjajaran University, Indonesia*
[2]*Oral Medicine Residency Program, Faculty of Dentistry, Padjadjaran University, Indonesia*
[3]*Oral Medicine Clinic, Kota Prabumulih General Hospital, South Sumatra, Indonesia*
[4]*Department of Oral Medicine, Faculty of Dentistry, Mahasaraswati University, Indonesia*

Correspondence should be addressed to Irna Sufiawati; irna.sufiawati@fkg.unpad.ac.id

Academic Editor: Paolo Giacomo Arduino

Introduction. Oral lichen planus (OLP) is a chronic inflammatory disease of the oral mucosa with unknown etiology. Suggested predisposing factors for the development of OLP include genetic factors, viral infections, psychological stress, trauma, drug intake, and some systemic diseases. This serial case aimed to evaluate the psychological stress in triggering various types of OLP and its management. *Case Report.* Six patients, four females and two males with an age range from 23 to 57 years, came to an oral medicine clinic with chief complaints of chronic pain and burning sensations in the oral cavity. All cases showed typical clinical features of OLP on the oral mucosa, including reticular, plaque-like, erosive, and ulcerative lesions. An incisional biopsy was performed in some cases and the histopathology features confirmed the diagnosis of OLP with no signs of dysplasia/malignancy. According to the Depression, Anxiety, Stress Scale (DASS)-21, the patients had different levels of depression ranging from mild to severe; 3 patients were considered to have moderate anxiety and others had severe anxiety; and 5 patients experienced mild stress and 1 patient had moderate stress. The patients were given corticosteroids, supportive therapy, and psychological counseling. All patients experienced significant improvement of the lesions after treatment. *Conclusion.* Psychological stressors play an essential role as a risk factor in the development of OLP. Therefore, management of OLP encompasses not only an appropriate treatment of the lesions but also psychological intervention.

1. Introduction

Oral lichen planus (OLP) is a chronic inflammatory disease of unknown etiology affecting the oral mucosa. The estimated prevalence of OLP in adults is roughly 0.5–2%. The ratio for this disease in males and females is 2 : 1 and the average age of onset is 30–60 years old [1, 2]. OLP is a potentially malignant disorder despite the lingering controversy regarding the potential of OLP malignant transformation; however, the chance of OLP malignant transformation is only 0–12.5% [3–5]. The diagnosis of OLP is usually made by clinical and histological examinations. The clinical features of OLP are bilateral with symmetrical patterns and distinctive buccal mucosa. Other commonly affected sites are the tongue, gingiva, and labial mucosa [6]. On the other hand, an uncommon OLP lesion may also affect the palate, floor of the mouth, and lips. There are six clinical subtypes of OLP that can be observed: reticular, plaque-like, atrophy, erosive/ulcerative, papule, and bullous. The most common subtypes of OLP are reticular, erosive/ulcerative, and plaque-like [7, 8]. The risk factors of OLP are genetic, viral infections, psychological stress, trauma, and the association of systemic diseases that often be one of the complaints in OLP patients [9, 10].

Psychological stressors have been shown to be contributory to the pathogenesis of OLP since OLP patients often experience depression and anxiety [1, 2, 11–13]. Many studies suggest that psychological stress can alter the innate and adaptive immune

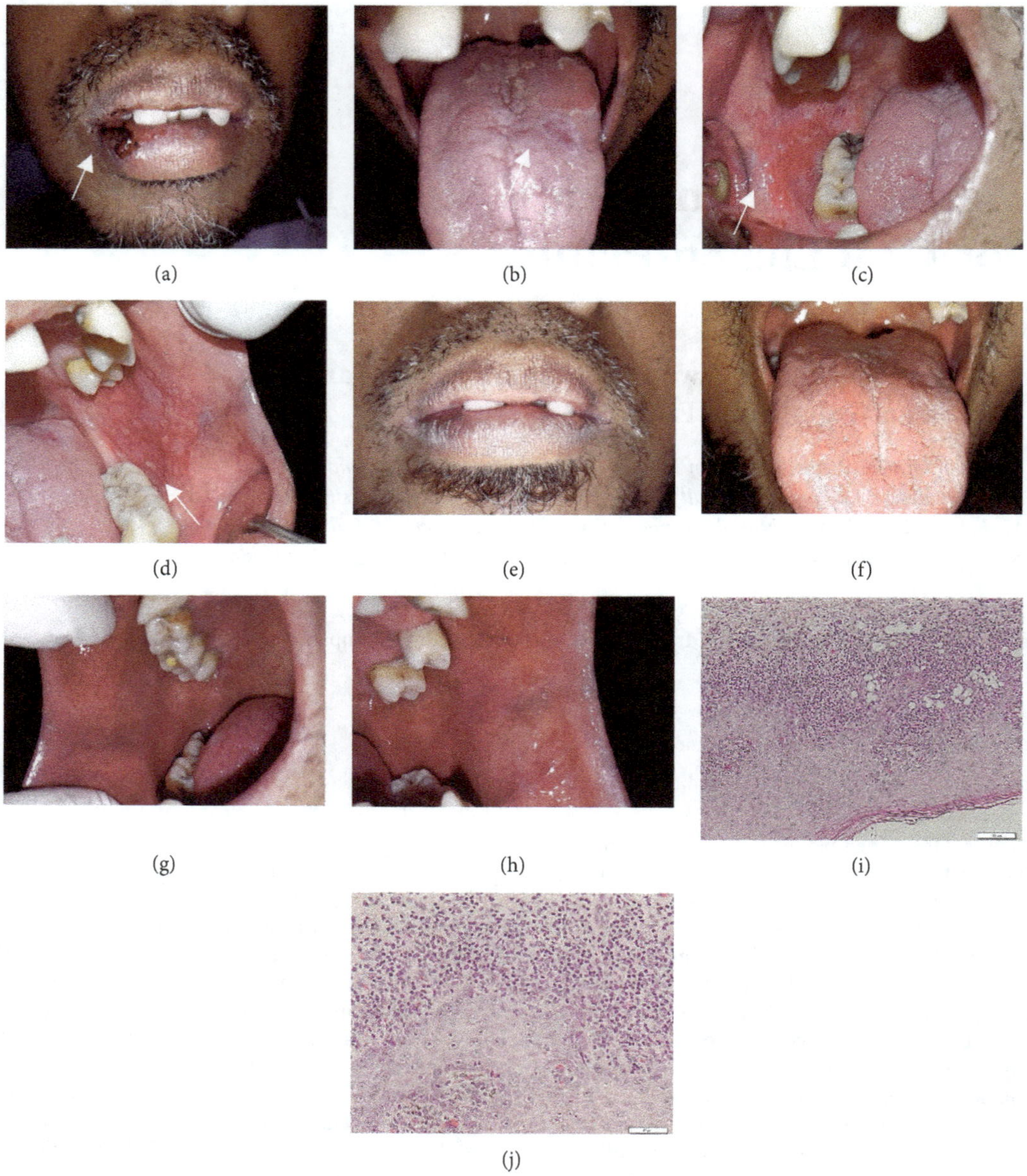

FIGURE 1: The clinical features of OLP in a 42-year-old man; (a) hemorrhagic crust, erosive surrounded by radiating white striae (Wickham striae) on the lower lip; (b). Erosive lesion surrounded by Wickham striae on the left dorsum of the tongue; (c) and (d). Erosive and ulcerative lesions on the right and left buccal mucosa; (e)–(h) Lesions on the lips, dorsum of the tongue, and the buccal mucosa completely healed after two months of treatment; (i) and (j) Histopathological features of the lesion with 100x and 400x magnification.

systems. These alterations are primarily mediated by a neuroendocrine mediator from the hypothalamic-pituitary-adrenal (HPA) and sympathetic adrenal axis, through peripheral neuropeptide release and the sympathetic nervous system [14]. Thus, stress and anxiety can be some of the risk factors for OLP.

The purpose of this case report is to evaluate psychological stress as a possible trigger of OLP and a multidisciplinary therapeutic approach in these presented cases.

2. Case Report

2.1. Case 1. A 42-year-old man visited the oral medicine clinic with a complaint of painful ulcers on the right and left inner cheeks for the last 3 months. He has no history of any systemic disease, but he was often stressed by his job as a contractor. The patient had visited a dentist and was prescribed aloe vera mouthwash and lip ointment, but there was no improvement. The patient stated that he was quite stressed because of his job.

Extraoral examination showed hemorrhagic crust, erosive lesions surrounded by radiating white striae (Wickham striae) on the lower lips. Intraoral examination showed an erosive lesion with radiating white striae (Wickham striae) on the dorsum of the tongue, and also erosive/ulcerative lesions on the right and left buccal mucosa. Based on the clinical features, the suspected diagnosis for this case was the reticular, ulcerative, and erosive type of OLP (Figure 1(a)–1(d)).

A depression test was carried out using the Depression, Anxiety, and Stress Scale (DASS)-21 questionnaire. The result of the test showed that the patient was in a state of

Table 1: DASS test results.

Case number	Depression		Anxiety		Stress	
	Before treatment	After treatment	Before treatment	After treatment	Before treatment	After treatment
1	Moderate	Mild	Severe	Mild	Mild	Mild
2	Severe	Moderate	Severe	Mild	Mild	Mild
3	Moderate	Moderate	Severe	Mild	Mild	Normal
4	Severe	Moderate	Moderate	Mild	Moderate	Mild
5	Mild	Normal	Moderate	Mild	Mild	Normal
6	Mild	Mild	Moderate	Mild	Mild	Mild

moderate depression, severe anxiety, and mild stress (Table 1). An incisional biopsy from the right buccal mucosa was performed to confirm the diagnosis. The histopathological features of the lesion showed a layer of stratified squamous epithelium that underwent a lichenoid reaction in the form of damage to basal cells and interface dermatitis. In the subepithelial cells, a massive inflammatory cell of lymphocytes, plasma cells, eosinophils, and histiocytes along the upper lamina propria can be seen forming a band-like pattern. The melanin pigment can also be seen. There was no sign of malignancy. These histopathological findings are in line with OLP (Figures 1(i)–1(j)).

The patient was administered moderate systemic corticosteroid (prednisone 30 mg/day for 14 days and then tapered), supportive therapy (multivitamin), and oral hygiene instruction (OHI). The patient was also referred to a psychological clinic to manage the stress level. In two months, the prednisone dose was reduced after each visit. Moreover, the pain in the oral cavity disappeared and the patient was able to eat normally. Intraoral examination showed that all lesions were improved after two months (Figures 1(g) and 1(h)). No pain or other symptoms were present. The patient has no longer felt as anxious as before. He was recalled and psychological tests were performed; the DASS-21 results showed decreasing scores of depression and anxiety (Table 1).

2.2. Case 2. A 31-year-old man complained of ulcer and discomfort when eating for the last three months. The man had visited several doctors and was prescribed antibiotics, analgesics, and mouthwash, but there was no improvement. The patient admitted to having family and work issues for the past few months. On intraoral examination, we found characteristics of Wickham striae with erosive areas on the lower labial mucosa and on both sides of buccal mucosa (Figures 2(a)–2(c)). The results of the DASS test revealed a severe score of depression and anxiety and a moderate level of stress (Table 1). There was no histopathological examination because the patient refused to get a biopsy. Based on the clinical examination, the patient was diagnosed with OLP with erosive and reticular type. The patient was initially administered moderate systemic corticosteroid (30 mg prednisone/day orally) for 2 weeks, multivitamins, and OHI. The patient was also referred to a psychologist for stress management. At the second visit, the lesions had subsided, and the patient was given a combination of lowered-dose prednisone and azathioprine. The oral lesion was completely healed after five months of treatment (Figures 2(d)–2(f)). The patient felt comfortable while eating and no longer felt depression after five months. We recently recalled the patient to do a psychological test using DASS-21, and the results showed that the levels of depression and anxiety were reduced compared to the first visit (Table 1).

2.3. Case 3. A 23-year-old woman complained of a painful ulcer on her tongue that caused discomfort while eating for the last three weeks. The patient had consulted a dentist and was prescribed aloe vera mouthwash, but no improvement could be seen. The patient admitted to having work issues for the past few months. Intraoral examination revealed a yellowish pseudomembranous surrounded by a well-defined erythematous with irregular borders on the ventral side of the tongue (Figures 3(a) and 3(b)). White plaques with striae surrounded by erythematous can be seen on the left and right buccal mucosa (Figures 3(c) and 3(d)). The DASS test results revealed that the patient was considered to have moderate depression, severe anxiety, and mild stress (Table 1). Histopathological examination was not carried out since the patient had refused to do a biopsy. Based on the clinical examination, the patient was diagnosed OLP with reticular and erosive type. The patient was treated with systemic corticosteroid, supportive therapy, and OHI. The patient was also referred to a psychological clinic for stress management. The oral lesion showed a significant improvement within two months of therapy. After three months of treatment, the oral lesion completely healed (Figures 3(e)–3(h)). The patient has no complaint of pain while eating and no longer felt anxious as before. Recently, the DASS-21 was carried out again and the results showed that the levels of anxiety and stress were reduced (Table 1).

2.4. Case 4. A 32-year-old woman complained of white patches and numbness on her tongue. The patient also had a habit of smoking and using over-the-counter mouthwash regularly. The patient admitted to having business issues for the past few months. Intraoral examination revealed multiple round white plaques with clear and irregular borders on the dorsum of the tongue. White plaques with striae surrounded by erythematous could also be seen on the left and right buccal mucosa (Figures 4(a)–4(c)). The DASS test results revealed that the patient had severe depression, moderate anxiety, and moderate stress (Table 1). Histopathological examination was not carried out since the patient had refused to do a biopsy. Based on the clinical examination, the patient was diagnosed OLP with reticular and plaque-

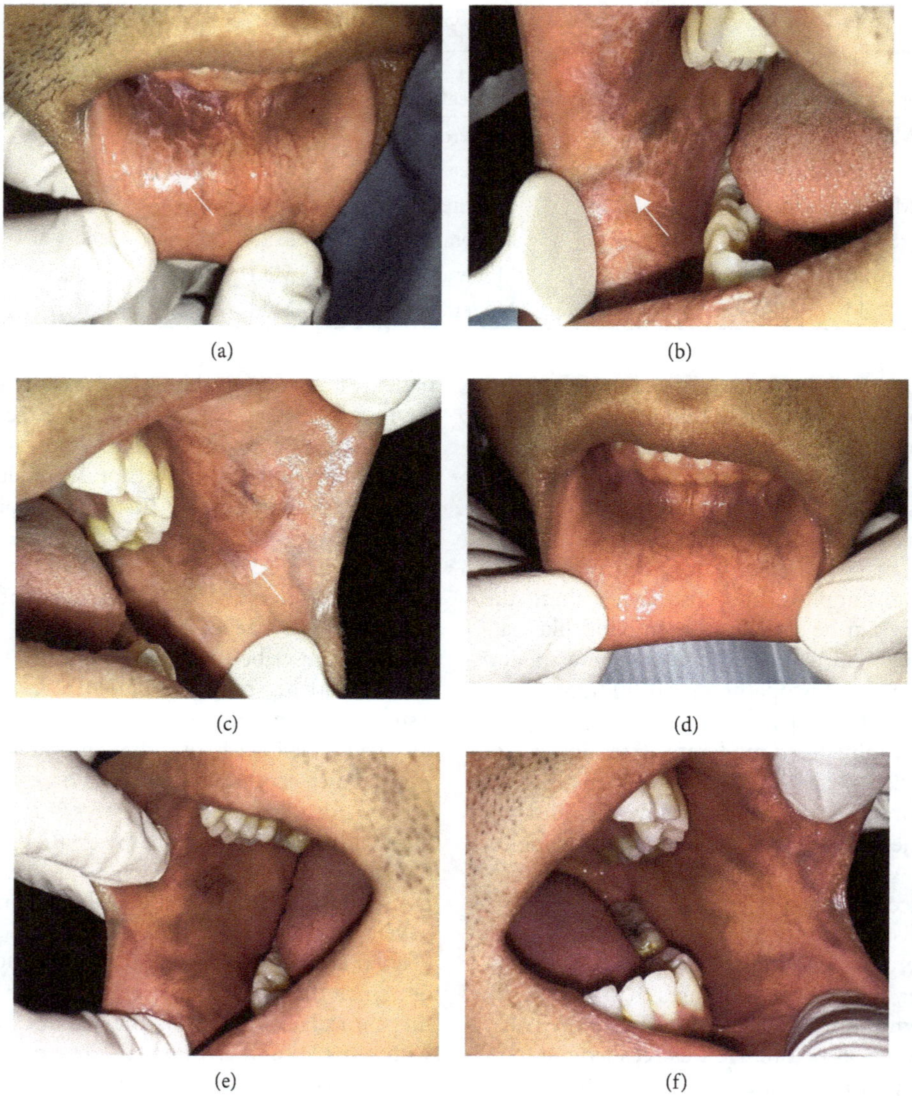

Figure 2: The clinical features of OLP in a 31-year-old man; (a)–(c). Wickham striae on the lower labial mucosa and on the right and left buccal mucosa; (d)–(f). Oral lesion completely healed after five months of treatment.

like type. The patient was administered corticosteroid mouthwash, supportive therapy, and OHI. The patient was referred to the Department of Psychology for stress management. After three months of therapy, the lesion showed a significant improvement (Figures 4(d)–4(f)). The patient felt no numbness of taste and was anxious anymore. The DASS-21 was done and the levels of depression were lower compared to the first visit (Table 1).

2.5. Case 5. A 54-year-old woman visited the oral medicine clinic with a complaint of pain and burning sensation throughout the oral cavity for the past three months. The patient also felt some discomfort when eating or drinking which resulted in lethargy and lack of motivation. The patient had no record of allergies. The patient admitted to feeling extremely anxious due to family issues for the past few months. Intraoral examination revealed white plaques on the right and left buccal regions which formed a bilateral pattern similar to Wickham striae with multiple erosive (Figures 5(a)–5(d)). The DASS-21 test revealed that the patient experienced mild depression, moderate anxiety, and moderate stress (Table 1). Histopathological examination showed the presence of stratified squamous epithelium with inflammatory cells in the epidermis and cell nucleus but still within normal limits. No signs of malignancy can be found (Figures 5(i) and 5(j)). Based on the clinical and histopathological examination, the patient was diagnosed OLP with reticular and erosive type.

The patient was administered systemic corticosteroid, supportive therapy, and OHI. The patient was also referred to a psychological clinic for stress management. The lesion on the labial mucosa dan buccal mucosa showed a significant improvement after two months of treatment (Figures 5(e)–5(h)). The patient has no longer burning sensation in her mouth and no longer felt anxiety as before. The DASS-21 was performed again. She was considered to have only mild anxiety, while the scores of depression and stress were reduced to normal levels (Table 1).

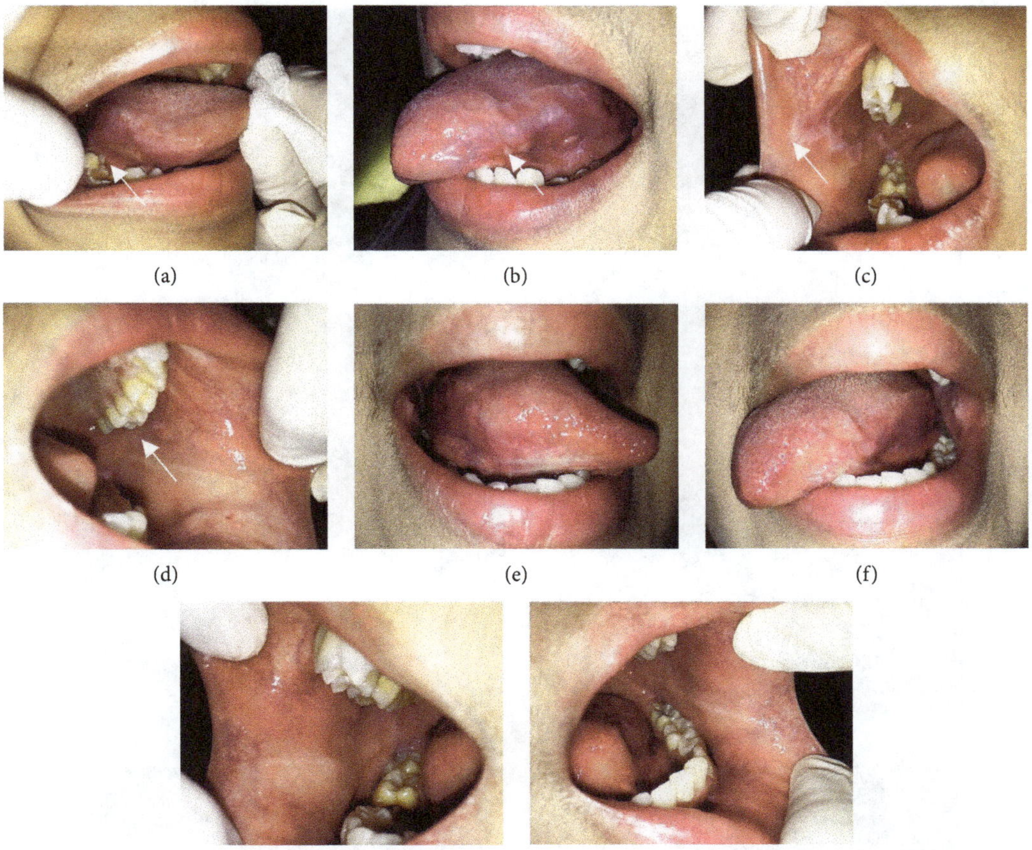

(a) (b) (c) (d) (e) (f) (g) (h)

FIGURE 3: The clinical features of OLP in a 23-year-old woman; (a) and (b) yellowish pseudomembranous on the ventral of the tongue; (c) and (d) white plaques with striae surrounded by erythematous on the right and left buccal mucosa; (e)–(h) Oral lesion showed a significant improvement after two months of treatment.

2.6. Case 6. A 57-year-old woman visited the oral medicine clinic with complaints of pain and burning sensation throughout the oral cavity for the last four months. The patient complained that these conditions had worsened over the last few weeks. The patient was extremely uncomfortable with the conditions and believed that they were symptoms of oral cancer. The DASS-21 test results showed that the patient had mild depression, moderate anxiety, and mild stress (Table 1). Extraoral examination revealed the presence of Wickham striae on the right lower lip. Intraoral examination revealed bilateral white striae on the right and left buccal mucosa (Figures 6(a)–6(d)). Histopathological examination revealed hyperkeratosis of stratified squamous epithelium, but the nucleus was still within normal limits (Figures 6(i) and 6(j)). Based on the clinical and histopathological examination, the patient was diagnosed OLP with reticular and erosive type.

The patient was administered systemic corticosteroid, supportive therapy, and OHI. The patient was also referred to a psychologist for stress management. After two months, the pain and burning sensation in the oral cavity had disappeared. The patient was able to eat without any discomfort and no longer felt as anxious as before. Based on the intraoral examination, the Wickham striae on the right and left buccal mucosa had improved, leaving diffuse erythematous on the affected areas (Figures 6(e)–6(h)). Systemic corticosteroid was still administered at a lower dose. The DASS-21 was recently performed again and the results indicated that the levels of depression and anxiety were reduced to mild, but she still experienced mild stress (Table 1).

The characteristic of the patients, clinical profile of OLP, and their treatment were summarized in Table 2. The results of the DASS-21 test before and after the treatment can be seen in Table 1.

3. Discussion

Based on the six OLP cases above, all the patients experienced some sort of psychological stress. The DASS-21 scores revealed different levels of psychological stress for each patient. Stress was experienced due to family problems, work-related issues, pressure, fear of possible malignancy, and fear of unsuccessful treatments. Pain, anxiety, and fear can cause some changes in the metabolic and endocrine systems, causing physiological side effects such as increased cortisol. Cortisol is glucocorticoid 21-carbon secreted by the adrenal cortex to regulate the metabolism of protein, carbohydrate, fat, and water that can affect the nervous system sensitivity and stress responses [14, 15].

According to the relationship between stress and OLP, stressful life changes play an important role in the onset or reactivation of OLP, depending on each person's ability to

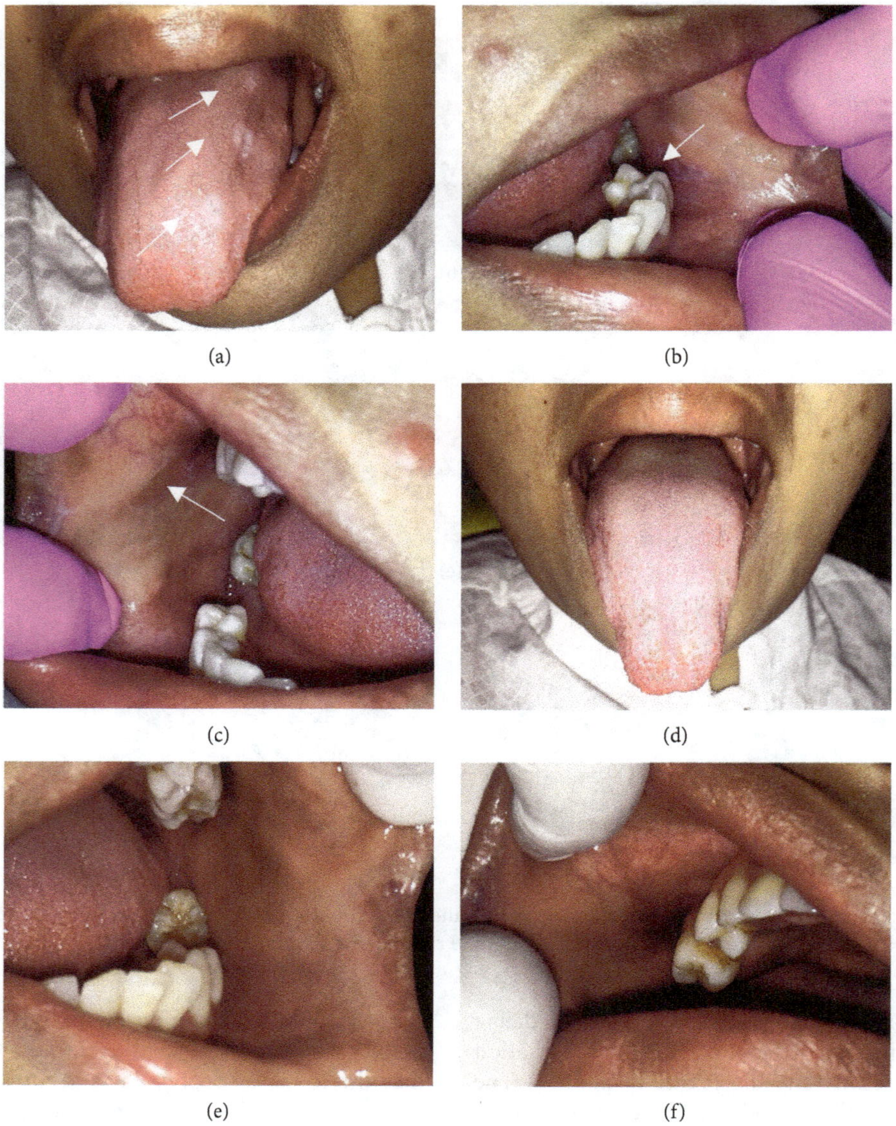

Figure 4: The clinical features of OLP in a 32-year-old woman; (a) multiple white plaques on the dorsum of the tongue; (b) and (c) erosive lesions surrounded by Wickham striae on the right and left buccal mucosa; (e)–(g) oral lesion was completely healed after three months of treatment.

cope and their particular reaction to stress [11]. Psychological conditions such as anxiety, depression, and stress tend to be more prevalent in OLP patients. Karthikeyan et al. (2016) found that serum, saliva, and urine cortisol levels in the OLP group were significantly higher than in the control group, indicating that the level of psychological stress was higher in the study group compared to the control group [12]. Based on these studies, it can be concluded that psychological stress is indicated to have a role in the manifestation of OLP.

The pathogenesis of OLP is quite complex. OLP is a cell-mediated autoimmune reaction in which CD4+ and CD8+ T lymphocytes induce the apoptosis of epithelial basal cells [16]. Patients with lichen planus experience a stressful event before the onset of the disease and major stressful events can exacerbate lichen planus. Psychological stress can trigger autoimmune disorders or skin disorders through neuroendocrine and neuroimmune dysregulation [17]. Immunological abnormalities lead to delayed growth of mucosa epithelial, which is responsible for hyperkeratosis [18].

From the higher psychological test scores in patients with OLP, it is not possible to determine whether the observed psychological changes are a direct cause of OLP or a consequence of OLP and its lesions. OLP patients who have a susceptibility to stress are also often concerned about the possibility of malignancy, which may contribute to the further potentiation of anxiety. OLP patients also report a poorer sleep quality due to a painful condition in their mouth that increases depression [19]. Therefore, OLP patients with psychological stress require a combination of OLP therapy and psychotherapy. OLP can be improved by regulating mood through medication and psychological counseling [20].

All the cases were treated with corticosteroids. Corticosteroids can be administered systemically or topically. The dose of corticosteroids was gradually reduced based on the

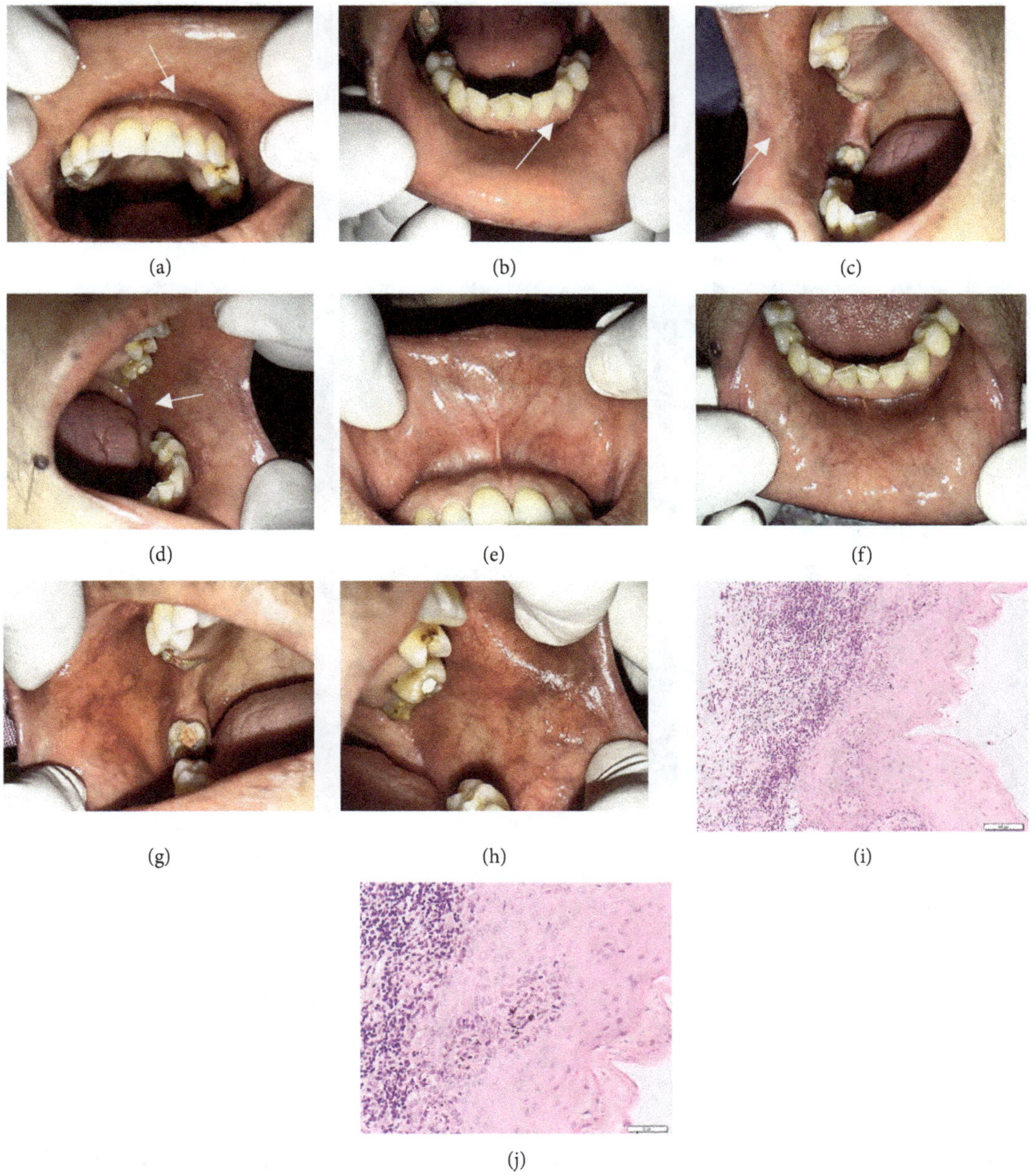

FIGURE 5: The clinical features of OLP in a 54-year-old woman; (a) and (b) erythema with radiating white striae on the upper and lower labial mucosa; (c) and (d) Wickham striae on the lower left labial mucosa and on the left buccal mucosa; (e)–(h) lesion on the upper and lower labial mucosa and the right and left buccal mucosa showed a significant improvement; (i) and (j) histopathological features of the lesion with 100x and 400x magnification.

severity of the lesion. Corticosteroids are endogenous steroid hormones produced from the adrenal cortex. Corticosteroids are also synthetically produced hormones used for pharmacotherapy. Corticosteroids have been widely used as anti-inflammatory drugs to combat autoimmune disorders. Systemic corticosteroids work by affecting lipid, carbohydrate, protein, calcium, and electrolyte. Glucocorticoids suppress all types of inflammation and allergic reactions by inhibiting the activity of plasminogen and reducing the inflammatory mediators such as prostaglandins and leukotrienes [21, 22].

The release of glucocorticoid compounds would increase the levels of corticotrophin-releasing hormone (CRH) and arginine vasopressin (AVP). Both of these hormones will activate the sympathetic nervous system and the hypothalamic-pituitary-adrenal (HPA) axis. Moreover, the hippocampus and amygdala, which regulate specific stress responses, also have glucocorticoid receptors. The translocation of steroid receptor complexes to the nucleus and the presence of glucocorticoid receptors can alter gene transcription. These changes will produce neurotransmitters including dopamine, serotonin, and neuropeptides, namely somatostatin and beta-endorphins [22, 23]. Indirectly, the release of endogenous glucocorticoids can regulate psychological stress responses such as depression and anxiety.

The limitation of this study is that the number of patients is too small so that the results cannot be generalized.

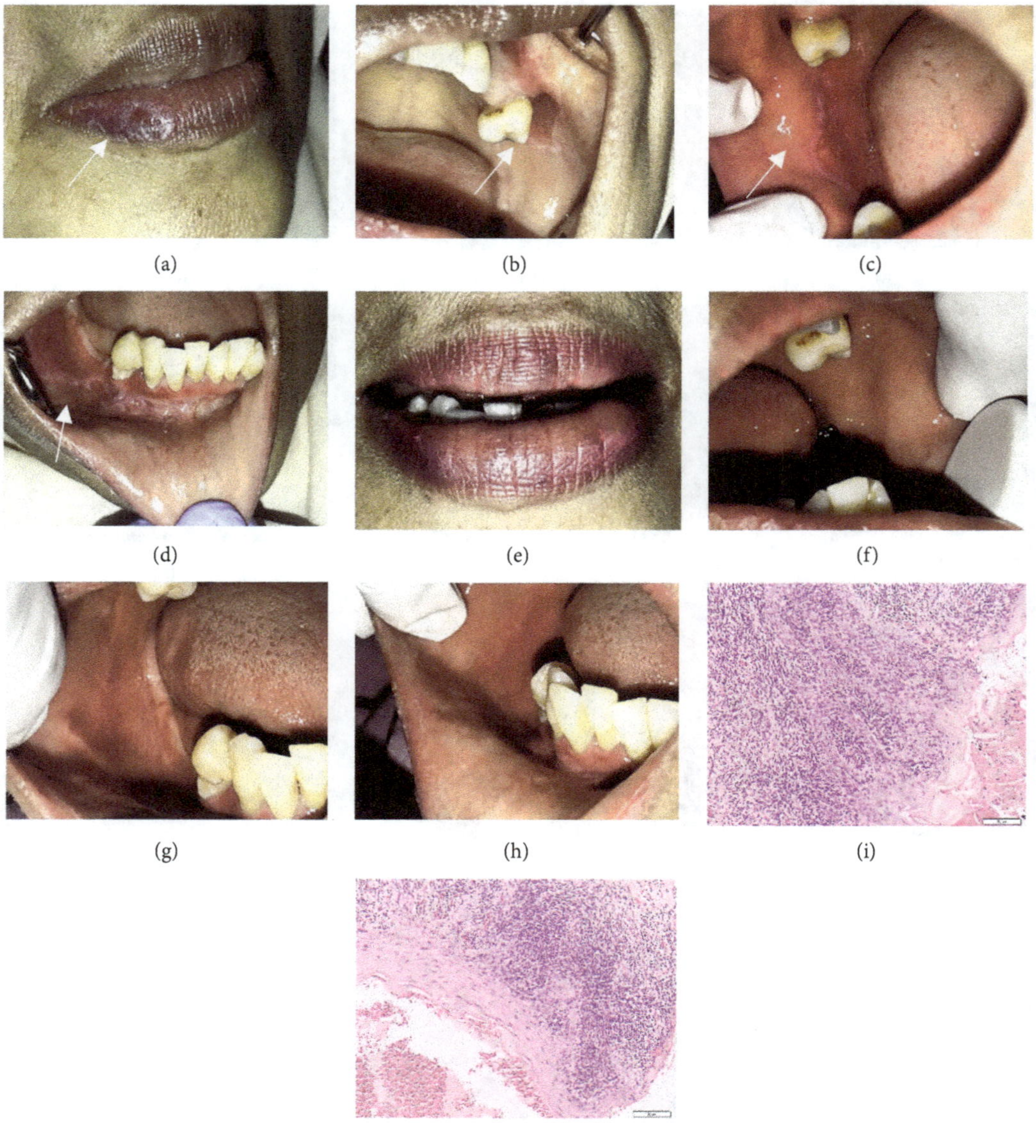

(a) (b) (c) (d) (e) (f) (g) (h) (i) (j)

Figure 6: The clinical features of OLP in a 57-year-old woman; (a) erosive lesion and Wickham striae on the right lower lip; (b)–(d) bilateral erosive lesion surrounded by Wickham striae on the right and left buccal mucosa; (e)–(h) lesions showed improvement after 2 months of treatment; (i) and (j) microscopic appearance of the lesion with 100x and 400x magnification.

Table 2: The characteristic of the patients, clinical profile of OLP, and the treatment.

Case number	Sex	Age (years old)	Location	Type of OLP	Treatment
1	Male	42	Lip, dorsum of the tongue, right and left buccal mucosa	Reticular, erosive, and ulcerative	Systemic corticosteroid
2	Male	31	Lower labial mucosa, right and left buccal mucosa	Reticular	Systemic corticosteroid
3	Female	23	Right and left buccal mucosa, right and left side of the tongue	Reticular and erosive	Systemic corticosteroid
4	Female	32	Dorsum of the tongue, right and left buccal mucosa	Reticular and plaque-like	Topical corticosteroid
5	Female	54	Upper and lower labial mucosa, right and left buccal mucosa	Reticular and erosive	Systemic corticosteroid
6	Female	57	Lip, gingiva and vestibule of mandibular, right and left buccal mucosa	Reticular and erosive	Systemic corticosteroid

Further longitudinal studies using larger samples need to be carried out.

4. Conclusion

Psychological stressors may play an essential role as a risk factor in the development of OLP. Therefore, dentists should consider the mental problems of OLP patients. This report may psychological interventions are a vital component of the collaborative care approach in the treatment of OLP.

Consent

Informed consent has been obtained from the patient for this publication.

Acknowledgments

The authors thank the patients, academic staff, residents of Oral Medicine Residency Program, and workers of Dental Clinic of Hasan Sadikin General Hospital and Dental Hospital of Universitas Padjadjaran for their support.

References

[1] E. Ruoppo, M. D. Mignogna, S. Leuci, M. Amato, M. Aria, and D. Adamo, "Sleep disturbances, anxiety and depression in patients with oral lichen planus: a case-control study," *Journal of the European Academy of Dermatology and Venereology*, vol. 29, no. 2, pp. 291–297, 2014.

[2] L. Gavic, L. Cigic, D. Biocina Lukenda, V. Gruden, and J. S. Gruden Pokupec, "The role of anxiety, depression, and psychological stress on the clinical status of recurrent aphthous stomatitis and oral lichen planus," *Journal of Oral Pathology & Medicine*, vol. 43, no. 6, pp. 410–417, 2014.

[3] E. A. Rosa, A. M. Hurtado-Puerto, D. P. Falcão, A. P. Brietzke, D. A. P. Franceschi, and F. F. Cavalcanti Neto, "Oral lichen planus and malignant transformation: the role of p16, Ki-67, Bub-3 and SOX4 in assessing precancerous potential," *Experimental and Therapeutic Medicine*, vol. 15, no. 5, pp. 4157–4166, 2018.

[4] M. Tampa, C. Caruntu, M. Mitran et al., "Markers of oral lichen planus malignant transformation," *Disease Markers*, vol. 2018, 13 pages, 2018.

[5] H. B. Margono and I. Sufiawati, "The challenge in predicting malignant transformation of oral lichen planus. Case rep," *Dent*, pp. 1–14, 2018.

[6] A. Alsarraf, K. Mehta, and N. Khzam, "The gingival oral lichen planus: a periodontal-oral medicine approach," *Case Reports in Dentistry*, vol. 2019, 3 pages, 2019.

[7] M. Glick, *Burket's Oral Medicine*, People's Medical Publising House, 12th edition edition, 2015.

[8] H. H. Elsabagh, Y. Y. Gaweesh, J. K. Ghonima, and M. Gebril, "A novel comprehensive scoring system for oral lichen planus: a validity, diagnostic accuracy, and clinical sensitivity study," *Oral Surgery, Oral Medicine, Oral Pathology, Oral Radiology*, vol. 131, no. 3, pp. 304–311, 2021.

[9] M. Garma, W. Hasni, B. Annabi, B. Sriha, S. Boudegga, and A. Boughzella, "Isolated lichen planus of the lips: cases reports and literature review," *Journal of Oral Medicine and Oral Surgery*, vol. 26, no. 2, pp. 14–16, 2020.

[10] R. Puri, "Lichen planus. A case report," *Journal of Case Reports in Dental Medicine*, vol. 2, no. 2, pp. 25–28, 2020.

[11] M. Čanković, B.-B. Marija, and N. Zdenka, "Stressful life events and personality traits in patients with oral lichen planus," *Acta Dermatovenerologica Croatica*, vol. 23, no. 4, pp. 270–276, 2015.

[12] P. Karthikeyan and N. Aswath, "Stress as an etiologic co-factor in recurrent aphthous ulcers and oral lichen planus," *Journal of Oral Science*, vol. 58, no. 2, pp. 237–240, 2016.

[13] L. K. Nadendla, "Association of salivary cortisol and anxiety levels in lichen planus patients," *Journal of Clinical and Diagnostic Research*, pp. 10–13, 2014.

[14] N. A. S. M. Azmi, N. Juliana, S. Azmani, N. M. Effendy, I. F. Abu, N. I. M. F. Teng et al., "Cortisol on circadian rhythm and its effect on cardiovascular system," *International Journal of Environmental Research and Public Health*, vol. 18, no. 2, pp. 1–15, 2021.

[15] P. Lopez-Jornet, C. A. Cayuela, A. Tvarijonaviciute, F. Parra-Perez, D. Escribano, and J. Ceron, "Oral lichen planus: salival biomarkers cortisol, immunoglobulin A, adiponectin," *Journal of Oral Pathology & Medicine*, vol. 45, no. 3, pp. 211–217, 2016.

[16] Z. B. Kurago, "Etiology and pathogenesis of oral lichen planus: an overview," *Oral Surgery, Oral Medicine, Oral Pathology, Oral Radiology*, vol. 122, no. 1, pp. 72–80, 2016.

[17] N. S. Sawant, N. A. Vanjari, U. Khopkar, and S. Adulkar, "A study of depression and quality of life in patients of lichen planus," *Scientific World Journal*, vol. 2015, pp. 1–6, 2015.

[18] S. Sagari, S. Sanadhya, M. Doddamani, and R. Rajput, "Molecular markers in oral lichen planus: a systematic review," *Journal of Oral and Maxillofacial Pathology*, vol. 20, no. 1, pp. 115–121, 2016.

[19] B. Manczyk, J. Gołda, A. Biniak et al., "Evaluation of depression, anxiety and stress levels in patients with oral lichen planus," *Journal of Oral Science*, vol. 61, no. 3, pp. 391–397, 2019.

[20] X. Song, X. Wu, C. Wang, S. Sun, and X. Zhang, "Case report: treatment of oral lichen planus with a focus on psychological methods. front," *Psychiatry*, vol. 12, p. 731093, 2021.

[21] G. Lodi, M. Manfredi, V. Mercadante, R. Murphy, M. Carrozzo, and Cochrane Oral Health Group, "Interventions for treating oral lichen planus: corticosteroid therapies," *Cochrane Database of Systematic Reviews*, vol. 2020, no. 2, p. CD001168, 2020.

[22] M. S. Kiran, S. Vidya, G. S. Aswal, V. Kumar, and V. Rai, "Systemic and topical steroids in the management of oral mucosal lesions," *Journal of Pharmacy & Bioallied Sciences*, vol. 9, no. 1, pp. S1–S3, 2017.

[23] D. Cruz-Topete and J. A. Cidlowski, "One hormone, two actions: anti- and pro-inflammatory effects of glucocorticoids," *Neuroimmunomodulation*, vol. 22, no. 1–2, pp. 20–32, 2014.

Maxillary Fungal Osteomyelitis Mimicking and Treated as Endodontic Pathosis

Sarang Suresh Hotchandani, Feroze Ali Kalhoro, Priya Rani Harjani, and Mahwish Memon

Department of Operative Dentistry, Liaquat University of Medical & Health Sciences, Jamshoro, Pakistan

Correspondence should be addressed to Sarang Suresh Hotchandani; hotchandaniss@hotmail.com

Academic Editor: Sivakumar Nuvvula

Fungal osteomyelitis is a lethal opportunistic infection that affects only a small percentage of patients present to endodontists. It is a highly contagious infection that requires urgent treatment. We discuss three cases in which endodontic pathology was initially recognized but subsequent follow-up revealed severe osteolytic fungal infection of the maxilla manifesting as acute apical abscesses in the maxillary canine region. CBCT demonstrated osteolytic abnormalities, and further histology confirmed the illness was caused by mucormycosis in patients with uncontrolled diabetes mellitus and exposure to COVID-19.

1. Introduction

Mucormycosis is a rare but severe fungal infection caused by a group of molds known as mucoromycetes. It is quite uncommon. Mucormycosis is more prevalent in individuals with preexisting health problems or those who take medications that decrease the immune system's ability to fight infection and disease. Diabetes patients are at an increased risk of developing mucormycosis, an invasive fungal infection that can be fatal if it spreads to other areas of the body. Individuals with hematological malignancies or who require a solid-organ transplant are at a higher risk of receiving it [1]. Mucormycosis is most frequently found in the nose, eye, and brain of those who contract it. The diagnosis may take so long due to the scarcity of symptoms. Any nonbacterial sinusitis in diabetics, even if ketoacidosis is not present, should increase the risk of mucormycosis [2].

Globally, the incidence of mucormycosis is increasing, but it is increasing at an alarming rate in India and China among people with uncontrolled diabetes mellitus. However, according to figures from the early COVID-19 times, there are 14 cases per 100,000 people in Pakistan. Cases are on the rise due to underreporting and dentists' misunderstanding of their presentation in endodontic clinics [3]. Here, three cases are reported in which patients initially complained of endodontic problems and were treated accordingly but were later diagnosed with fungal osteomyelitis masquerading as endodontic pathosis.

2. Case Presentations

2.1. Case 1

2.1.1. Presenting Complaint. A 45-year-old well-educated gentleman was referred by his general dentist to the Department of Operative Dentistry and Endodontics with the complaint of persistent pain in his upper and lower anterior teeth following nonsurgical endodontic treatment of his teeth from tooth number 6 to 11 and pus discharge with swelling on his upper posterior region.

2.1.2. History of Presenting Complaint and Past Treatments. The patient stated that he had been experiencing soreness in his upper and lower anterior teeth for one month and had seen his family dental practitioner. His previous dental practitioner diagnosed pulp necrosis in all his maxillary anterior teeth from tooth number 6 to 11 and initiated root canal treatment, which took approximately 20 days to complete. A few teeth remain untreated, but due to the persistence of pain, he was referred to the endodontic department for further evaluation and management. The patient had a history of dengue virus infection, which resulted in a low platelet count, and was hospitalized for many days. Apart from that, he is asymptomatic and has no significant medical history. The patient stated that he had no history of diabetes.

2.1.3. Lab Workup and Results. His most recent complete blood work revealed a normal platelet count. His chemical pathology report showed C-reactive protein 3.341 mg/dl. Apart from that, he is asymptomatic and has no significant medical history. However, when glycated hemoglobin (HBA1c) was determined, the result was 6.53 percent.

2.1.4. Extraoral Clinical Examination. Extraoral clinical examination revealed an obese patient with a normal gait and an excellent sense of spatial and temporal orientation. He has broad diffuse edema on the right side of his face; his temporomandibular joint testing is normal. There was no cervical lymphadenopathy.

2.1.5. Intraoral Clinical Examination. Intraoral examination revealed multiple wear facets on the incisal edge of the maxillary anterior teeth, a supernumerary maxillary right lateral incisor, ulcer with swelling on the attached gingiva of the maxillary right canine, and widespread diffuse gingival swelling over the maxillary anterior teeth. Periodontal examination indicated grade two movement between the maxillary right third molar and the maxillary left canine, as well as grade three mobility in the maxillary right second molar, with deep probing depths. The gingiva of the maxillary right buccal region was found to be damp, spongy, and wrinkled, with pus discharge from the cervices. The palatal surface revealed a deep palate with tooth-colored restorations from tooth number 7 to 11, as well as temporary, white-colored restorations on the maxillary right supernumerary lateral incisor and tooth number 6. There were buccal and palatal swelling on the right side, with a bulbous interdental papilla between tooth number 5 and 6, and stained crack lines on the tooth number 4 and 5. The pulp tests did not result in response on the cold and electronic pulp tester (Figure 1).

2.1.6. Radiographic Examination. Two OPGs were exposed to the patient by the referring clinician: one at the time of presentation to the general dentist and another after 20 days. The initial OPG revealed no notable results. The second OPG reveals a radiolucent line on the mesial surface of tooth number 2 and periapical radiolucency on adjacent teeth. Tooth numbers 6 and 7 exhibit obturation with restoration; however, only radiopaque restoration with empty canals is seen from tooth number 8 to 11. Multiple periapical radiographs revealed intracanal medicament in other canals that seemed empty on OPG (Figure 2). In 3D reconstruction, cone beam computed tomography (CBCT) images revealed a patchy osteolytic appearance of the maxilla from the right side of the alveolus to the left premolar area of the alveolus. Axial views revealed full haziness in the right maxillary sinus, as well as a moth-eaten aspect to the right maxilla (Figures 3 and 4).

The patient was then referred to the department of oral and maxillofacial surgery for evaluation and treatment. A computed tomography scan of the face and neck with contrast was obtained by a maxillofacial surgeon which showed mucosal thickening, resulting in partial opacification of the bilateral maxillary sinus. There was also significant erosion of the inferior wall of the maxillary sinus and the entire alveolar process of the maxilla. Additionally, a linear pathological fracture of the right maxillary alveolar process was observed along with the premolar tooth socket. The findings showed a severe maxillary sinus infection caused by a fungal infection.

2.1.7. Management. The tooth number 2 was extracted, and an incisional biopsy sample was collected via intrasocket debridement. Histopathological examination was obtained. After enquiring from the oral and maxillofacial department, the patient was on the intravenous treatment of amphotericin B and was planned for future maxillectomy.

2.1.8. Histopathology. Histopathological examination revealed minute fragments of extensively inflamed and ulcerated squamous mucosa, profuse granulation tissue, and necrotic bone chips. In the intrabony zones, scattered fungal hyphae were observed. Most hyphae were slender and aseptate in shape. However, the report also stated wide, ribbon-like, and aseptate hyphae. These data suggested a mixed fungal infection containing mucor.

2.2. Case 2

2.2.1. Presenting Complaint. This 36-year-old male patient arrived for a follow-up appointment after initiating endodontic treatment in his tooth number 11 for pulp necrosis with persistent apical abscess.

2.2.2. History of Presenting Complaint. This case was initiated by a postgraduate resident at the Operative Dentistry and Endodontics Department. The case was initially diagnosed as pulp necrosis with chronic apical abscess, and nonsurgical root canal therapy was planned and initiated in two visits in tooth number 11, with one visit pulpectomy followed by biomechanical preparation of canal after determining working length and intracanal calcium hydroxide placed for 15 days. However, at the follow-up visit, the patient still reported pus discharge from the same place as before. This patient was then referred to the author for additional evaluation and management. After referral, a history was obtained, and the patient claimed no major past or present medical history. The patient was prescribed by the previous resident, capsule doxycycline 100 mg for 5 days, but the pus did not cease. The patient reported COVID-19 symptoms around a month ago and is currently COVID-19 PCR-negative. He is otherwise asymptomatic and healthy with no history of diabetes.

2.2.3. Clinical Examination. Clinical examination revealed obvious plaque on the maxillary posterior teeth, as well as

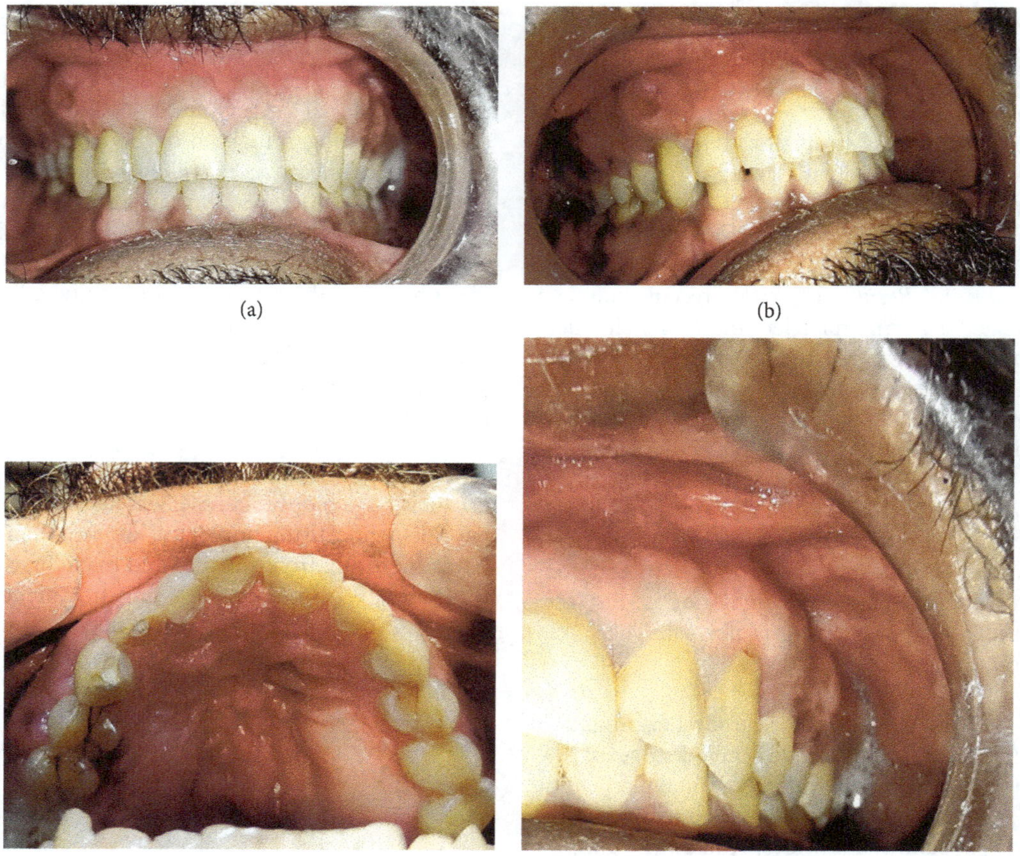

(a) (b)

(c) (d)

Figure 1: Clinical photographs of case 1: (a) frontal view, (b) right maxillary view showing the ulcer, (c) palatal view, and (d) right maxillary view showing normal gingiva.

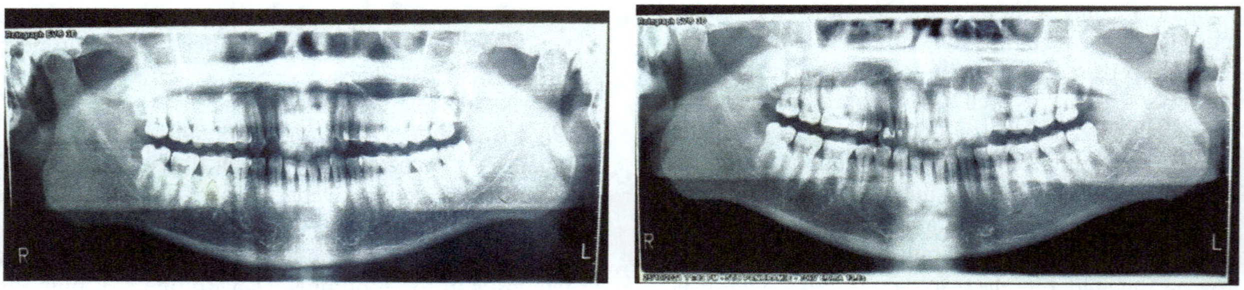

(a) (b)

Figure 2: OPG of case 1 obtained at 15 days' gap.

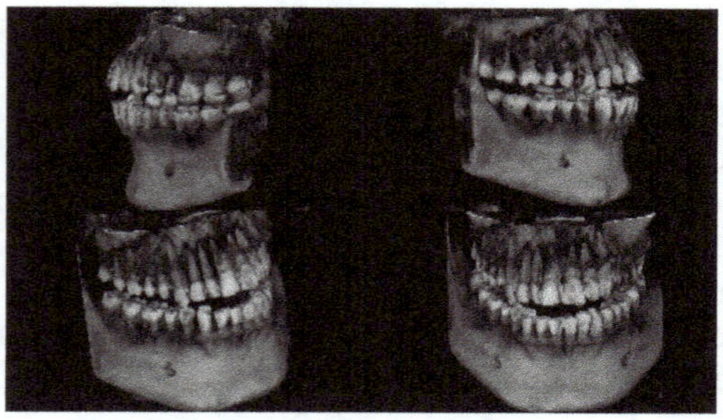

Figure 3: 3D CBCT view of case 1 showing resorption over the maxillary alveolus region on the right side.

yellowish pus discharge from the attached gingiva between tooth numbers 5 and 6 (Figure 5).

2.2.4. Radiographic Examination. The OPG indicated osteolytic alterations in the maxillary right posterior area and a significant cystic lesion in the maxillary left anterior region. A CBCT scan was obtained to evaluate the 3-dimensional alterations in the maxillary region (Figure 6). CBCT indicated significant osteolytic alterations in the front maxilla, as well as the involvement of the right maxillary sinus and bony sequestrum.

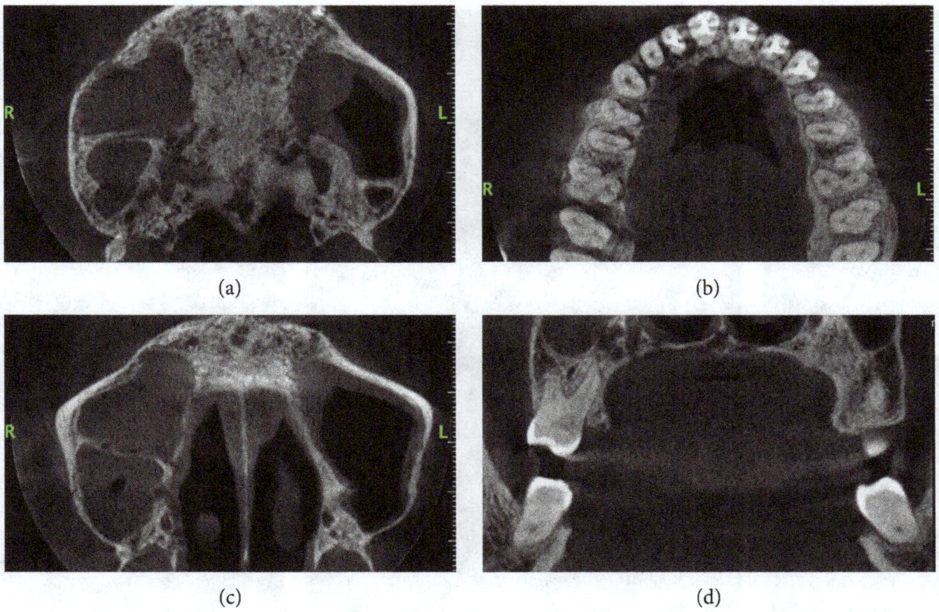

FIGURE 4: CBCT of case 1: (a–c) axial views; (d) cross-sectional view. (a) Osteolytic change in the posterior area. (b) Radiopaque obturating material in maxillary anterior teeth with resorption of alveolar process. (c) Haziness in the maxillary sinus on the right side. (d) Osteolytic changes on the palatal alveolar region on the maxillary 1st molar.

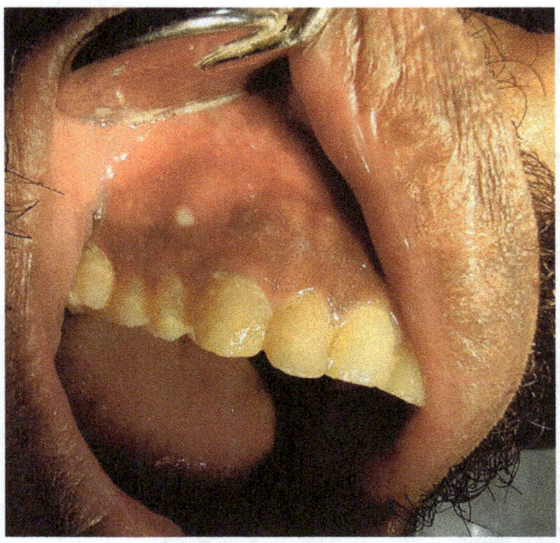

FIGURE 5: Clinical picture of case 2 showing yellowish pus discharge apical to the maxillary 1st premolar.

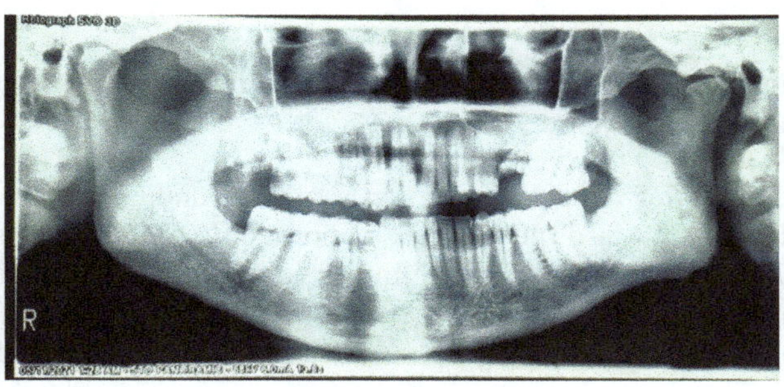

FIGURE 6: OPG of case 2.

2.2.5. Lab Reports and Results. A blood biochemical analysis revealed a normal total blood picture with elevated neutrophils and erythrocyte sedimentation rate and HBA1c of 10.9 percent.

2.2.6. Management. This patient was then referred to a physician for diabetes care. After a few days, the pus discharge ceased, and histology revealed that the patient had fungal osteomyelitis. The patient refused surgical therapy in favor of medicinal treatment (Figures 7 and 8).

2.3. Case 3

2.3.1. Presenting Complaint. This 65-year-old retired officer was referred to the author for the diagnosis and treatment of persistent swelling over the gingiva in the maxillary anterior area.

2.3.2. History of Presenting Complaint. This patient appeared to his family dentist with a complaint of several swellings above the tooth number 5 and 6, as well as pain while eating. After a diagnosis of pulp necrosis and symptomatic apical periodontitis, nonsurgical root canal therapy was commenced in the tooth number 6 and 7. The root canal treatment was scheduled to be completed in two visits, with pulpectomy and intracanal medicament for 15 days, calcium hydroxide. However, the pain subsided after 15 days, but the swellings did not, and another enlargement on the palatal region emerged after 7 days. The patient was subsequently referred to the author for diagnosis and care. On questioning about the patient's background, there is no history of trauma, and the patient is a regular visitor to his family dentist. He is otherwise healthy and stable right now.

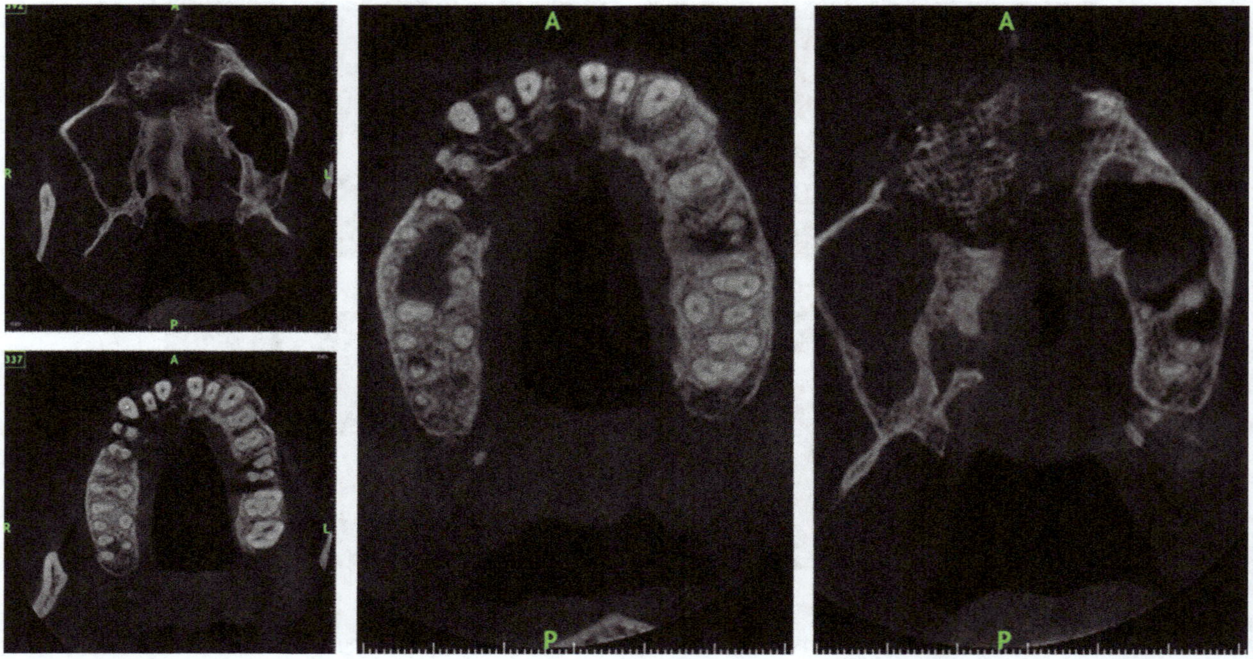

FIGURE 7: CBCT axial views of case 2 showing gross osteolytic changes with bony sequestrum with haziness on the right maxillary sinus.

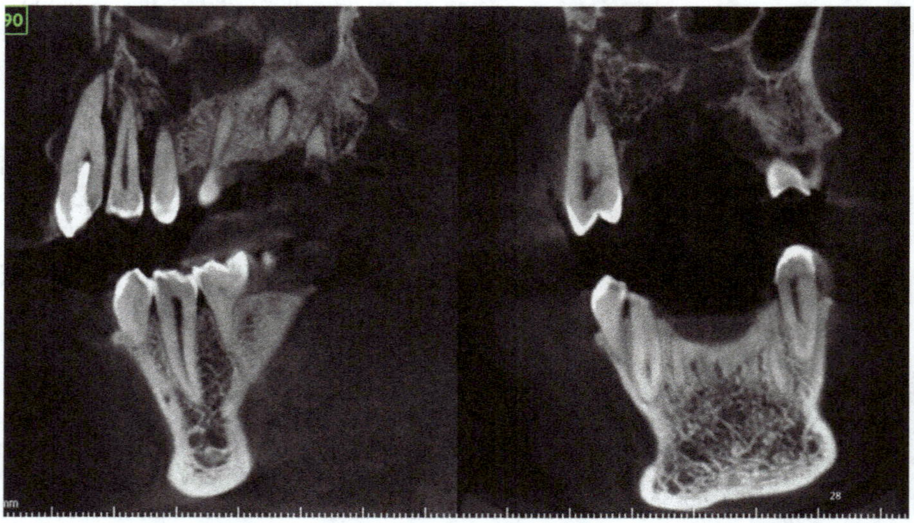

FIGURE 8: CBCT sagittal and coronal views of case 2 showing bony sequestrum with gross osteolytic changes infiltrating the floor of the maxillary sinus.

2.3.3. Lab Results. The patient had a history of type 2 diabetes maintained with normal laboratory tests; current whole blood HBA1c is 5.0 percent, serum creatinine 1.1 mg/dl, eGFR > 60 ml/min/1.73, normocytic normochromic blood profile, and ESR 75 mm/1Hr, and lipid profile values are normal. He sees his doctor regularly and takes his medication as prescribed.

2.3.4. Clinical Examination. Clinical examination indicated plaque from tooth number 4 to 8, four swellings in the attached gingiva, and a cervical lesion on the tooth number 4. From the tooth number 4 through 8, there was grade 1 mobility with soft swelling in the palatal region not crossing the midline (Figure 9).

2.3.5. Radiographic Examination. Periapical and OPG examinations revealed no notable abnormalities; nevertheless, CBCT was performed, which indicated osteolytic alterations in the anterior maxilla on the right side extending from the tooth number 4 through 8, as well as haziness in the left maxillary sinus.

2.3.6. Management. The patient was referred to a maxillofacial surgeon and histopathology diagnosed as fungal osteomyelitis; he is under medical treatment now (Figure 10).

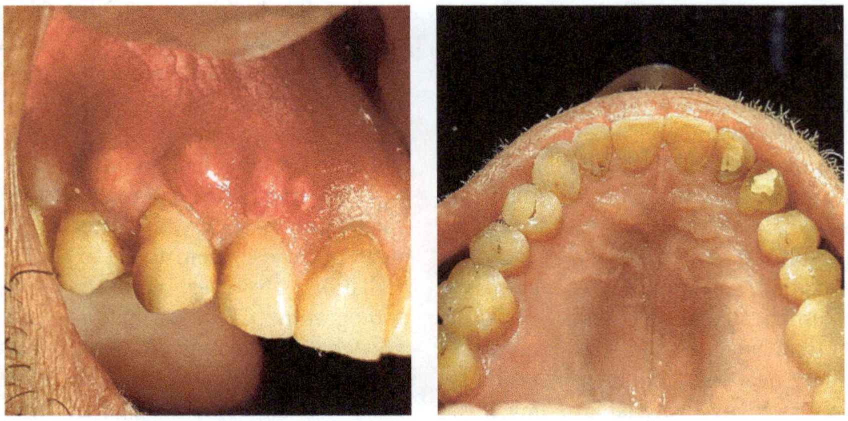

(a) (b)

Figure 9: Clinical photograph of case 3 showing multiple swellings apical to the maxillary right lateral incisor and maxillary canine, with palatal swelling indicated with an arrow.

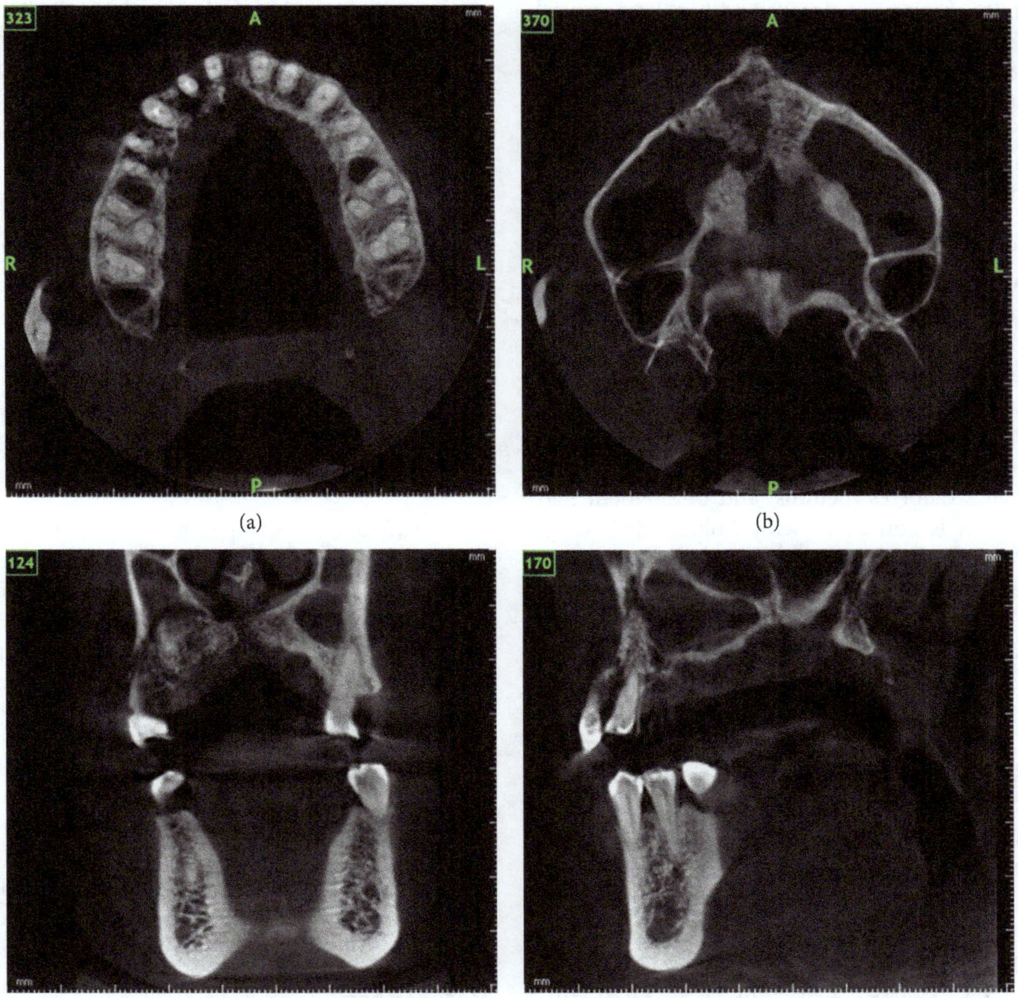

(a) (b)

(c) (d)

Figure 10: CBCT images of case 3 showing (a, b) axial views with osteolytic changes in the alveolus and palate with perforating sinus floor as seen in coronal views and sagittal views (c, d).

3. Discussion

The phrase osteomyelitis comes from the Greek words osteon, myelo, and itis, which means inflammation. In 1844, Nelaton invented the term osteomyelitis. Osteomyelitis is a bone inflammation that starts in the medullary cavity and ends in the periosteum. Trauma, surgical therapy, bacteremia, fungal infection, and systemic disorders that reduce host defense mechanisms such as diabetes, cancer, anemia, radiation, malnutrition, osteoporosis, osteopetrosis, and Paget's disease are all implicated in the disease [4]. Osteomyelitis is the most frequently encountered cause of intraoral necrosis (maxillary necrosis). Maxillary necrosis is a condition that can be caused by bacterial osteomyelitis, herpes zoster, trauma, surgical infections, or fungal infections such as mucormycosis and aspergillosis. Mucormycosis is a fungal infection of the nasal cavity and paranasal sinuses caused by Mucorales fungus. It is disseminated via breathed fungus spores, swallowed fungus spores, or infected mucosa or skin. It is highly contagious and has the potential to be lethal in immunocompromised, handicapped, or diabetic patients [5, 6].

Candida osteomyelitis is a condition that can be exacerbated by diabetes. If fungus is not identified and treated promptly, it can cause wound healing to be impaired [7]. Diabetic patients are more likely to contract uncommon infections and have slower healing wounds. Macrophages' chemotaxis, phagocytosis, and cytokine release are all affected by diabetes' chronic hyperglycemic condition, which alters the cell-mediated immune system. Furthermore, in patients with diabetic ketoacidosis (DKA), phagocyte dysfunction results from reduced intracellular oxidative and nonoxidative killing of pathogens [8, 9]. In our cases, two patients had no history of diabetes before the authors seeking a lab report that revealed the presence of undetected uncontrolled type 2 diabetes mellitus, and one patient had stable diabetes. This is consistent with Ankita's [6] study, which found that uncontrolled hyperglycemia was a factor in 40% of instances of fungal osteomyelitis of the maxilla.

COVID-19 causes immunological dysregulation, which increases the likelihood of opportunistic fungal infection. It can also cause cytokine bursts in the body, resulting in vascular damage and reduced blood flow, which results in bone necrosis [10]. Two of our three patients had a history of diagnosed COVID-19, while the third had a probable but unconfirmed diagnosis. It is possible that glucocorticoid medication results in insulin resistance and diabetes, as well as dysregulation of the vascular system, in COVID-19. Both COVID-19 and diabetes have been linked to an increased risk of mucormycosis.

A wide range of imaging modalities may be required to accurately identify osteomyelitis in some cases. First, conventional radiography should be utilized since it provides a complete picture of the bone and soft tissue architecture and disease of the region. Because of the low sensitivity and specificity of plain radiography for the early diagnosis of acute osteomyelitis [11], our patient's OPGs and periapical radiographs returned no meaningful results. Up to 80% of patients will have a normal radiograph in the first two weeks following the start of the infection. Plain films cannot reveal the earliest indications of bone marrow edema [12]. Positron emission tomography (PET), single-photon emission computed tomography (SPECT), and magnetic resonance imaging are all good ways to find osteomyelitis. None of the tests had an advantage over the other in terms of how accurate they were at diagnosing people. It is easier for people to get an MRI because it is more common and does not cause them to be exposed to dangerous ionizing radiation. However, we used cone beam computerized tomography (CBCT), which is used a lot in dental work, to see what was going on. After we started the endodontic treatment, we used CBCT to find out what was causing the sinus drainage even though the endodontic treatment was good.

The patients were referred to an oral and maxillofacial surgeon for histopathology for confirmation and subsequent management due to the multidisciplinary nature of mucormycosis treatment, which includes the use of antifungal medications, surgical debridement, and management of underlying pathology that may contribute to the development of the fungal infection. The first line of therapy for this illness is liposomal amphotericin B. On the other hand, medical therapy alone will not cure the problem, and rigorous surgical treatment will eventually be necessary to augment the efficacy of antifungal drugs.

When detected early, this fungal infection can be treated medically with minor surgical debridement. Patients with a history of diabetes and COVID-19 should be screened with CBCT if they present with an intraoral lesion that looks like a periapical abscess due to the limited sensitivity of conventional routine radiographs used in endodontics to diagnose fungal osteomyelitis.

4. Conclusions

In the case of a diabetic patient with pulp necrosis and apical pathosis without potential localized cause in the maxillary canine and premolar region and a history of suspected or confirmatory COVID-19 infection, cone beam computed tomography should be performed to rule out osteomyelitis to avoid delayed treatment of this highly aggressive illness.

Consent

Written informed consent was obtained from the patients for capturing their photographs which could be used for publication in the journal without identifiable data in the publication.

References

[1] M. Khanna, S. Challa, A. S. Kabeil et al., "Risk of mucormycosis in diabetes mellitus: a systematic review," *Cureus*, vol. 13, no. 10, article e18827, 2021.

[2] I. Mahalaxmi, K. Jayaramayya, D. Venkatesan et al., "Mucormycosis: an opportunistic pathogen during COVID-19," *Environmental Research*, vol. 201, no. October, p. 111643, 2021.

[3] B. K. Ghazi, S. Rackimuthu, U. U. Wara et al., "Rampant increase in cases of mucormycosis in India and Pakistan: a serious cause for concern during the ongoing COVID-19 pandemic," *The American Journal of Tropical Medicine and Hygiene*, vol. 105, no. 5, pp. 1144–1147, 2021.

[4] R. Arani, S. N. H. Afsar Shareef, and H. M. Khuthija Khanam, "Mucormycotic osteomyelitis involving the maxilla: a rare case report and review of the literature," *Case Reports in Infectious Diseases.*, vol. 2019, pp. 1–6, 2019.

[5] D. Mendhe, P. Wankhede, M. Wanjari, and S. Alwadkar, "Mucormycotic osteomyelitis of maxilla post-COVID patient: a case report," *The Pan African Medical Journal*, vol. 39, p. 275, 2021.

[6] A. Srivastava, M. Mohpatra, and A. Mahapatra, "Maxillary fungal osteomyelitis: a review of literature and report of a rare case," *Annals of Maxillofacial Surgery*, vol. 9, no. 1, pp. 168–173, 2019.

[7] G. M. Torrence and B. M. Schmidt, "Fungal osteomyelitis in diabetic foot infections: a case series and comparative analysis," *The International Journal of Lower Extremity Wounds*, vol. 17, no. 3, pp. 184–189, 2018.

[8] J. Casqueiro, J. Casqueiro, and C. Alves, "Infections in patients with diabetes mellitus: a review of pathogenesis," *Indian Journal of Endocrinology and Metabolism*, vol. 16 Suppl 1, pp. S27–S36, 2012.

[9] L. M. Frydrych, F. Fattahi, K. He, P. A. Ward, and M. J. Delano, "Diabetes and sepsis: risk, recurrence, and ruination," *Frontiers in Endocrinology*, vol. 8, p. 271, 2017.

[10] G. Song, G. Liang, and W. Liu, "Fungal co-infections associated with global COVID-19 pandemic: a clinical and diagnostic perspective from China," *Mycopathologia*, vol. 185, no. 4, pp. 599–606, 2020.

[11] A. Llewellyn, J. Jones-Diette, J. Kraft, C. Holton, M. Harden, and M. Simmonds, "Imaging tests for the detection of osteomyelitis: a systematic review," *Health Technology Assessment*, vol. 23, no. 61, pp. 1–128, 2019.

[12] Y. J. Lee, S. Sadigh, K. Mankad, N. Kapse, and G. Rajeswaran, "The imaging of osteomyelitis," *Quantitative Imaging in Medicine and Surgery*, vol. 6, no. 2, pp. 184–198, 2016.

11

Clinicoradiographic Features and Histopathologic Variations of Intraosseous Lipoma: Report of a Case and Review of the Literature

Saede Atarbashi-Moghadam,[1] **Ali Lotfi**,[1] **Mohammad Mehdizadeh**,[2] **and Fazele Atarbashi-Moghadam**[3]

[1]*Department of Oral and Maxillofacial Pathology, School of Dentistry, Shahid Beheshti University of Medical Sciences, Tehran, Iran*
[2]*Department of Oral and Maxillofacial Surgery, School of Dentistry, Qom University of Medical Sciences, Qom, Iran*
[3]*Department of Periodontics, School of Dentistry, Shahid Beheshti University of Medical Sciences, Tehran, Iran*

Correspondence should be addressed to Fazele Atarbashi-Moghadam; dr.f.attarbashi@gmail.com

Academic Editor: Giovanni Mergoni

Intraosseous lipoma is a very rare lesion, and the jaw is its least common bone location. Fibrolipoma is a microscopic variant of lipoma which is characterized by a significant fibrous component intermixed with lobules of fat cells. Intraosseous fibrolipoma of the jaw is a rare lesion, and to the best of our knowledge, only two cases have been reported from 1948 in English literature. This paper presents a 39-year-old man with a chief complaint of tooth displacement in the anterior region of the mandible. Radiographic evaluation revealed a unilocular radiolucent lesion with sclerotic borders located between the left lateral incisor and canine. Histopathologic evaluation after an excisional biopsy confirmed the diagnosis of intraosseous fibrolipoma. We also reviewed the literature on this rare lesion.

1. Introduction

Intraosseous lipoma (IOL) is the rarest benign primary bone neoplasm and accounts for about 0.1% of all bone tumors. Its commonest location is the metaphysis of the long bones and the calcaneus [1]. It is often discovered incidentally during radiographic examinations, although it may be associated with pathological fractures. IOLs are almost always solitary but multiple lesions have also been reported [2]. IOLs of long bones show discrete osteolytic lesions, often with sclerotic border and radioopacities in the center due to fatty necrosis and calcification [1]. There is no sex predilection in IOLs of long bone [2].

There are few reports of IOL in the jaw, and the cause of this lesion is not known [1, 3–8]. It is usually asymptomatic; although pain, swelling, and paraesthesia have been reported [1, 4]. It is found incidentally on radiographs that show a well-defined radiolucency [4]. This lesion has clinical similarities with several other radiolucent jaw lesions, and its definitive diagnosis needs histopathologic examination [4, 5]. Recurrence or malignant transformation of IOL in the maxillofacial region has not been reported in the literature. Fibrolipoma is a variant of conventional lipoma composed of mature fat cells intermixed with fibrous connective tissue. Conservative surgery is the treatment of choice [3]. This paper presents a case of intraosseous fibrolipoma of the mandible afflicting a 39-year-old man and reviews the literature on this rare lesion.

2. Case Report

A 39-year-old man with a chief complaint of tooth displacement in the mandibular left lateral incisor and canine area was referred to a private dental clinic (Tehran, Iran) in November 2019. There was neither a history of medical problems nor trauma. Extraoral examination was within normal limits and the intraoral examination revealed no expansion or inflammation. The displaced teeth were vital. Cone-beam computed tomography (CBCT) revealed an

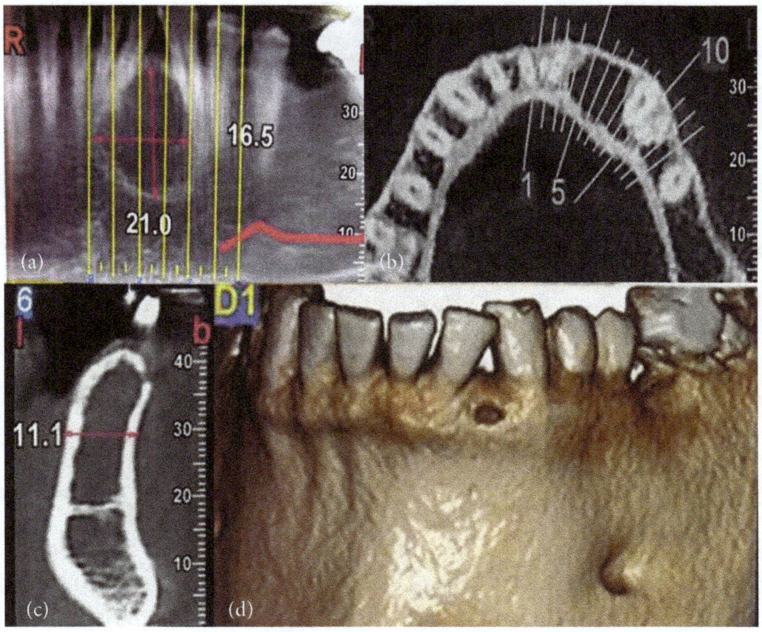

Figure 1: Cone beam computed tomography assessment of the lesion: (a) a well-defined radiolucent lesion with root separation in panoramic view; (b) mesiodistal extension of the lesion in axial view; (c) cross-sectional view; (d) 3D assessment.

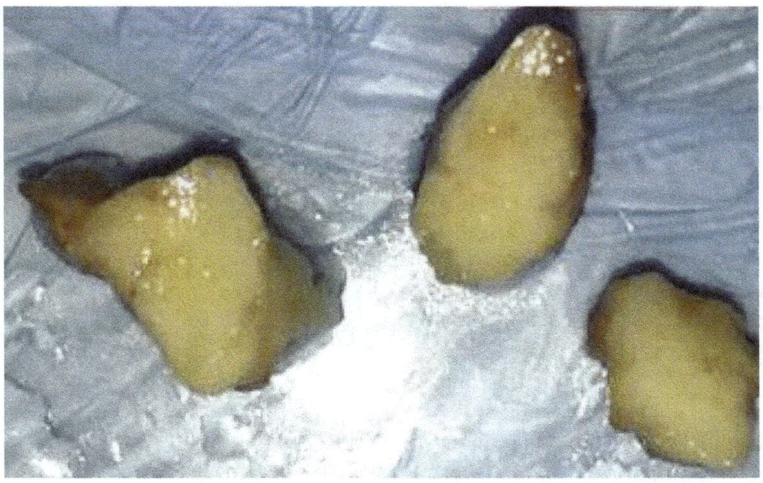

Figure 2: Gross of the lesion with solid and yellow cut surface.

approximately 2 cm, unilocular radiolucent lesion with sclerotic borders located between the mandibular left lateral incisor and canine which causes root divergence of the involved teeth (Figure 1). There was no evidence of root resorption.

Lateral periodontal cyst, odontogenic keratocyst, and central giant cell granuloma were considered as differential diagnoses. To make a final diagnosis, an excisional biopsy was performed under local anesthesia in the same month. The gross of the specimen showed a well-defined, solid, yellow lesion with soft consistency (Figure 2). Microscopic examination showed a well-defined mass composed of mature fat cells intermixed with fibrous connective tissue (Figure 3). The histopathological features in combination with radiologic findings were consistent with the diagnosis of intraosseous fibrolipoma. The patient has been under follow-up and free of disease until now.

3. Discussion

Although lipocytes are present throughout the bone marrow, intraosseous type of lipoma rarely occurs [6]. IOL is divided into intramedullary and intracortical groups [4]. Our literature review of IOL in the PubMed database (with sufficient information) from 1948 to November 2020 resulted in 29 cases. The demographic, clinical, and radiographic features of these cases and the present case are summarized and presented in Table 1. According to this review, the female to male ratio was equal. However, previous studies stated a male predilection or equal tendency for both sexes [6, 7]. IOL of the jaws, like long bone IOL, can develop in almost any age group with a mean age of 42.66 ± 14.28 (ranging from 15 to 65 years) but occurs most often in the 6th decade of life.

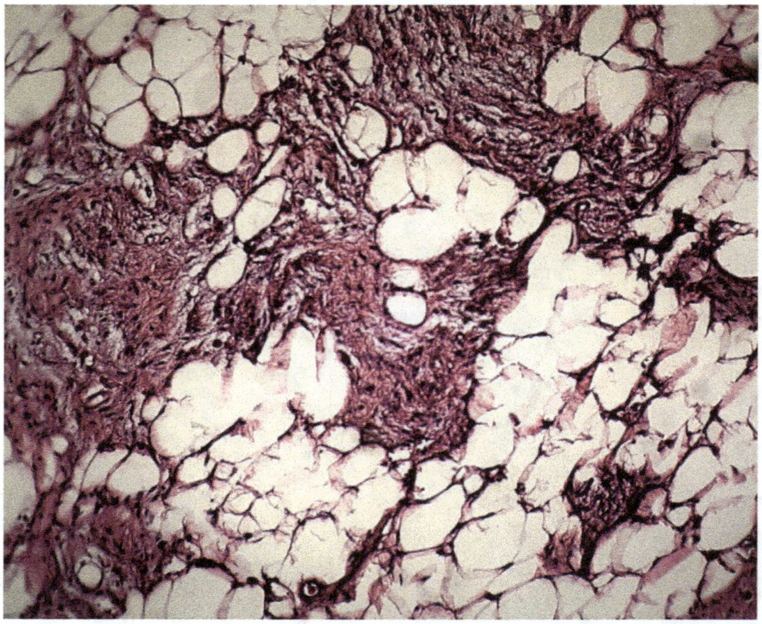

FIGURE 3: The proliferation of fatty tissue intermixed with fibrous connective tissue (H&E, 100x).

The mandible was more afflicted than the maxilla (86.66%). All maxillary cases were in the posterior region; moreover, there is a posterior predilection for mandibular lesions (Figure 4). About 46.66% of IOLs were asymptomatic, although swelling, pain, chin numbness, hypoesthesia, trismus, and periodontal signs are also reported [9–13]. Burić et al. [6] mentioned that the symptoms of the IOL are mostly related to the location and size of the lesion. The present case showed root divergence of adjacent teeth without signs of resorption (Figure 1). Almost all cases were intramedullary (93.33%), while one periosteal case and one parosteal case were reported [11, 14]. The majority of lesions were radiolucent, though 6.66% of cases showed mixed radiolucent/radiopaque radiography [4, 15]. IOL usually shows uncharacteristic radiography and demonstrates a cyst-like lesion with increased radiolucency surrounded by a sclerotic rim [3]. A multilocular lesion was also reported [13]. Therefore, microscopic examination is mandatory for diagnosis [6].

Histopathologic examination of IOL shows mature adipocytes without atypia and hematopoietic tissue that may be encapsulated [8]. Fibrolipoma is a variant of conventional lipoma composed of mature fat cells intermixed with fibrous connective tissue [3]. In the current review, the most common subtype was angiolipoma (16.66%), followed by fibrolipoma (10%) and spindle cell lipoma (3.33%). Spindle cell lipoma is also rare among all soft tissue lipomas and accounts for about 1.5% of cases [9]. The etiology of IOL is not clear; however, the role of factors such as trauma, infarction, inflammation, and nutritional problems has been suggested [1, 3, 6]. In the presented case, there was not any history of trauma or tooth extraction in this region. In addition, Burić et al. [6] considered the chronic bacterial infection of retained roots as a causative factor by creating a bone defect in the periapical region, which allows the easy accumulation of fat cells and the formation of a lipoma in the bone. In our case, the adjacent teeth were vital without any symptoms of pulpitis or periapical infection. Moreover, some of the IOLs were found in the ramus area without any relationship to the teeth [3, 8]. In the study of Barker and Sloan [7], patients were over 50 years old; therefore, they suggested that these findings represented fatty degeneration of the bone marrow. However, in the

TABLE 1: Demographic, clinical, and radiographic data of patients reported with intraosseous lipoma described in the literature and present case.

Variables	
Patients (n)	30
Male (%)/female (%)	15 (50)/15 (50)
Age (years), mean ± SD (min-max)	42.66 ± 14.28 (15-65)
Position (%)	
Maxilla	4 (13.33)
Mandible	26 (86.66)
Clinical feature	
Asymptomatic (%)	14 (46.66)
Symptomatic (%)	16 (53.33)
Radiographic feature	
Radiolucent	27 (90)
Mixed	3 (10)
Pathological diagnosis	
Lipoma	21 (70)
Angiolipoma	5 (16.66)
Fibrolipoma	3 (10)
Spindle cell lipoma	1 (3.33)

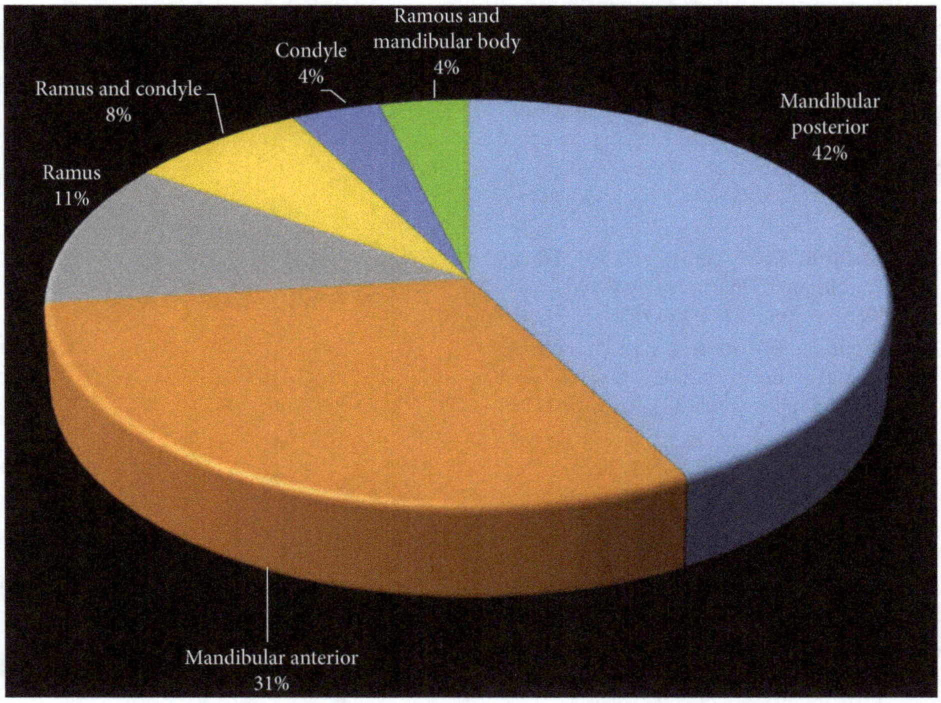

FIGURE 4: Frequency of intraosseous lipoma in different regions of the mandible in patients reported with intraosseous lipoma described in the literature and present case.

present literature review, about 43.33% of patients were under 40 years old; thus, fatty degeneration of bone marrow can be ruled out. Conservative surgery is the treatment of choice, and recurrence or malignant transformation of IOL in the maxillofacial region has not been reported in the literature [3]. However, malignant transformation of IOL in other sites has been reported [16].

4. Conclusion

As IOL is infrequent, each new case must be documented. To the best of our knowledge, only three cases of intraosseous fibrolipoma of the mandible (including our case) have been reported since 1948. IOLs of the jaws affect both genders equally, and it occurs most often in the 6th decade of life. The majority of cases are asymptomatic, although swelling, pain, paresthesia, and root divergence may be encountered.

Acknowledgments

The authors are grateful to Dr. Yaser Safi, Associate Professor of the Oral and Maxillofacial Radiology, Department of Shahid Beheshti University of Medical Sciences, for his help in interpreting and selecting the radiographic images.

References

[1] S. Cakarer, F. Selvi, S. C. Isler, M. Soluk, V. Olgac, and C. Keskin, "Intraosseous lipoma of the mandible: a case report and review of the literature," *International Journal of Oral and Maxillofacial Surgery*, vol. 38, no. 8, pp. 900–902, 2009.

[2] D. Dammerer, J. Neugebauer, D. Putzer, and B. Henninger, "Multiple intraosseous lipomatosis - a case report and a review of the literature," *In Vivo*, vol. 35, no. 2, pp. 959–964, 2021.

[3] A. Castellani, G. Bocchialini, and L. Ferrari, "A rare case of intraosseous fibrolipoma of the mandible: diagnosis and treatment," *Case reports in dentistry*, vol. 2015, 519824 pages, 2015.

[4] S. Basheer, J. Abraham, P. Shameena, and A. Balan, "Intraosseous lipoma of mandible presenting as a swelling," *Journal of oral and maxillofacial pathology*, vol. 17, no. 1, pp. 126–128, 2013.

[5] S. Hemavathy, S. Roy, and A. Kiresur, "Intraosseous angiolipoma of the mandible," *Journal of Oral and Maxillofacial Pathology*, vol. 16, no. 2, pp. 283–287, 2012.

[6] N. Burić, D. Krasić, M. Visnjić, and V. Katić, "Intraosseous mandibular lipoma: a case report and review of the literature," *Journal of Oral and Maxillofacial Surgery*, vol. 59, no. 11, pp. 1367–1371, 2001.

[7] G. R. Barker and P. Sloan, "Intraosseous lipomas: clinical features of a mandibular case with possible aetiology," *The British Journal of Oral & Maxillofacial Surgery*, vol. 24, no. 6, pp. 459–463, 1986.

[8] A. Sanjuan, A. Dean, B. Garcia, F. Alamillos, E. Roldan, and A. Blanco, "Condylar intramedullary intraosseous lipoma: contribution of a new case and review of the literature," *Journal of clinical and experimental dentistry*, vol. 1, no. 9, pp. e498–e502, 2017.

[9] T. J. Cooper, T. Lincoln, D. T. James, and S. Borgna, "Intraosseous spindle cell lipoma of the mandible: case report," *The British Journal of Oral & Maxillofacial Surgery*, vol. 55, no. 8, pp. 839-840, 2017.

[10] L. M. González-Pérez, J. L. Pérez-Ceballos, and A. Carranza-Carranza, "Mandibular intraosseous lipoma: clinical features of a condylar location," *International Journal of Oral and Maxillofacial Surgery*, vol. 39, no. 6, pp. 617–620, 2010.

[11] Z. Sun, L. Sun, Z. Zhang, and X. Ma, "Ossifying parosteal lipoma of the mandible: a case report and review of the literature," *Dento Maxillo Facial Radiology*, vol. 42, no. 1, p. 57852073, 2013.

[12] W. B. Miller, J. E. Ausich, R. K. McDaniel, and J. J. Longo, "Mandibular intraosseous lipoma," *Journal of Oral and Maxillofacial Surgery*, vol. 40, no. 9, pp. 594–596, 1982.

[13] D. M. Lewis, R. B. Brannon, B. Isaksson, and A. Larsson, "Intraosseous angiolipoma of the mandible," *Oral Surgery, Oral Medicine, and Oral Pathology*, vol. 50, no. 2, pp. 156–159, 1980.

[14] M. Steiner, A. R. Gould, J. Rasmussen, and D. LaBriola, "Parosteal lipoma of the mandible," *Oral Surgery, Oral Medicine, Oral Pathology*, vol. 52, no. 1, pp. 61–65, 1981.

[15] A. M. Manganaro, H. L. Hammond, and T. P. Williams, "Intraosseous angiolipoma of the mandible: a case report and review of the literature," *Journal of Oral and Maxillofacial Surgery*, vol. 52, no. 7, pp. 767–769, 1994.

[16] J. W. Milgram, "Malignant transformation in bone lipomas," *Skeletal Radiology*, vol. 19, no. 5, pp. 347–352, 1990.

12

Management of 3 Avulsed Permanent Teeth: Case Report of a 3-Year Follow-up

Soukaina El Kharroubi, Sofia Drouri, Bouchra Doumari, Sara Dhoum, and Hafsa El Merini

Department of Conservative Dentistry and Endodontics, School of Dentistry, Hassan II University of Casablanca, Morocco

Correspondence should be addressed to Soukaina El Kharroubi; soukainakrb44@gmail.com

Academic Editor: Tatiana Pereira-Cenci

Dental avulsion is one of the most serious dental injuries. When the tooth is knocked out, the blood supply to the pulp is interrupted and the periodontal ligament cells are exposed to injuries caused by the external environment. In recent years, research findings have shown the possibility of complete healing under favorable conditions: replanting the tooth according to the criteria required by the guideline such as the extra oral time which should be very short, the time of pulp removal after replantation, and the appropriate storage medium. This set of criteria may lead to a slower progression of the phenomenon of resorption with a better prognosis over time; however, there is a high risk of complications such as external root resorption which lies in late replantation. The research results of many research-groups around the world have given us a better understanding of healing and complications. Nowadays, even teeth that are replanted after a delay can be saved. The dentist remains the key person in the case of dental trauma, namely, dental avulsion as his role is the management of the emergency situations. The objective of this case study is to present a successful management of 3 avulsed permanent incisors, replanted and remained with no complications for over a period of 3 years.

1. Introduction

Tooth avulsion is a serious traumatic dental injury (total luxation, extrusion, or avulsion). It is a dental trauma that corresponds to the complete displacement of the tooth out of the alveolar bone socket [1–3]. Avulsion of permanent teeth varies from 0.5% to 16% of all traumatic injuries, as it is one of the rare and serious dental injuries. The young population is the most affected and the maxillary central incisors are the teeth most often involved due to their exposed position in the dental arch [4]. The risk of infection and root resorption can occur at any time after avulsion and dental replantation, which may influence the treatment outcome and survival rate including the prognosis of the teeth involved [5]. Besides, the consequences of dental avulsion are countless; they differ from patient to patient and may be related to the individuals' quality of life, psychological, and social problems, as well as the costs of treatment. [6]. In case of tooth avulsion, most periodontal ligament cells left on the root surface are due to the tearing of the alveolar-dental ligament; these cells must be hydrated to maintain the durability of the tooth while reducing the phenomenon of resorption and allowing healing. However, when the extraoral time increases, leaving the periodontal ligament dry, inflammatory resorption occurs [4]. The incidence of an external root resorption (inflammatory/replacement) remains high even in a correct management of replantation of the tooth. However, several criteria can lead to slow progression and a better prognosis over time if they are well respected.

[6] After all, the natural history of inflammatory and replacement resorption is important in order to detect the right prognosis of the replanted tooth. [6]

The aim of this study/case report is to present a successful replantation of 3 avulsed permanent maxillary incisors. No sign of resorption and ankylosis were seen over a period of 3 years.

2. Case Report

A 28-year-old female patient was referred to the Department of Conservative Dentistry and Endodontics at the School of Dentistry (Casablanca-Morocco) after an assault causing three avulsions of maxillary incisors after one hour of trauma. The patient was examined for extraoral signs of injury, including swelling and asymmetry of the face. No other oral injury was clinically detected. The patient reported that she has a history of periodontitis already treated and stabilized. The intraoral examination revealed that the maxillary permanent central incisors and lateral left incisor (tooth 11, 21, and 22) were avulsed with lacerations of soft tissue of gingiva (Figure 1). The avulsed teeth had been kept in whole milk, from the moment of trauma until emergency visit 60 minutes later. The crowns of the avulsed teeth were intact, and the roots had closed apexes (Figure 2).

Preoperative panoramic radiograph showed empty sockets of 11, 21, and 22 (Figure 3) The alveolar bone losses resulting from periodontal disease on these teeth and other teeth are also observed in this radiograph. The roots and sockets were cleaned gently with a saline rinse and the teeth replanted manually compressed to its original position under local anesthesia. Placement of teeth was confirmed radiographically before a flexible splint was placed for 4 weeks (Figure 4). Systemic antibiotic therapy was prescribed (penicillin 1 million units immediately, thereafter 2 million units daily for 6 days). A soft diet, good oral hygiene with the use of a soft- bristled toothbrush, and a 0.12% chlorhexidine mouth rinse were also prescribed for 2 weeks.

The patient was called after one-week postreplantation (Figure 5) for an intracanal placement of calcium hydroxide which was renewed for after 3 months, and the canals were obturated with Gutta-percha later (Figure 6). The splinting wire was removed after 4 weeks (Figure 7). Successive radiograph testing (periapical and CBCT) was performed in the follow-up period to disclose root resorption (Figures 8, 9, and 10) The radiographic tests showed no evidence of root resorption. A periodontal bone loss has been detected with absence of the gingival inflammation or bleeding on probing (absence of periodontal pocket); this represents a reliable indicator of periodontal stability.

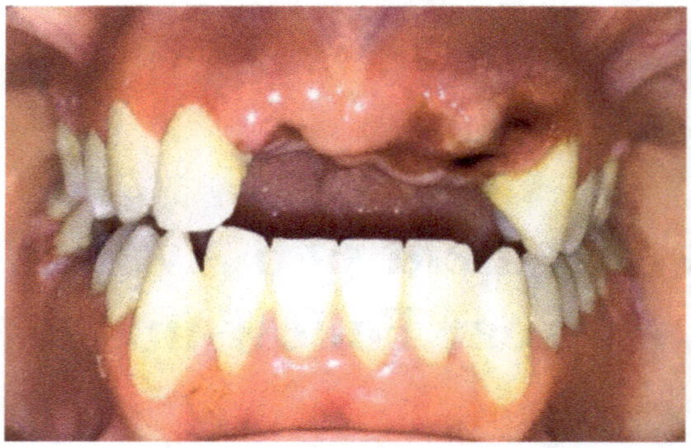

FIGURE 1: Intraoral view showing avulsion of teeth 11, 21, and 22.

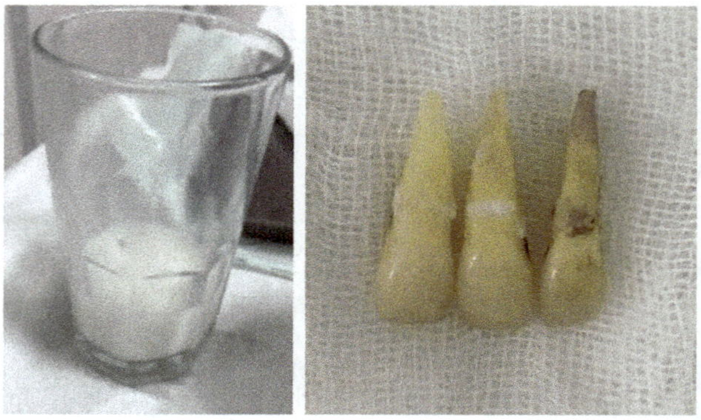

FIGURE 2: Avulsed teeth conserved in milk for 60 minutes—intact teeth.

3. Discussion

Dental avulsion mostly affects children and adolescents with a prevalence of 17.5%. It is mostly found among males than females [6].

3.1. The Different Criteria Affecting the Management of the Replanted Avulsed Teeth. The incidence of the external root resorption (inflammatory/replacement) can be high and varies between 59% and 80% in patients with so-called correct replantation [6]. Several studies have investigated the effect of dry storage that plays an important role in the viability of the periodontal ligament cells and may be responsible for the occurrence of inflammatory resorption. It has also been shown that the periodontal ligament cells can survive a drying time of 10 to 15 minutes, but the possibility of their survival beyond this time where the drying time exceeds 60 minutes may be very limited; as a result, the risk of early resorption increases [7]. Therefore, milk remains the correct balanced storage medium. It is the most relevant medium since it preserves the cells of the periodontal ligament for several hours and keeps them in a good condition until replantation. A balanced salt and saliva solution could also have the same indications effects as milk [8]. As in this present case, the avulsed teeth were kept in milk for 60 minutes from the moment of trauma until emergency visit and remained intact. The factors associated with avulsion injury show that an immature tooth develop more complications and have a lower survival rate than a mature tooth [9]. In this present clinical case, this factor is favorable, with three teeth closed apexes. Another study shows that the age of the patient can be a good factor to determine the progression of root resorption in teeth with an extended extra oral time. [6] Rightly as well, patients between 17 and 39 years old present higher rates at the time of the avulsion trauma in comparison to younger patients between 8 and 16 years old.

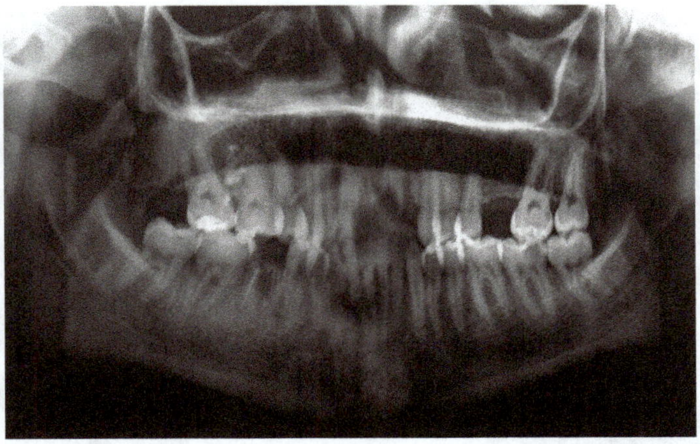

FIGURE 3: Preoperative panoramic radiograph showing empty sockets of 11, 21, and 22. No sign of fracture or contusion of the alveolar sockets.

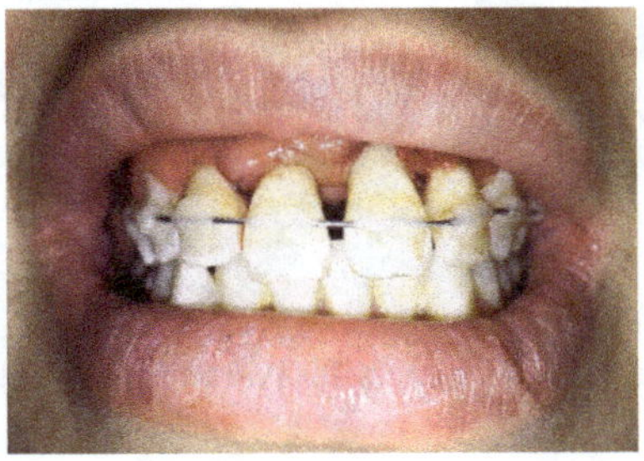

FIGURE 4: Immediate replanted and splinted teeth 11, 21, and 22. A flexible splint stabilized teeth for 4 weeks.

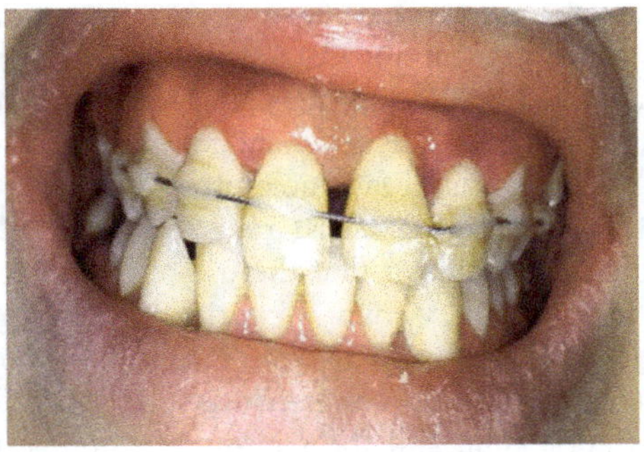

FIGURE 5: 1-week posttrauma.

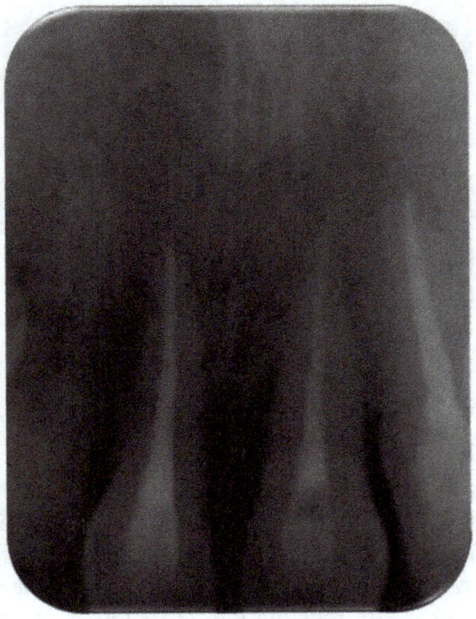

FIGURE 6: Obturation canals after 3-months medication with replanted calcium hydroxide treatment.

A recent study also shows that the risk of developing severe inflammatory resorption is related to the pulpectomy time. The timing of pulp extirpation after replantation is very important and it must be done promptly to reduce the risk of early complications [10]. Regarding our case, the pulpectomy was done after one-week postreplantation and the intracanal calcium hydroxide was placed for 3 months before the obturation canals. This aspect of the treatment of replanted teeth/a replanted tooth has been the most controversial and has undergone several changes over time. In the past clinical and experimental studies, endodontic treatment (biomechanical preparation followed by obturation with Gutta-percha and sealer) used to be performed extraorally before the replantation. [11] Nowadays, guidelines recommend endodontic treatment to be performed intraorally because it can minimize the extraoral time and reduce many risk factors [12]. As in our case, the canals' obturation with Gutta-percha and sealer was performed intraorally. From a previously reported clinical study of replanted teeth [13], the increase of the duration of the dry time can lead to the increase of the risk of ankylosis which is significantly higher with mature teeth that have closed apex than with immature teeth [13] [14]. Moreover, it has been shown that internal and external root resorption (inflammatory or replacement) have different incidences after dental avulsion and replantation [5]. As a result, it was found that the replacement root resorption is the most prominent, followed by the inflammatory external root resorption, then the surface root resorption, and finally, the internal root resorption which is the least common. Periodontal disease has been considered a contraindication to replantation. However, various studies have shown that periodontitis is no more an absolute contraindication to dental

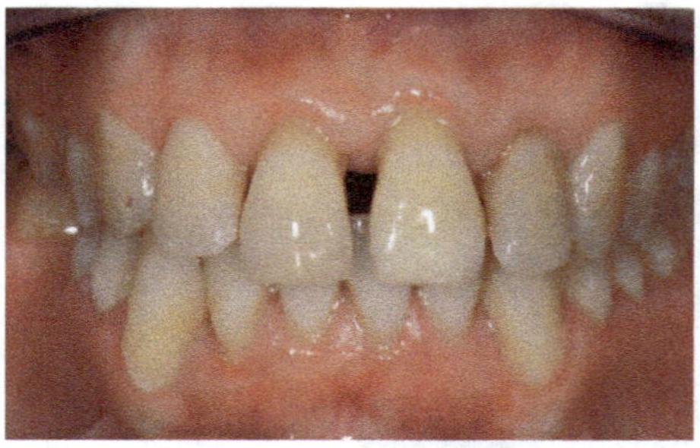

FIGURE 7: 4-week posttrauma.

FIGURE 8: 18-month follow-up of teeth.

replantation [15]. Teeth with one periodontal pocket >6 mm in patients under the age of 40 had a 2.5- and 2.6-fold lower risk of failure, compared to the teeth with more pockets and patients over the age of 40. These factors should be carefully observed for teeth replantation [15]. Other studies have shown that delayed replantation does not fully maintain the bone volume as the bone disappears with the tooth. In the anterior region of the maxilla, the buccal profile of the alveolar bone depends on teeth with a feasible periodontal ligament [16]. In our case study, the conditions for the replantation of the 3 teeth were favorable as the young patient had stable periodontitis that was successfully treated, and the maintenance phase of periodontal therapy performed since that time. The absence of inflammation and bleeding on probing can be used as predictors of the periodontal stability.

3.2. Prognosis. The prognosis of an avulsed replanted permanent tooth depends on different criteria as the amount of damage to the root surface, the degree of the root development of the avulsed teeth, and the extra-alveolar dry period and storage medium in which the tooth was kept prior to replantation. There are many factors that can affect the clinical success of a tooth replantation such as endodontic treatment, antibiotics prescription, age of the patient, type of the splinting used, and the time of the replantation, as well as

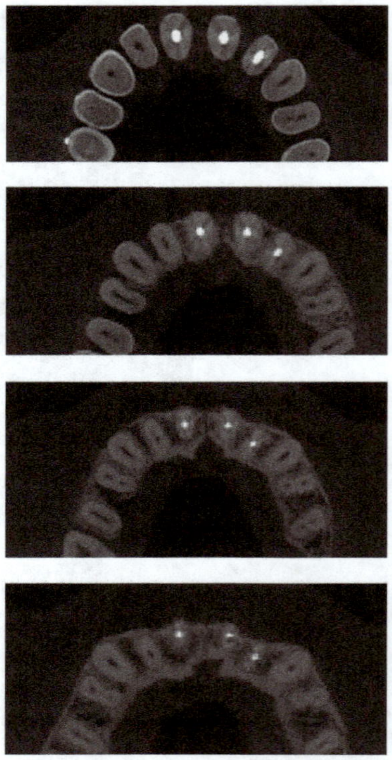

FIGURE 9: CBCT images—3 years after replantation.

the time kept for the storage [3]. There are reports of replanted teeth having favorable prognosis and could last for over 30 years. Some of them remain in function for 5 years or more, but most of them are lost due to root resorption or other complications like ankylosis. However, a good management of the infection may lead to a tissue regeneration and give a good environment for its healing [17]. It has been reported that a favorable prognosis of a replanted teeth with an arrested external root resorption after a 2-year follow-up has shown that the use of milk as a storage medium maintain the viability of periodontal ligament cells [18]. As for our case, the 3 replanted teeth have not shown any sign of root resorption or ankylosis for 3 years. The minimum extraoral time and the appropriate storage medium after avulsion are directly associated with good prognosis of a replanted tooth staying on the dental arch for a long-time. This may happen because of a minimal infection, maintenance of root cementum, and a periodontal ligament cell on root surface remained alive. [19]

Below are the different factors influencing the prognosis of the avulsed tooth [20]:

(i) The type and the timing of the treatment

(ii) Pulp removal (root canal treatment) after tooth replantation within 7-14 days showed a significantly higher survival rate

(iii) Contraindications to replantation: uncooperative patient, many severe caries, advanced and untreated periodontal diseases, and serious general pathology (immunosuppression, severe cardiac conditions)

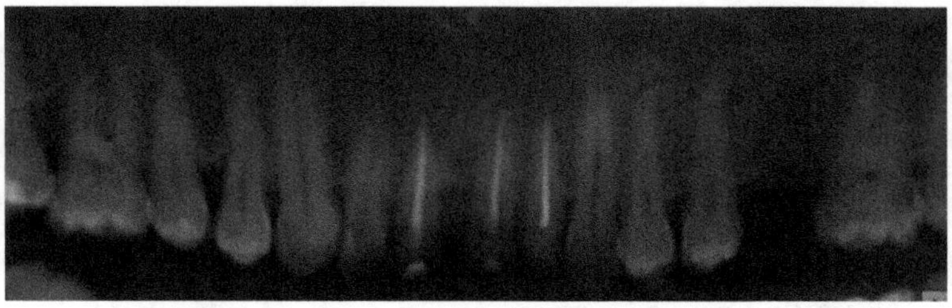

FIGURE 10: No pathology and resorption. 3-year radiograph examination.

(iv) Immature root (open apex) exhibits more complications and usually has worse prognosis compared to mature root (closed apex) with a lower survival rate

(v) Appropriate storage media increase the success rate of replantation

(vi) better treatment outcome lies in the immediate replantation of the avulsed tooth

(vii) The prognosis of replanted teeth is determined by the patient's compliance (postreplantation management and follow-up appointments).

Therefore, it can be concluded that tooth avulsion remains a severe dental injury with an unpredictable prognosis.

4. Conclusion

Although tooth avulsion is one of the most complicated types of teeth traumas. We were able to maintain a 3-year follow-up of the 3 replanted teeth with no sign of root resorption or ankylosis. Our treatment can be considered a successful one with a favorable prognosis.

A regular clinical and radiographic examination follow-up every year is fundamental.

Consent

An informed and written consent from the patient for publication of the case report was obtained.

References

[1] D. Finucane and M. J. Kinirons, "External inflammatory and replacement resorption of luxated, and avulsed replanted permanent incisors: a review and case presentation," *Dental Traumatology*, vol. 19, no. 3, pp. 170–174, 2003.

[2] M. de Lourdes Vieira Frujeri and E. D. Costa Jr., "Effect of a single dental health education on the management of permanent avulsed teeth by different groups of professionals," *Dental Traumatology*, vol. 25, no. 3, pp. 262–271, 2009.

[3] D. D. Müller, R. Bissinger, M. Reymus, K. Bücher, R. Hickel, and J. Kühnisch, "Survival and complication analyses of avulsed and replanted permanent teeth," *Scientific Reports*, vol. 10, no. 1, p. 2841, 2020.

[4] M. Singh, N. Singh, R. K. Dhiman, and D. Kumar, "External replacement resorption in an avulsed reimplanted permanent incisors," *Journal of the International Clinical Dental Research Organization*, vol. 5, no. 1, p. 27, 2014.

[5] B. D. M. Souza, K. L. Dutra, M. M. Kuntze et al., "Incidence of root resorption after the replantation of avulsed teeth: a meta-analysis," *Journal of Endodontics*, vol. 44, no. 8, pp. 1216–1227, 2018.

[6] M. Mazur, R. Marasca, L. Ottolenghi et al., "Different resorptive patterns of two avulsed and replanted upper central incisors based on scanning electron microscopy and stereomicroscopic analysis: a case report," *Applied Sciences*, vol. 10, no. 10, p. 3551, 2020.

[7] M. Trope, "Clinical management of the avulsed tooth: present strategies and future directions," *Dental Traumatology*, vol. 18, no. 1, pp. 1–11, 2002.

[8] M. Donaldson and M. Kinirons, "Factors affecting the time of onset of resorption in avulsed and replanted incisor teeth in children," *Dental Traumatology*, vol. 17, no. 5, pp. 201–205, 2001.

[9] B. Petrovic, D. Markovi'c, T. Peric, and D. Blagojevic, "Factors related to treatment and outcomes of avulsed teeth," *Dental Traumatology*, vol. 26, no. 1, pp. 52–59, 2010.

[10] A. M. Mavridou, E. Hauben, M. Wevers, E. Schepers, L. Bergmans, and P. Lambrechts, "Understanding external cervical resorption patterns in endodontically treated teeth," *International Endodontic Journal*, vol. 50, no. 12, pp. 1116–1133, 2017.

[11] J. O. Andreasen and E. Hjorting-Hansen, "Replantation of teeth. I. Radiographic and clinical study of 110 human teeth replanted after accidental loss," *Acta Odontologica Scandinavica*, vol. 24, no. 3, pp. 263–286, 1966.

[12] M. T. Flores, L. Andersson, J. O. Andreasen et al., "Guidelines for the management of traumatic dental injuries. II. Avulsion of permanent teeth," *Dental Traumatology*, vol. 23, no. 3, pp. 130–136, 2007.

[13] E. Lauridsen, J. O. Andreasen, O. Bouaziz, and L. Andersson, "Risk of ankylosis of 400 avulsed and replanted human teeth in relation to length of dry storage: a re-evaluation of a long-term clinical study," *Dental Traumatology*, vol. 36, no. 2, pp. 108–116, 2020.

[14] K. M. Campbell, M. J. Casas, and D. J. Kenny, "Ankylosis of traumatized permanent incisors: pathogenesis and current approaches to diagnosis and management," *Texas Dental Journal*, vol. 71, no. 10, pp. 596–601, 2005.

[15] S.-Y. Cho, S.-J. Lee, and E. Kim, "Clinical outcomes after intentional replantation of periodontally involved teeth," *Journal of Endodontics*, vol. 43, no. 4, pp. 550–555, 2017.

[16] M. Tsukiboshi and T. Tsukiboshi, "Bone morphology after delayed tooth replantation - case series," *Dental Traumatology*, vol. 30, no. 6, pp. 477–483, 2014.

[17] K. S. Nene and V. Bendgude, "Prognosis of replanted avulsed permanent incisors: a systematic review," *International Journal of Pedodontic Rehabilitation*, vol. 3, no. 2, p. 87, 2018.

[18] A. Al-Kahtani, "Avulsed immature permanent central incisors obturated with mineral trioxide aggregate: a case report," *Journal of International Oral Health: JIOH*, vol. 5, no. 3, pp. 88–96, 2013.

[19] N. BrierDe, D. A. Zideman, and E. De Buck, "Storage of an avulsed tooth prior to replantation: a systematic review and meta-analysis," *Dental Traumatology*, vol. 36, no. 5, pp. 453–476, 2020.

[20] J. Kim, "Avulsed Permanent Teeth," *Dental Traumatology*, vol. 26, pp. 52–59, 2010.

13

Unusual Variant of Unicystic Ameloblastoma with CEOT-Like Areas: A Rare Case Report with Review of Literature

Venkata Ramanand Oruganti,[1] **Shylaja Sanjeevareddygari**,[1] **Manay Srinivas Munisekhar**,[2] **Sharath Kumar Reddy Eppalapalli**,[1] **Raghu Vamshi Vishwakarma**,[1] **Kiran Kumar Ganji**,[3] **Kiran R. Halkai**,[4] **and Rahul Halkai**[4]

[1]*Department of Oral Pathology, SVS Institute of Dental Sciences, Mahabubnagar, Telangana, India*
[2]*Oral Pathology Division, Department of Preventive Dentistry, College of Dentistry, Jouf University, Sakaka, Al Jouf, Saudi Arabia*
[3]*Periodontics Division, Department of Preventive Dentistry, College of Dentistry, Jouf University, Sakaka, Al Jouf, Saudi Arabia*
[4]*Department of Conservative Dentistry and Endodontics, Al-Badar Dental College and Hospital, Kalaburgi, Karnataka, India*

Correspondence should be addressed to Manay Srinivas Munisekhar; dr.srinivas.manay@jodent.org

Academic Editor: Tommaso Lombardi

Ameloblastoma is an epithelial odontogenic neoplasm with clinical and histological diversity. They are locally invasive tumors with 3 clinical variants such as solid, unicystic, and peripheral ameloblastomas, and the unicystic variant constitutes only 13%. Histologically, it shows diverse microscopic patterns that may occur isolated or in combination with other patterns. The granular cell variant accounts for 3.5% of all ameloblastoma cases. The eosinophilic granules seen in the cytoplasm of the tumor are thought to be lysosomes and presumably contribute to the pathogenesis of the tumor. Although such a phenomenon is rare in unicystic ameloblastoma, granular cell differentiation in solid multicystic ameloblastoma is a well-established phenomenon. In this paper, we present a unique case of unicystic ameloblastoma with granular cell differentiation with a brief review.

1. Introduction

Ameloblastoma is a true benign odontogenic tumor of epithelial origin containing enamel organ-like tissue without any hard tissue formation. It was defined by Robinson as "unicentric, nonfunctional, intermittent in growth, anatomically benign and clinically persistent" tumor [1]. It is a locally invasive tumor accounting for 11% among odontogenic tumors in Caucasians [2]. Histologically, plexiform and follicular variants are the two chief patterns, and when certain changes like granular transformation and squamous metaplasia may be noted, they are referred to as granular cell and acanthomatous variants, respectively [3]. The granular cell variant is the least common, but the most aggressive histological type with higher incidence of malignant transformation and distant metastasis [4]. WHO clinically categorized ameloblastomas into solid multicystic, unicystic, desmoplastic, and peripheral ameloblastomas. However, they are similar histologically. Rarely do they present interesting variations microscopically. However, unicystic ameloblastoma (UA) rarely presents with a myriad of histopathological patterns. In this article, an interesting case of UA is presented along with a literature review relevant to its unique microscopic features [5].

2. Case Report

A 45-year-old female patient reported with a swelling in the mandibular anterior region since 4 years. It began as a peanut-sized swelling which progressed to about 6 cm and has increased rapidly during the last two months. Extraoral examination revealed that there was facial asymmetry (Figure 1) with the swelling extending from the right

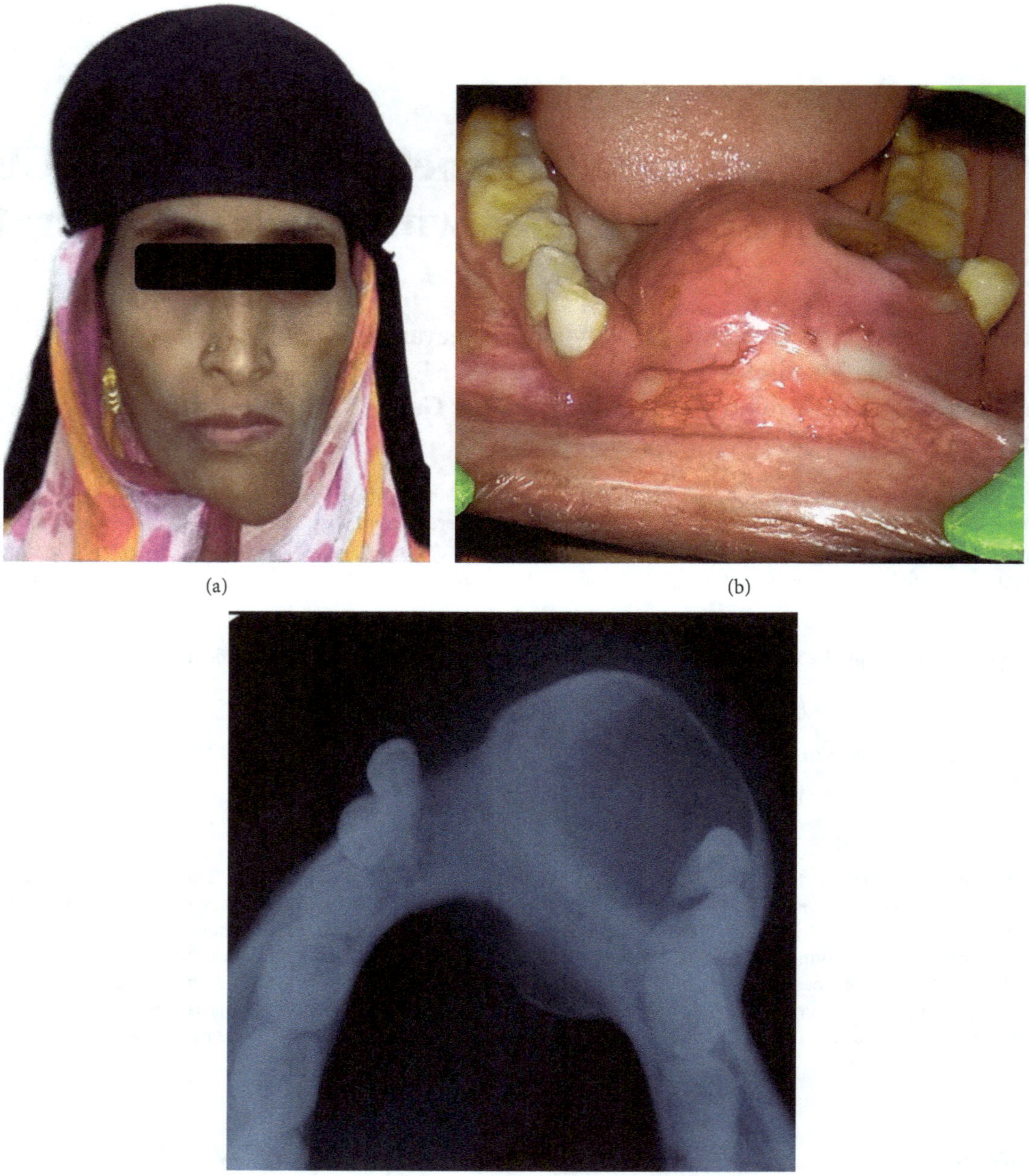

(a) (b) (c)

Figure 1: (a) Extraoral swelling; (b) intraoral ulcerated mass with obliteration of labial vestibule; (c) radiographic presentation showing the expansion of cortical plates.

parasymphysis to the left parasymphysis region anterio-posteriorly and superio-inferiorly from the lower lip to the inferior border of the mandible. The skin over the swelling was smooth and was of the same color as the adjacent skin. On intraoral examination, it is approximately 6 × 7 cm in size extending from 43 to 34 obliterating labial and lingual vestibules (Figure 1(b)).

The mandibular left premolars were displaced, and the swelling presented an ulcerated surface on the left side. On palpation, it was hard and nontender. Orthopantamograph (OPG) revealed unilocular radiolucency extending from the mesial aspect of 43 to the mesial aspect of 34, and the occlusal view showed an expansion of labial and lingual plates with intact cortical bone (Figure 1(c)). Sections of the incisional biopsy specimen stained with hematoxylin (H) and eosin (E) revealed odontogenic tumor epithelial cells arranged in sheets, cords, and follicles exhibiting tall columnar peripheral cells with central star-shaped cells resembling the stellate reticulum. The intervening connective tissue was predominantly fibrous. Areas of the lining epithelium were evident made of the parakeratinized stratified squamous epithelium overlying a fibrocellular connective tissue with few chronic inflammatory cells. It was diagnosed as plexiform ameloblastoma followed by surgical removal.

Under all aseptic conditions, GA was administered through naso-endochondral intubation. The patient's face

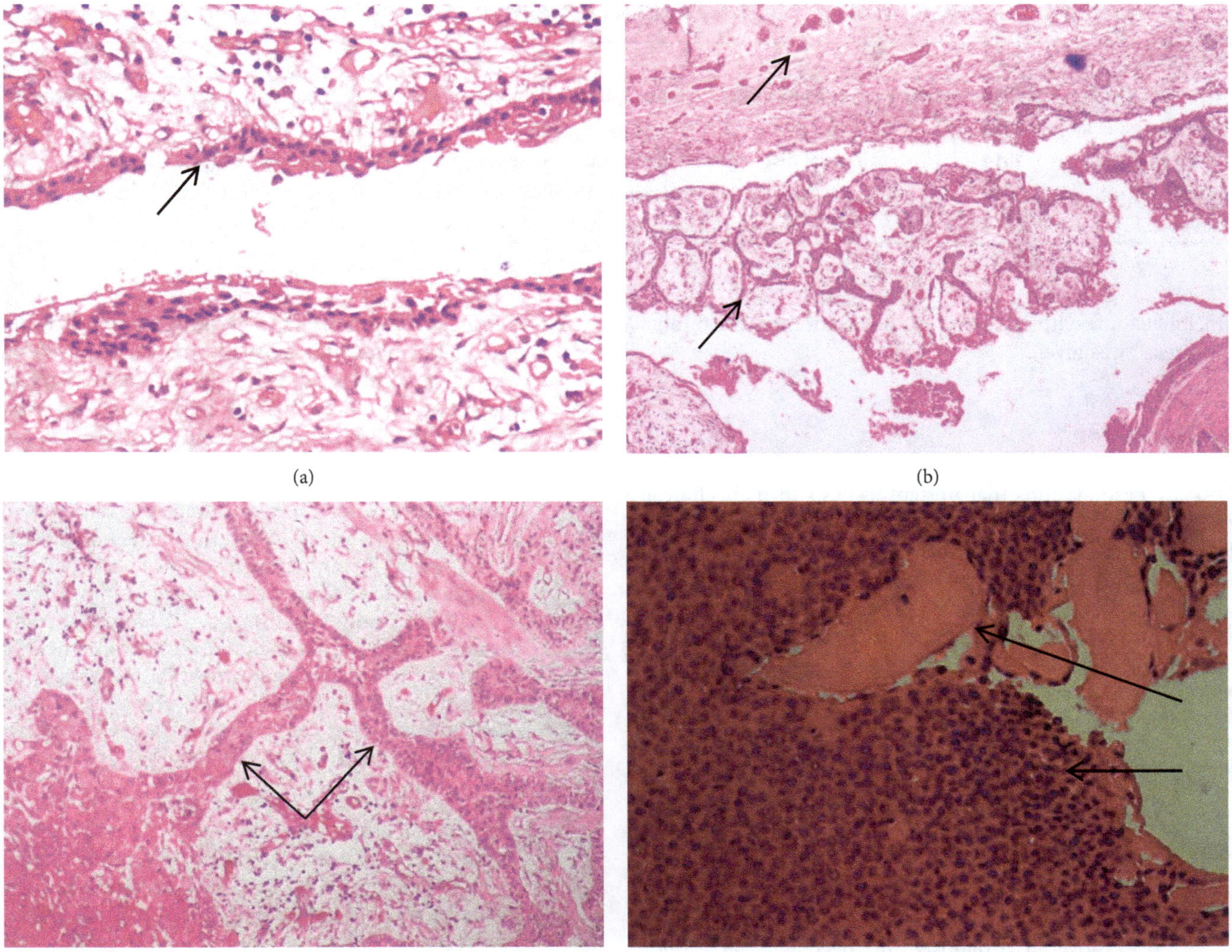

(a) (b) (c) (d)

Figure 2: (a) H&E-stained section showing the cystic lumen lined by a thin nonkeratinized stratified squamous epithelium with columnar basal cells at focal areas (×100). (b) H&E-stained section showing epithelial proliferations into both the cystic lumen and the connective tissue wall (×40). (c) H&E-stained section showing odontogenic epithelial cells arranged in interconnecting strands and sheets with granular cells located centrally (×100). (d) H&E-stained section showing darkly stained polygonal cells arranged in sheets with homogenous eosinophilic deposits resembling CEOT-like areas.

and oral cavity were painted with povidine-iodine and draped. LA with adrenaline 1 : 80,000 was administered as a bilateral inferior alveolar nerve block and mental nerve block. Incision was placed from 46 to 36, and subperiosteal dissection was done bilaterally up to the premolar region both buccally and lingually. Supraperiosteal dissection was done over the anterior mandibular region to expose the tumor. Tumor borders were osteotomized with the help of osteotomes, and the lesion was separated from the mandible. Lingually, genioglossus and geniohyoid muscles were found to be attached to the genial tubercles and were secured. Curettage along with chemical cauterization using Carnoy's solution was done at the lesion site. Hemostasis was achieved. Thorough intraoral irrigation was done. Primary closure was done using 3-0 vicryl with horizontal mattress sutures. Tongue stitch was placed to prevent fall back of the tongue immediately postoperatively and secured extraorally. Ryle's tube was placed, and no intraoral complications were noted. The patient was extubated and shifted to the postoperative ward uneventfully. The healing was uneventful with no recurrence till date.

The H&E-stained sections of the excisional biopsy specimen revealed a well-defined cystic lumen lined by a nonkeratinized stratified squamous epithelium with basal tall columnar ameloblast-like cells and superficial stellate reticulum-like tissue satisfying Vickers and Gorlin criteria (Figure 2(a)). The epithelial lining showed mural proliferations and proliferations into the cystic lumen in the form of interconnecting strands and cords, with stellate reticulum-like tissue exhibiting granular cell differentiation with eosinophilic granules in the cytoplasm (Figures 2(b) and 2(c)). The intervening connective tissue showed delicate collagen fibers. In some areas, eosinophilic polygonal cells with prominent nuclei and amorphous eosinophilic material resembling calcifying epithelial odontogenic tumor (CEOT) were noticed (Figure 2(d)). A diagnosis of "unicystic granular cell

Table 1: List of cases reported.

Authors	Year	Cases reported
Abaza et al. [18]	1989	Granular cell odontogenic cyst: a unicystic ameloblastoma with late recurrence as a follicular ameloblastoma
Thillaikarasi et al. [9]	2010	Cystic granular cell ameloblastoma
Ponce et al. [11]	2014	Unusual histological patterns and hyaline ring granulomas in a unicystic ameloblastoma
Motahhary et al. [19]	2014	Granular cell type of a unicystic ameloblastoma: an unusual case and review of the literature
Jain et al. [5]	2017	Unicystic ameloblastoma of the mandible with an unusual diverse histopathology

ameloblastoma with calcifying epithelial odontogenic tumor-like areas" was given.

3. Discussion

UAs are cystic lesions that present as cysts in their clinical, radiographic, and gross features but histologically have features resembling ameloblastoma-like areas in the lining epithelium of the cystic cavity [6]. Depending upon the histological location of the tumor nodules within the lesional tissue, they have been categorized as intraluminal, luminal, and mural variants [7]. Though it resembles conventional ameloblastoma histologically, it has been separated from it as it differs from it in the following characteristics.

(a) It is relatively common in younger individuals

(b) It is more commonly associated with impacted mandibular third molars and hence resembles a dentigerous cyst on a radiograph

(c) It is less aggressive in its biological behavior with better overall prognosis and decreased recurrence rate [8]

Although granular cell differentiation has been a documented phenomenon in conventional ameloblastomas, such a feature has been infrequently appreciated in UA [9]. According to Broca, they account for 1 to 2% of all jaw tumors and cysts. It is common in the posterior mandibular region (third molar). However, it was noted in the lower anterior region in our case. It is uncommon in fourth and fifth decades with no sex predilection [10]. Ponce et al. reported UA demonstrating histological patterns such as granular cell, basal cell, and acanthomatous patterns and hyaline ring granuloma [11]. However, in our case, granular cell changes and those resembling CEOT were identified. Since such changes are rare (Table 1), the impact of such findings on its biologic behavior is unknown and documentation of few more similar cases may shed light on its pathogenesis and nature [5]. Granular cell ameloblastoma (GCA) is characterized by islands of odontogenic tumor epithelial cells containing peripheral ameloblast-like cells with centrally large oval to polyhedral cells with abundant coarse granules within the cell displacing the nucleus to the periphery of the cells. Electron microscopy revealed that these granules are lysosomes [3]. However, the probable reasons for their occurrence have been speculated as follows:

(1) During amelogenesis, in the synthetic and postsecretory stages, ameloblasts usually show an increase in autophagic lysosomes. Similarly, in ameloblastoma, the odontogenic epithelial cells show granular changes due to either lysosomal insufficiency or excessive production of unused materials [9]

(2) Aging theory: since granular change was observed in ameloblastomas after two decades of the initial onset of the tumor, it was assumed that aged components get accumulated within the tumor cells and that there is decreased ability of lysosomes to dispose them with increasing age [12]. Thus, increased lysosomes within the tumor cells might indicate enhanced activity to digest the unwanted compounds. However, Neville et al. did not consider it an aging change since it was found in younger patients also [13]

(3) Electron microscopy observed apoptotic cell fragments of compact nuclei in granular cells, which were removed by neighboring granular cells, implying that increased tumor cell apoptosis accompanied by phagocytosis could be leading to cytoplasmic granularity [14]

(4) However, another electron microscopic study showed that the nuclei of the granular cells were normal without any degenerative changes, and therefore, it was suggested that the presence of numerous lysosomes is indicative of active function and does not represent an aging change [9]

Differential diagnosis for GCA includes granular cell tumor, granular cell myoblastoma, granular cell odontogenic tumor, congenital epulis, and granular cell ameloblastic fibromas. Though the morphology of the granular cells is similar in all these tumors, their histogenesis differs. Secondly, GCA is epithelial in origin and the others are mesenchymal. Immunohistochemistry may help in distinguishing GCA from these tumors [15]. The treatment of ameloblastoma is controversial, and hence, comprehensive history, routine radiographs, proper clinical examination, advanced imaging, and representative biopsy should be considered. It is an established fact that UAs are less aggressive as compared to solid ameloblastomas and are treated successfully with enucleation or curettage [16]. However, since granular cells are associated with aggressive nature with higher incidence of malignancy and metastasis, it would be more appropriate to plan a more radical approach [17].

4. Conclusion

In the present case, though incisional biopsy report suggested it to be a plexiform ameloblastoma, enucleation was done as the patient preferred a more conservative approach and its healing was uneventful without any evidence of recurrence till date. Since the excisional biopsy report showed the presence of granular cells and CEOT-like areas, the idea that does it warrant an additional surgery that is more invasive is still questionable. Unless few more such cases are reported, the precise treatment protocols for such lesions cannot be established.

References

[1] B. Sivapathasundharam, *Shafer's Textbook of Oral Pathology E-Book*, S. B. RR, Ed., New Delhi, Elsevier Health Sciences, 2020.

[2] S. Arora, A. Mujhib, G. Diwakar, and V. Amberker, "Granular cell ameloblastoma : A case report with a brief note on review of literature," *Egyptian Journal of Ear, Nose, Throat and Allied Sciences*, vol. 15, no. 3, pp. 267–269, 2014.

[3] L. M. Cherian, A. Sood, and R. Heera, "Granular cell ameloblastoma: report of an unusual case and review of literature," *Oral & Maxillofacial Pathology Journal*, vol. 5, no. 2, 2014.

[4] S. Hunasgi, A. Koneru, D. S. Chauhan, and Y. Guruprasad, "Rare giant granular cell ameloblastoma: a case report and an immunohistochemical study," *Case Reports in Dentistry*, vol. 2013, Article ID 372781, 5 pages, 2013.

[5] K. Jain, G. Sharma, P. Kardam, and M. Mehendiratta, "Unicystic ameloblastoma of mandible with an unusual diverse histopathology: a rare case report," *Journal of Clinical and Diagnostic Research*, vol. 11, no. 4, 2017.

[6] Z. Chaudhary, U. S. Pal, V. Sangwan, and P. Sharma, "Unicystic ameloblastoma: a diagnostic dilemma," *National Journal of Maxillofacial Surgery*, vol. 2, no. 1, pp. 89–92, 2011.

[7] P. A. Reichart and H. P. Philipsen, *Odontogenic tumors and allied lesions*, Quintessence Pub, 2004.

[8] R. Rajendran, *Shafer's Textbook of Oral Pathology*, Elsevier India, 2009.

[9] R. Thillaikarasi, J. Balaji, B. Gupta et al., "Cystic granular cell ameloblastoma," *Journal of Maxillofacial and Oral Surgery*, vol. 9, no. 3, pp. 310–313, 2010.

[10] Y. Martin, M. Sathyakumar, J. Premkumar, and K. Magesh, "Granular cell ameloblastoma," *Journal of Oral and Maxillofacial Pathology*, vol. 21, no. 1, p. 183, 2017.

[11] J. Ponce, H. Lima, M. Rodrigues, F. Souza, and V. Lara, "Unusual histological patterns and hyaline ring granulomas in a unicystic ameloblastoma," *Hippokratia*, vol. 18, no. 1, p. 83, 2014.

[12] S. Patankar and A. Mehtha, "Granular cell ameloblastoma: a case report," *International Journal of Oral & Maxillofacial Pathology*, vol. 2, no. 4, pp. 63–67, 2011.

[13] B. Neville, D. Damm, C. Allen, and A. Chi, *Oral and Maxillofacial Pathology*, Elsevier Health Sciences, United States, 2015.

[14] H. Kumamoto and K. Ooya, "Immunohistochemical and ultrastructural investigation of apoptotic cell death in granular cell ameloblastoma," *Journal of Oral Pathology & Medicine*, vol. 30, no. 4, pp. 245–250, 2001.

[15] N. Afroz, S. Qadri, N. Shamim, and S. Qadri, "Granular cell ameloblastoma of maxilla: masquerading as pyogenic granuloma," *Oral and Maxilofacial Pathology Journal*, vol. 6, no. 1, pp. 568–571, 2015.

[16] V. Kattimani, J. Sumanti, and L. Prasad, "Granular cell ameloblastoma: a case report and literature review," *Journal of Dental Problems and Solutions*, vol. 2, pp. 031–033, 2014.

[17] T. L. Yogesh and S. Sowmya, "Granules in granular cell lesions of the head and neck: a review," *ISRN Pathology*, vol. 2011, Article ID 215251, 10 pages, 2011.

[18] N. A. Abaza, L. Gold, and E. Lally, "Granular cell odontogenic cyst: a unicystic ameloblastoma with late recurrence as follicular ameloblastoma," *Journal of Oral and Maxillofacial Surgery*, vol. 47, no. 2, pp. 168–175, 1989.

[19] P. Motahhary, A. Etebarian, and F. Asareh, "Granular cell type of a unicystic ameloblastoma: an unusual case and review of the literature," *Journal of Oral and Maxillofacial Pathology*, vol. 18, no. 2, p. 331, 2014.

Clinical and Immunohistochemical Features of Oral Angioleiomyoma: A Comprehensive Review of the Literature and Report of a Case in a Young Patient

Amerigo Giudice ,[1,2] Francesco Bennardo ,[2] Caterina Buffone,[1] Ylenia Brancaccio,[1] Francesca Maria Plutino,[3] and Leonzio Fortunato[1,2]

[1]*School of Dentistry, Magna Graecia University of Catanzaro, Italy*
[2]*Department of Health Sciences, Magna Graecia University of Catanzaro, Italy*
[3]*Istituto Clinico De Blasi, Reggio Calabria, Italy*

Correspondence should be addressed to Amerigo Giudice; a.giudice@unicz.it

Academic Editor: Pablo I. Varela-Centelles

Angioleiomyoma (AL) is an uncommon benign soft tissue neoplasia arising from the tunica media of the smooth muscle cells. AL appears as a solitary and slow-growing mass and seldom is observed in oral tissues. We reported a rare case of AL involving the cheek of a 17-year-old young woman. A review of the English-language literature was performed entering the keywords "angioleiomyoma" and "oral" in the search fields of PubMed. 70 results were identified. Excluded were cases that were not in the oral cavity or not compatible with the AL diagnosis or report lacking immunohistochemical analysis. According to the exclusion criteria, we selected 30 studies that included 63 cases of AL. The results of the review showed an average age of 42.97 years with a prevalence between the fourth and fifth decade of life with a male-to-female ratio of 1.95 : 1. The most affected sites were palate, buccal mucosa of the cheek, lip, tongue, and gingiva. Surgical excision was the treatment of choice, and diagnosis was possible through histopathological and immunohistochemical analysis. SMA, vimentin, CD34, desmin, and S-100 were the most common markers to guide the histopathological diagnosis of oral AL. In conclusion, oral AL is a rare entity, especially in adolescence as in the reported case of AL of the cheek in a 17-year-old woman. The clinical aspects of AL did not allow clinicians to make a correct presumptive diagnosis. A scrupulous histopathological analysis and immunohistochemical examinations are fundamental to differentiate AL from other lesions.

1. Introduction

Leiomyoma is a circumscribed benign smooth muscle neoplasia that frequently occurs on the skin, especially on the lower extremities, in the gastrointestinal tract and female genital tract. Given the low presence of smooth muscle cells in the oral cavity, leiomyoma rarely localizes in the mouth: it develops from smooth muscle cells of tunica media or excretory ducts of salivary glands [1, 2].

In relation to the prevailing histological pattern, it can be classified into three types: solid leiomyoma, vascular leiomyoma (angioleiomyoma), and sporadic form of epithelioid leiomyoma (leioblastoma) [3].

Angioleiomyoma (AL) is the most common microscopic pattern affecting the oral cavity. Nevertheless, oral AL is a rare benign tumor. Typically, it occurs in middle-aged man between the fourth and sixth decades of life [4].

AL was found in the cheek, lips, tongue, mandible, palate, and gingiva. AL is commonly present as well circumscribed and slow-growing asymptomatic lesion [5–7].

The clinical aspects of AL are similar to many other lesions of the oral cavity. Therefore, the differential diagnosis of AL in the oral cavity includes other benign conditions of the salivary glands as mucocele, pleomorphic adenoma, mesenchymal tumors, lymphangioma, pyogenic granuloma, and schwannoma [8, 9].

The diagnosis is possible after histopathological and immunohistochemical analysis due to its nonspecific clinical features. Surgical excision is the treatment of choice of AL, and recurrences are very rare [9].

We report a rare case of AL in a 17-year-old woman and an extensive review of the literature on oral AL.

2. Case Report

A 17-year-old woman was referred to our Oral Pathology Unit by her family dentist to evaluate a solitary asymptomatic, mobile, and well-circumscribed mass in her left cheek.

The patient reported a swelling in the left cheek in the last two months. Her family and medical histories were irrelevant; she was not following any drug therapy; she did not smoke or usually consume alcohol.

Clinically, we observed a palpable hard-elastic mass, measuring 1.5×1.0 cm approximately, in the submucosal layer of the left cheek. The patient did not report pain; the skin and the covering mucosa were normal. An ultrasound scan (US) was prescribed and showed a hypoechoic homogenous mass with well-defined margins.

The patient underwent an excisional biopsy under local anesthesia (Figure 1) after received an antibiotic prophylaxis therapy with 2 grams of amoxicillin 60 minutes before the surgery. She continued antibiotic therapy with 1 gram of amoxicillin every 12 hours until the 4th postoperative day. As analgesic therapy, the patient received paracetamol 500 mg immediately after the surgery.

The specimen was stored in a tube containing formalin 10% and sent to a laboratory for histopathological analysis.

The tumor was well circumscribed with a thin fibrous capsule, and a sample obtained was firm, sharply circumscribed, yellow-white round to ovoidal nodule (1×0.6 cm in dimension). It was composed of uniform spindle smooth muscle cells with pale eosinophilic cytoplasm and blunt-ended or cigar-shaped nuclei, with slightly wavy contour, vesicular chromatin, and occasionally small nucleolus; in cross-sections, nuclei appeared surrounded by a clear halo as contained in boxes. Mitotic figures were very rarely seen (1/20 hpf). The cells were arranged in uniform interlacing bundles, with interposition of the low amount of fibrous connective tissue, and distributed around numerous small tortuous "slit-like" vessels, with virtual lumen and lined by normal-appearing endothelium but with no elastic lamina present, resembling a solid or capillary subtype appearance (closely compacted smooth muscle bundles), in contrast to venous (vessels have thick muscular walls that merge with smooth muscle bundles) and cavernous (dilated vascular channels with minimal smooth muscle that merges with smooth muscle bundles) subtypes; they have no clinical significance [1].

Necrosis, atypical mitoses, and pleomorphism were not observed in the histological examinations (Figure 2).

In addition to the histopathological analysis, immunohistochemical staining of the sample with α-smooth muscle actin (SMA), CD34, desmin, and vimentin was performed: the proliferating spindle cells were diffusely and strongly immunoreactive for SMA, desmin, and vimentin; the vascular spaces were consistently CD34-positive staining (Figure 3).

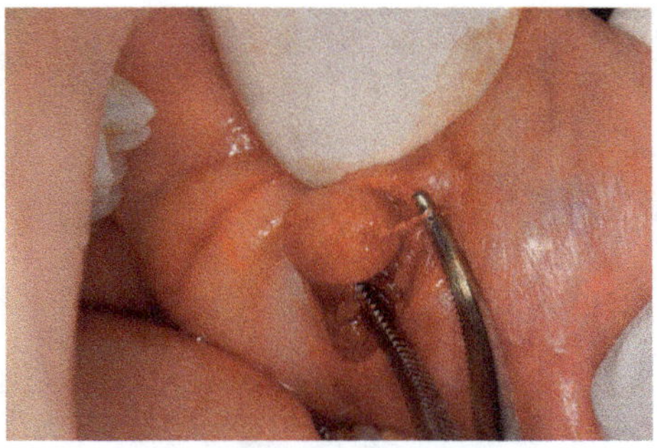

FIGURE 1: Surgical excision of the lesion.

The histopathological and immunohistochemical analysis suggested the diagnosis of AL.

Follow-up examinations at 1 week, 4 weeks, and 6 months showed mucosal integrity and no sign of recurrence.

3. Review of the Literature

A review of the English-language literature was performed. The keywords "angioleiomyoma" and "oral" were entered in the search fields of PubMed. The research was conducted by considering the articles published until August 2018. 70 results were identified. Excluded were cases that were not in the oral cavity or not compatible with the AL diagnosis or report lacking immunohistochemical analysis.

According to the exclusion criteria, we selected 30 studies [3, 4, 8–34] that included 63 cases of AL. We analyzed patient's age, gender, tumor location, size, and immunohistochemical markers. The principal features and data pertaining the selected cases and those of the reported case are compiled in Table 1.

Age data were available in all selected studies, except for 14 cases described by Aitken-Saavedra et al. that reported only the mean age of 45.2 [34].

In our study, the average age was 42.97 years (range 2 months-79 years old) with a prevalence between the fourth and fifth decade of life.

All studies included in our review, except one, reported the gender of the subjects. The analysis of the data collected suggested a male predilection with a male-to-female ratio of 1.95 : 1 (63 cases: 41 M, 21 F, and1 not reported). A graph of the age and gender distribution is reported in Figure 4.

In 63 cases reviewed, the analysis of localization in the oral cavity showed 19 in the lip (30%; 11 in the upper lip, 17.4%; 8 in the lower lip, 12.6%), 16 cases in the buccal mucosa of the cheek (or buccal space; 25.3%), 12 in the palate (19%), 5 in/on the tongue (7.9%), 5 in the gingiva (7.9%), and 3 in the mandible (4.7%). One lesion was observed in the retromolar area (1.58%). Other localizations were in the lower left back tooth region (1.58%) and in the lingual mucosa of the mandible (1.58%).

Size data were available in 46 of 63 cases. As reported in the literature, the size of the tumor can be very variable with a range from 0.5×0.5 to $3.5 \times 3.3 \times 2.0$ cm.

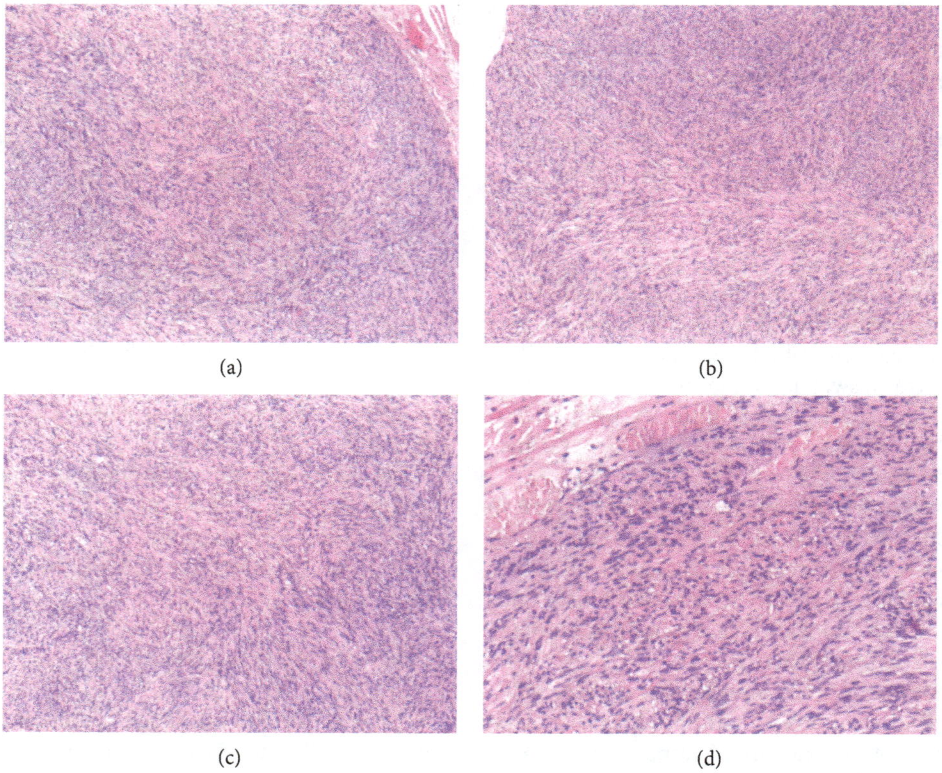

FIGURE 2: Histological findings of the case of angioleiomyoma reported. (a, b, c) The tumor is well circumscribed and shows an admixture of bundles of smooth muscle cells surrounding the blood vessels (4x); (d) AL: high-power view (10x).

The immunohistochemical analysis was performed for the differential diagnosis in all studies considered. This investigation revealed that the specimens were reactive to SMA (95.2%), desmin (73%), CD34 (44.4%), vimentin (42.8%), S-100 (7.9%), HHF-35 (7.9%), factor VIII (4.7%), h-caldesmon (1.58%), CD31 (1.58%), and NSE (1.58%).

Radiological investigations were not been prescribed in most cases considered; however, the investigations commonly described by many authors in the literature were MRI, CT, and US.

4. Discussion

Leiomyoma is described by the World Health Organization as a tumor of the soft tissue that arises from smooth muscle. It can be found in sites rich in smooth muscles such as the gastrointestinal tract, the myometrium, and the skin. Leiomyoma originating from smooth muscle cells of vessels lying on deep soft tissue is rare. Due to the lack of smooth muscle in the oral cavity, leiomyoma is relatively rare or uncommon. The possible sources of smooth muscle in the oral cavity include blood vessels, circumvallate papillae, and heterotopic smooth muscle [1, 2, 35].

In oral cavity, its origin is not well elucidated, but minor trauma, venous stasis, hormonal changes, and genetic translocation have been postulated as possible causes [36].

Leiomyoma is classified in three different types/major groups according to the prevailing histological pattern: the most common is the vascular form defined as AL (75%), followed by the solid form defined as leiomyoma (24%), and some cases of an epithelioid form defined as leiomyoblastoma are reported in the literature (<1%) [5, 37].

AL is a benign tumor resulting from the tunica media of smooth muscle cells of arterial and venous walls [37].

In the literature, it has been reported that AL accounts for 5% of all benign soft tumors and represents 3-3.9% of neoplasms that occur in the oral cavity [29, 36]. The incidence of AL in the oral cavity is rare and has been estimated to be roughly 0.065% [3].

Morimoto proposed a subclassification of AL describing solid, cavernous, and venous types [38]. On the authors' knowledge, only few authors have followed this subclassification reporting cases of intraoral AL: Liu et al. in a series of 21 tumors reported 5 solid, 6 venous, 9 cavernous, and 1 venous-cavernous AL [28]; Aitken-Saavedra et al. described 8 solid type, 4 cavernous type, and 2 venous type of AL [34].

Most of the AL are diagnosed between the fourth and sixth decade of life [38, 39], even if several studies have documented the tumor occurrence in subjects from 1 month to 84 years old [9]. There is only one study that reported a congenital tumor [21]. When AL occurs in this population, it is called leiomyomatous epulis, which clinically mimics a congenital granular cell tumor [28]. AL was rarely found during infancy and adolescence: only 6 reported cases of AL (5 males, 1 female) were diagnosed in patients younger than 20 years of age (Figure 4).

Conversely to extraoral localization, intraoral AL has a male predilection as reported in the literature by several authors [6, 24, 28, 34]. The results of our review of 63 cases confirm this with a 1.95 : 1 male-to-female ratio.

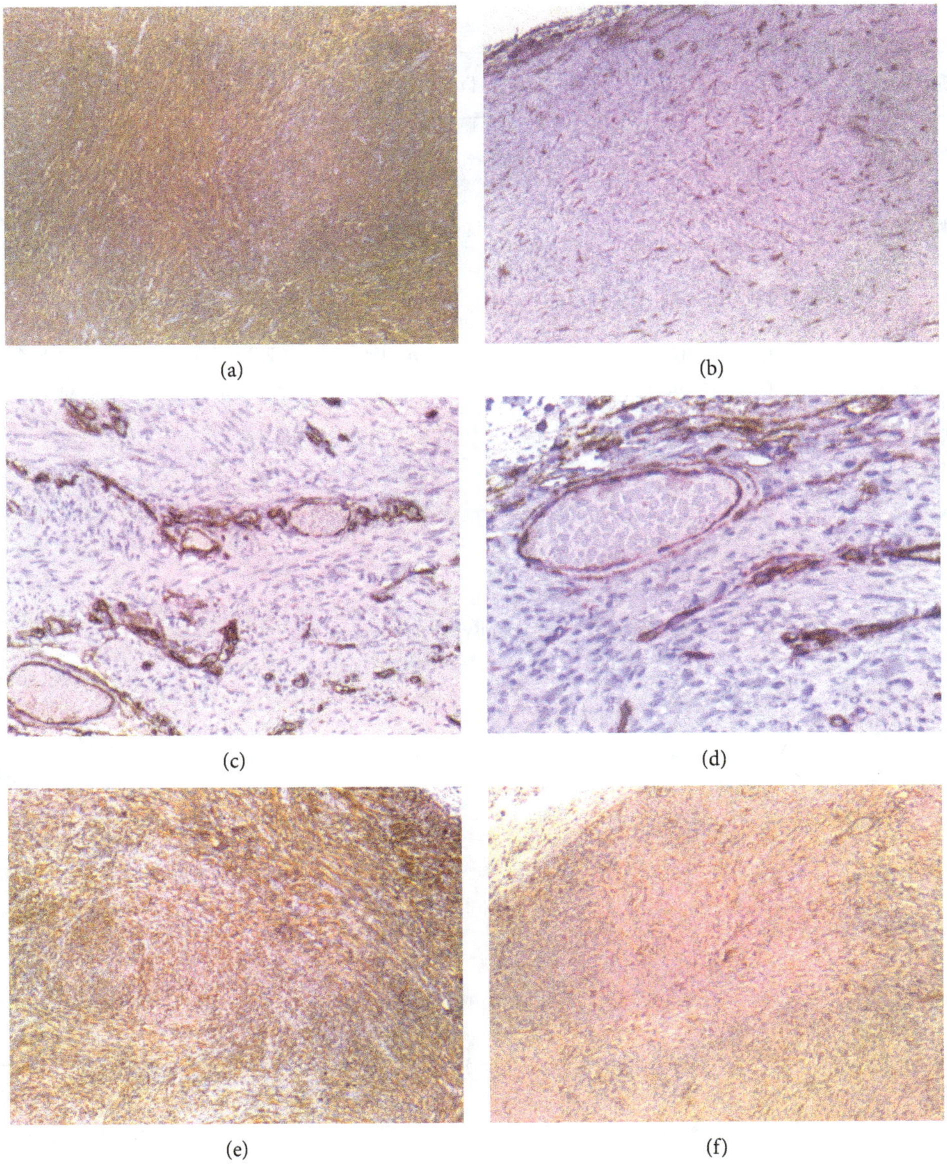

FIGURE 3: Immunohistochemical findings of the case of angioleiomyoma reported. (a) The tumor cells show strong and diffuse SMA expression (4x); (b) blood vessels endothelium marked with CD34 immunostaining (4x); (c) blood vessels endothelium marked with CD34 immunostaining at high magnification (10x); (d) blood vessels endothelium marked with CD34 immunostaining at high magnification (20x); (e) the tumor cells show strong and diffuse desmin expression (4x); (f) uniformly staining for vimentin (4x).

Many reports describe the lips as the most affected site with a frequency of 49%, followed by the palate, the buccal space, the mandible, the tongue, and the gingiva. Rare cases of intraosseous tumors are reported in the literature [25, 29]. The cheek was not the most frequent site of AL in the oral cavity, and the 16 cases reported in our review were observed in adult patients (age > 21). Therefore, we can consider our case rare of AL of the cheek reported in a young 17-year-old female teenager.

At clinical examination, AL appears in the oral cavity as a small, solitary, slowly developing mass [37], most commonly painless, and well localized. It presents as a palpable soft mass or elastic firm mass beneath the mucosa. The color of the mucous surface can be very variable, from normal to rosy or red [6].

Radiological investigations potentially useful for the diagnosis of AL are MRI, CT, and US. Yanagi et al., analyzing the usefulness of dynamic contrast-enhanced MRI in the differential diagnosis of AL in the buccal space, observed a very high signal intensity on T2WI and extremely high enhancement on Gd-T1WI; the inner aspect was homogeneous on T1WI and T2WI [40]. On CT images, AL appeared as a well-defined mass, heterogeneously well enhanced after the dye injection [22]. US revealed general hypoechogenicity with well-defined margins; in power Doppler mode, vascularity varies in density from low to high [41].

It is difficult to distinguish AL from the other solid lesions of the oral cavity, such as lymphangioma, hemangioma, fibroma, lipoma, pyogenic granuloma, and some other malignant lesions like angioleiomyosarcoma. AL is a benign

Table 1

Study (year of publication)	*N* of cases	Age (years)	Gender	Tumor location	Size (cm)	Immunohistochemical markers
(1) Maeda et al. (1989) [10]	1	37	M	Upper lip	0.7 × 0.8	Vimentin+, desmin+, factor VIII+ S-100^{-}, NSE+
(2) Maeda and Osaki (1989) [11]	1	49	F	Cheek	2.0 × 2.0	Vimentin+, desmin+, factor VIII+ S-100^{-}
(3) Anastassov and Damme (1995) [12]	1	51	M	Upper lip	1.5 × 1.0	SMA+, factor VIII-
(4) Toida et al. (2000) [13]	1	10	M	Lower lip	2.0 × 1.5	SMA+, S-100^{-}
(5) Marden et al. (2004) [14]	1	25	M	Tongue	3.2 × 3.0 × 1.2	SMA+, CD34^{+}, CD31^{+}
(6) Manor et al. (2007) [15]	1	39	M	Buccal mucosa	3.5 × 3.3 × 2.0	SMA+
(7) Scheper et al. (2007) [16]	1	67	M	Palate	5.0 × 5.0	SMA+
(8) Suresh et al. (2007) [17]	1	51	F	Mandible	1.7 × 1.5	SMA+, vimentin+, CD34^{-}, S-100^{-}
(9) Cepeda et al. (2008) [18]	5	39	F	Retromolar area	0.9 × 0.6 × 1.0	SMA+, vimentin+, desmin+, CD34^{-}, S-100^{-}
		27	F	Mandible	1.4 × 1.3 × 1.0	SMA+, vimentin+, desmin+, CD34^{-}, S-100^{-}
		43	F	Lower lip	0.7 × 0.5 × 0.4	SMA+, vimentin+, desmin+, CD34^{-}, S-100^{-}
		36	M	Upper lip	1.5 × 1.0 × 1.0	SMA+, vimentin+, desmin+, CD34^{-}, S-100^{-}
		48	M	Upper lip	1.7 × 1.0 × 1.0	SMA+, vimentin+, desmin+, CD34^{-}, S-100^{-}
(10) Keerthi et al. (2009) [19]	1	32	M	Cheek	4.5 × 4.0	SMA+
(11) Grossman et al. (2009) [20]	1	35	F	Palate	1.0 × 1.0 × 0.5	SMA+, vimentin+, desmin+, S-100^{-}, HHF-35+, AE1/AE3-
(12) Kim et al. (2010) [21]	1	2 months	Not reported	Tongue	2.5 × 2.0	SMA+, vimentin-, desmin+, S-100^{-}
(13) Kim et al. (2010) [22]	1	51	M	Buccal space	3.0 × 3.0	SMA+, CD34^{-}, S-100^{-}
(14) Nonaka et al. (2011) [23]	1	39	M	Tongue	2.0 ∅	SMA+
(15) Gueiros et al. (2011) [24]	3	54	M	Lower lip	1.0 × 1.0	SMA+, desmin+, CD34^{+}, S-100^{+}, HHF-35+, D2-40-
		66	M	Upper lip	Not reported	SMA+, desmin+, CD34^{+}, S-100^{-}, HHF-35+, D2-40-
		54	M	Upper lip	0.8 × 0.5 × 0.5	SMA+, desmin+, CD34^{+}, S-100^{+}, HHF-35+, D2-40-
(16) Patil et al. (2011) [25]	1	57	M	Lower left back tooth region	3.0 × 1.5 × 1.0	SMA+, vimentin+, desmin+, S-100^{-}
(17) Menditti et al. (2012) [26]	1	14	M	Lingual mucosa of mandible	1.0/2.0 ∅	SMA+
(18) Eley et al. (2012) [27]	1	39	M	Palate	2.0 ∅	Desmin+, actin+
(19) Liu et al. (2014) [28]	14	62	F	Buccal mucosa	1.5 ∅	SMA+, vimentin+, desmin+, CD34^{+} in all cases S-100^{+} only in 3 cases (not specified)
		49	M	Buccal mucosa	2.0 ∅	
		36	F	Buccal mucosa	2.0 ∅	
		51	F	Buccal mucosa	1.0 ∅	
		49	F	Palate	1.0 ∅	
		10	F	Mandible	3.5 ∅	
		30	F	Buccal mucosa	3.0 ∅	
		20	M	Gingiva	2.5 ∅	

Table 1: Continued.

Study (year of publication)	N of cases	Age (years)	Gender	Tumor location	Size (cm)	Immunohistochemical markers
		60	M	Palate	1.5 ∅	
		34	M	Palate	1.0 ∅	
		58	M	Lip	6.0 ∅	
		18	M	Palate	3.5 ∅	
		19	M	Tongue	3.5 ∅	
		47	M	Buccal mucosa	2.0 ∅	
(20) Tsuji et al. (2014) [3]	1	79	M	Palate	1.5 × 1.5	SMA+, desmin+
(21) Ishikawa et al. (2014) [29]	1	51	M	Tongue	1.1 ∅	SMA+, vimentin+, desmin+, CD34$^-$, S-100$^-$, HHF-35+
(22) Ranjan and Singh (2014) [30]	1	45	F	Gingiva	3.0 × 3.0	SMA+
(23) Inaba et al. (2015) [31]	1	45	F	Cheek	Not reported	SMA+, factor VIII+
(24) Osano et al. (2015) [9]	1	45	M	Cheek	2.0 ∅	SMA+, vimentin+, desmin+, CD34$^-$, S-100$^-$
(25) Arpağ et al. (2016) [32]	2	25	M	Gingiva	0.5 × 0.5	SMA+
		55	F	Gingiva	1.5 × 2.0	SMA+
(26) Bajpai et al. (2016) [33]	1	39	M	Gingiva	3.0 × 3.0	SMA+, vimentin+, desmin+
(27) Hassona et al. (2017) [4]	1	52	F	Upper lip	Not reported	SMA+
(28) Rawal and Rawal (2017) [8]	1	70	M	Palate	2.0 × 1.5	SMA+
(29) Matiakis et al. (2018) [7]	1	51	M	Labial mucosa of the upper lip	0.8 ∅	SMA+, h-caldesmon+
(30) Aitken-Saavedra et al. (2018) [34]	14	Total mean 45.2	Male = 8 Female = 6	Lower lip	Not reported	SMA+, AE1/AE3-, CD68$^-$, desmin+, S-100$^-$ in all cases CD34$^+$ only in 10 cases (not specified)
				Lower lip	Not reported	
				Lower lip	Not reported	
				Lower lip	Not reported	
				Upper lip	Not reported	
				Upper lip	Not reported	
				Upper lip	Not reported	
				Buccal mucosa	Not reported	
				Buccal mucosa	Not reported	
				Buccal mucosa	Not reported	
				Buccal mucosa	Not reported	
				Soft palate	Not reported	
				Soft palate	Not reported	
				Hard palate	Not reported	
Case report	1	17	F	Cheek	1.5 × 1.0	SMA+, vimentin+, desmin+, CD34$^+$

tumor with a low rate of malignant transformation, and definitive diagnosis needs histopathological analysis. The presence of cellular atypia, pleomorphism, and necrosis at histological analysis is common in both AL and angioleiomyosarcoma, while the number of mitosis is the main criterion to establish the malignancy. Tumors that have 4-10 mitosis for 10 high-power fields (HPF) should be considered as potentially malignant, while those with at least 5 mitosis for 10 HPF as malignant [6, 19, 42].

The prognosis of AL also depends on surgical treatment, in fact the complete surgical excision represents the best strategy of treatment of AL [25].

In such cases, recurrence of AL occurs mainly due to incomplete excision of the lesion: in literature, recurrence have been reported in a few cases [19]. It is important to perform a complete tumor resection and a long-term follow-up observation [3].

Immunohistochemical analysis represents an essential tool in the diagnosis of AL. The most common markers assessed to confirm the diagnosis of AL are SMA, vimentin, CD34, desmin, and S-100 [28].

The results of this review reported a diffuse positivity to SMA in almost all cases. The markers vimentin, CD34, and desmin were reactive in about half of the cases. Only two

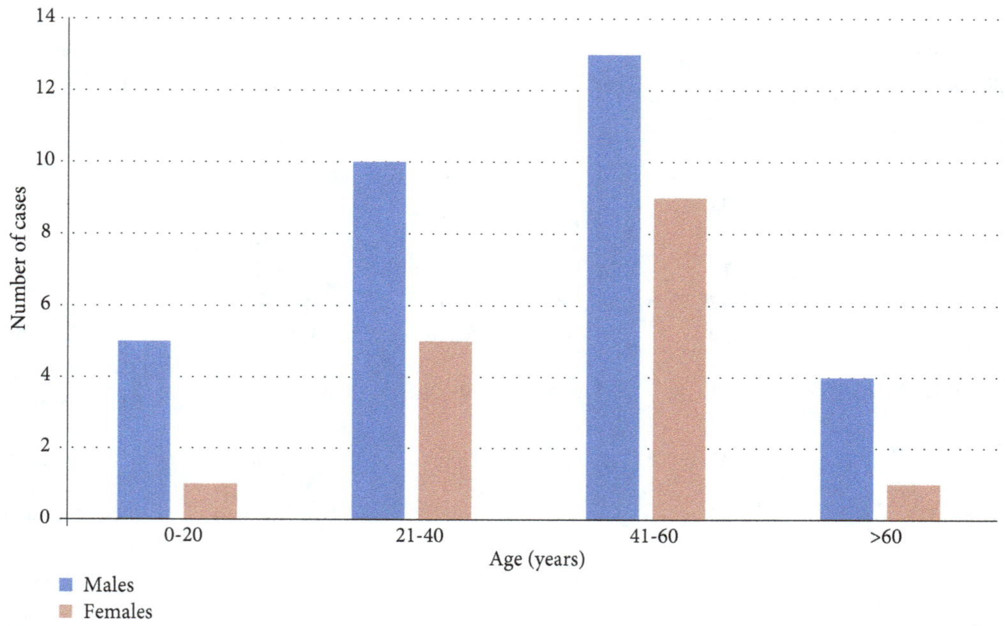

FIGURE 4: Distribution of age and sex in the 63 cases of angioleiomyoma of the oral cavity reviewed.

study showed S-100 positivity in small nerve fibers in five cases of AL [24, 28]. Matiakis et al. found the positivity of h-caldesmon in one case: they identified this marker as more specific for smooth muscle fibers than SMA and desmin, also to differentiate AL from myopericytoma [7].

Maeda et al. showed that vascular walls, hardly identified by hematoxylin eosin stain, became visible through factor VIII immunohistochemical staining [10, 11]. The factor VIII is synthesized by endothelial cells, and its expression has been reported in numerous vascular neoplasms [43].

Endothelial cells also express CD31; therefore, antibodies to CD31 have been used as a tool to identify the vascular origin of neoplasms [44].

Kim et al., Gueiros et al., and Ishikawa et al. described a positive staining for HHF-35 that, in addition to reactivity for SMA, vimentin, desmin, and S-100, can assist in the diagnosis as an adjunct to H&E staining [22, 24, 29].

Cepeda et al. emphasized the importance of immunohistochemical analysis in order to differentiate AL from other types of spindle cell tumor, including leiomyoma (CD34$^-$ and S-100$^-$), myopericytoma (desmin$^-$, CD34$^-$, and S-100$^-$), and myofibroma (desmin$^-$, CD34$^-$, and S-100$^{-/+}$) [18].

Kim et al. and Aitken-Saavedra et al. reported a negativity of the sample for AE1/AE3 and CD68 antibodies and showed that only SMA can be elected as a good marker for AL and be of help in the diagnosis of this lesion [22, 34].

Gueiros et al. immunohistochemical analysis showed a negativity of the sample for D2-40 and a positive staining for SMA, desmin, CD34, HHF-35, and S-100 in 2 cases [24].

Each marker is a characteristic of a specific tissue, but its detection is useful only in combination with clinical judgement and the measurement of other markers.

In conclusion, oral AL is a rare entity, especially in adolescence. We have reported a new rare case of AL of the cheek in a young woman. The clinical aspects of AL did not allow us to make a correct presumptive diagnosis. A scrupulous histopathological analysis made it possible to identify the pathological entity of the lesion. Immunohistochemical examinations are fundamental to differentiate AL from other lesions. SMA, vimentin, CD34, desmin, and S-100 are the most commonly investigated markers to guide histopathological diagnosis of oral AL.

References

[1] T. Hachisuga, H. Hashimoto, and M. Enjoji, "Angioleiomyoma. A clinicopathologic reappraisal of 562 cases," *Cancer*, vol. 54, no. 1, pp. 126–130, 1984.

[2] WHO, *Pathology and Genetics of Tumours of Soft Tissue and Bone*, C. D. M. Fletcher, K. K. Unni, and F. Mertens, Eds., IARC Press, 2002.

[3] T. Tsuji, K. Satoh, H. Nakano, and M. Kogo, "Clinical characteristics of angioleiomyoma of the hard palate: report of a case and an analysis of the reported cases," *Journal of Oral and Maxillofacial Surgery*, vol. 72, no. 5, pp. 920–926, 2014.

[4] Y. Hassona, F. Sawair, and C. Scully, "Angioleiomyoma of the upper lip," *BMJ Case Reports*, vol. 2017, article bcr-2016-219172, 2017.

[5] L. Barnes, J. W. Eveson, P. Reichart, and D. Sidransky, *Pathology and Genetics of Head and Neck Tumours, World Health Organization Classification of Tumours*, IARC Press, Lyon, France, 2005.

[6] J. K. Brooks, N. G. Nikitakis, N. J. Goodman, and B. A. Levy, "Clinicopathologic characterization of oral angioleiomyomas," *Oral Surgery, Oral Medicine, Oral Pathology, Oral Radiology, and Endodontology*, vol. 94, no. 2, pp. 221–227, 2002.

[7] A. Matiakis, P. Karakostas, A.-M. Pavlou, E. Anagnostou, and A. Poulopoulos, "Angioleiomyoma of the oral cavity: a case report and brief review of the literature," *Journal of the Korean Association of Oral and Maxillofacial Surgeons*, vol. 44, no. 3, pp. 136–139, 2018.

[8] S. Y. Rawal and Y. B. Rawal, "Angioleiomyoma (vascular leiomyoma) of the oral cavity," *Head and Neck Pathology*, vol. 12, no. 1, pp. 123–126, 2018.

[9] H. Osano, Y. Ioka, R. Okamoto et al., "Angioleiomyoma of the cheek: a case report," *Journal of Oral Science*, vol. 57, no. 1, pp. 63–66, 2015.

[10] Y. Maeda, J. Hirota, T. Osaki, K. Hayashi, H. Sonobe, and Y. Otsuki, "Angiomyoma of the upper lip: report of a case with electron microscopic and immunohistochemical observation," *British Journal of Oral and Maxillofacial Surgery*, vol. 27, no. 3, pp. 236–242, 1989.

[11] Y. Maeda and T. Osaki, "Angiomyoma of the cheek: a case report," *Journal of Oral and Maxillofacial Surgery*, vol. 47, no. 10, pp. 1090–1093, 1989.

[12] G. E. Anastassov and P. A. van Damme, "Angioleiomyoma of the upper lip: report of a case," *International Journal of Oral and Maxillofacial Surgery*, vol. 24, no. 4, pp. 301-302, 1995.

[13] M. Toida, H. Koizumi, and K. Shimokawa, "Painful angiomyoma of the oral cavity: report of a case and review of the literature," *Journal of Oral and Maxillofacial Surgery*, vol. 58, no. 4, pp. 450–453, 2000.

[14] F. A. Marden, G. C. Calilao, G. Guzman, and S. S. Roy, "Glossal angiomyoma: imaging findings and endovascular treatment," *Head & Neck*, vol. 26, no. 12, pp. 1084–1088, 2004.

[15] E. Manor, N. Sion-Vardy, M. Nash, and L. Bodner, "Angiomyoma of buccal vestibule: a rare case with a normal karyotype," *The Journal of Laryngology & Otology*, vol. 121, no. 12, pp. 1210–1212, 2007.

[16] M. A. Scheper, N. G. Nikitakis, and T. F. Meiller, "A stable swelling of the hard palate," *Oral Surgery, Oral Medicine, Oral Pathology, Oral Radiology, and Endodontology*, vol. 104, no. 4, pp. 461–464, 2007.

[17] L. Suresh, E. Matsumura, L. E. Calixto, E. Ruckert, and A. Aguirre, "Intraosseous angiomyoma of the mandible," *General Dentistry*, vol. 55, no. 2, pp. 132–135, 2007.

[18] L. A. Gaitan Cepeda, D. Quezada Rivera, F. Tenorio Rocha, E. R. Leyva Huerta, and E. R. Mendez Sanchez, "Vascular leiomyoma of the oral cavity. Clinical, histopathological and immunohistochemical characteristics. Presentation of five cases and review of the literature," *Medicina Oral Patologia Oral y Cirugia Bucal*, vol. 13, no. 8, pp. E483–E488, 2008.

[19] R. Keerthi, M. Nanjappa, S. S. Deora, and S. V. Kumaraswamy, "Angioleiomyoma of cheek: report of two cases," *Journal of Maxillofacial and Oral Surgery*, vol. 8, no. 3, pp. 298–300, 2009.

[20] S. d. M. C. Grossmann, A. C. R. Johann, W. H. Castro, H. Friedman, R. S. Gomez, and R. A. Mesquita, "Anterior midline nodule of the hard palate," *Oral Surgery, Oral Medicine, Oral Pathology, Oral Radiology, and Endodontology*, vol. 108, no. 6, pp. 808–811, 2009.

[21] Y.-H. Kim, Y.-W. Jang, H. Pai, and S.-G. Kim, "Congenital angiomyoma of the tongue: case report," *Dentomaxillofacial Radiology*, vol. 39, no. 7, pp. 446–448, 2010.

[22] H.-Y. Kim, S.-N. Jung, H. Kwon, W.-I. Sohn, and S.-H. Moon, "Angiomyoma in the buccal space," *Journal of Craniofacial Surgery*, vol. 21, no. 5, pp. 1634-1635, 2010.

[23] C. F. W. Nonaka, K. M. A. Pereira, and M. C. d. C. Miguel, "Oral vascular leiomyoma with extensive calcification areas," *Brazilian Journal of Otorhinolaryngology*, vol. 76, no. 4, p. 539, 2010.

[24] L. Gueiros, M. Romanach, A. Pires-Soubhia, F. Pires, O. Paes-De-Almeida, and P. Vargas, "Angioleiomyoma affecting the lips: report of 3 cases and review of the literature," *Medicina Oral Patología Oral y Cirugia Bucal*, vol. 16, no. 4, pp. e482–e487, 2009.

[25] K. Patil, V. Mahima, and H. Srikanth, "Recurrent oral angioleiomyoma," *Contemporary Clinical Dentistry*, vol. 2, no. 2, pp. 102–105, 2011.

[26] D. Menditti, L. Laino, L. Nastri, U. Caruso, P. Fiore, and A. Baldi, "Oral angioleiomyoma: a rare pathological entity," *In Vivo*, vol. 26, no. 1, pp. 161–163, 2012.

[27] K. A. Eley, S. Alroyayamina, S. J. Golding, R. N. Tiam, and S. R. Watt-Smith, "Angioleiomyoma of the hard palate: report of a case and review of the literature and magnetic resonance imaging findings of this rare entity," *Oral Surgery, Oral Medicine, Oral Pathology and Oral Radiology*, vol. 114, no. 2, pp. e45–e49, 2012.

[28] Y. Liu, B. Li, L. Li, Y. Liu, C. Wang, and L. Zha, "Angioleiomyomas in the head and neck: a retrospective clinical and immunohistochemical analysis," *Oncology Letters*, vol. 8, no. 1, pp. 241–247, 2014.

[29] S. Ishikawa, S. Fuyama, T. Kobayashi, Y. Taira, A. Sugano, and M. Iino, "Angioleiomyoma of the tongue: a case report and review of the literature," *Odontology*, vol. 104, no. 1, pp. 119–122, 2016.

[30] S. Ranjan and K. Singh, "Gingival angioleiomyoma-infrequent lesion of oral cavity at a rare site," *Journal of Oral and Maxillofacial Pathology*, vol. 18, no. 1, pp. 107–110, 2014.

[31] T. Inaba, M. Adachi, and H. Yagisita, "A case of angioleiomyoma in the buccal space," *Odontology*, vol. 103, no. 1, pp. 109–111, 2015.

[32] O. F. Arpağ, I. Damlar, S. Kılıç, A. Altan, Z. A. Taş, and T. Özgür, "Angioleiomyoma of the gingiva: a report of two cases," *Journal of the Korean Association of Oral and Maxillofacial Surgeons*, vol. 42, no. 2, pp. 115–119, 2016.

[33] M. Bajpai, N. Pardhe, and M. Kumar, "Angioleiomyoma of gingiva masquerading as pyogenic granuloma," *Journal of the College of Physicians and Surgeons Pakistan*, vol. 26, no. 7, pp. 631-632, 2016.

[34] J. Aitken-Saavedra, K. D. da Silva, A. P. N. Gomes et al., "Clinicopathologic and immunohistochemical characterization of 14 cases of angioleiomyomas in oral cavity," *Medicina Oral Patología Oral y Cirugia Bucal*, vol. 23, no. 5, pp. e564–e568, 2018.

[35] H. M. Cherrick, C. L. Dunlap, and O. H. King Jr, "Leiomyomas of the oral cavity: review of the literature and clinicopathologic study of seven new cases," *Oral Surgery*, vol. 35, no. 1, pp. 54–66, 1973.

[36] P. Ramesh, S. R. Annapureddy, F. Khan, and P. D. Sutaria, "Angioleiomyoma: a clinical, pathological and radiological review," *International Journal of Clinical Practice*, vol. 58, no. 6, pp. 587–591, 2004.

[37] F. M. Enzinger, R. Lattes, and H. Torloni, *Histological Typing of Soft Tissue Tumours*, World Health Organization, Geneva, Switzerland, 1969.

[38] N. Morimoto, "Angioleiomyoma [vascular leiomyoma]-a clinicopathologic study," *Medical Journal of Kagoshima University*, vol. 24, pp. 663–666, 1974.

[39] K.-W. Leung, D. Y.-K. Wong, and W.-Y. Li, "Oral leiomyoma: case report," *Journal of Oral and Maxillofacial Surgery*, vol. 48, no. 7, pp. 735–738, 1990.

[40] Y. Yanagi, J.-I. Asaumi, M. Hisatomi et al., "Usefulness of dynamic contrast-enhanced MRI in the differential diagnosis of angioleiomyoma in the buccal space," *European Journal of Radiology Extra*, vol. 48, no. 1, pp. 14–18, 2003.

[41] V. Gomez-Dermit, E. Gallardo, R. Landeras, F. Echevarría, and R. G. Barredo, "Subcutaneous angioleiomyomas: gray-scale and color Doppler sonographic appearances," *Journal of Clinical Ultrasound*, vol. 34, no. 2, pp. 50–54, 2006.

[42] R. Luaces Rey, F. Lorenzo Franco, G. Gómez Oliveira, B. Patiño Seijas, D. Guitián, and J. L. López-Cedrún Cembranos, "Oral leiomyoma in retromolar trigone. A case report," *Medicina Oral Patología Oral y Cirugia Bucal*, vol. 12, no. 1, pp. e53–e55, 2007.

[43] D. Little, J. W. Said, R. J. Siegel, M. Fealy, and M. C. Fishbein, "Endothelial cell markers in vascular neoplasms: an immunohistochemical study comparing factor VIII-related antigen, blood group specific antigens, 6-keto-PGF1 alpha, and Ulex europaeus 1 lectin," *The Journal of Pathology*, vol. 149, no. 2, pp. 89–95, 1986.

[44] D. V. Parums, J. L. Cordell, K. Micklem, A. R. Heryet, K. C. Gatter, and D. Y. Mason, "JC70: a new monoclonal antibody that detects vascular endothelium associated antigen on routinely processed tissue sections," *Journal of Clinical Pathology*, vol. 43, no. 9, pp. 752–757, 1990.

15

An Atypical Case of Oral Squamous Cell Carcinoma of Mandibular Alveolus

Seba Abraham, Bhagyalekshmi Mallika, Arunima Reshma, and ReejaMol Mohammed Kassim

PMS College of Dental Science and Research, India

Correspondence should be addressed to Bhagyalekshmi Mallika; bhagyalekshmirajesh511@gmail.com

Academic Editor: Ronald S. Brown

Oral squamous cell carcinoma is the most common type of oral malignant neoplasm. As per literature, squamous cell carcinomas of the alveolar ridge account for 9% of all the oral carcinomas. The oral squamous cell carcinoma shares clinical similarity with various forms of inflammatory gingival lesions and is often misdiagnosed in our routine dental practice. The dentist should have precise knowledge regarding the clinical manifestation of this deadly disease as early diagnosis and prompt treatment can reduce morbidity and mortality of the disease.

1. Introduction

Oral cancer accounts for the eleventh most common cancer worldwide [1]. Oral squamous cell carcinoma (OSCC) is the common oral carcinoma with varied clinical presentations. It accounts for more than 90% of all malignant lesions in the oral cavity [2]. The affected population group was <40 years of age in high-incidence countries such as India, Pakistan, and Sri Lanka [3]. Alveolar ridge SSC accounts for 9% of all cases with oral SCC [4]. Alveolar ridge SSC accounts for the second position, with the first being carcinoma of the tongue as per site specificity. As per local recurrence rate by site, mandibular alveolus carcinoma has the highest local recurrence rate (26/42), second being carcinoma of the tongue (20/47). Squamous cell carcinomas can occur in all areas of the body, but they are most common in the skin and oral cavity.

Oral squamous cell carcinoma of the mandibular region is found to have the lowest survival rate when compared with all other oral carcinomas [5]. Various aids used for assessing mandibular invasion include clinical examination, radiographic examination (OPG, CT dentascan, MRI, bone scans, ultrasound, and PET CT), and histopathological examination. Histopathologic analysis of squamous cell carcinoma reveals two basic patterns of tumor invasion: invasive pattern (infiltrative pattern) and erosive pattern (compressive patterns). In the invasive pattern, islands of tumor infiltrate cancellous spaces and have little osteoclastic activity and no intervening connective tissue. However, in the erosive pattern, the tumor advances as a broad front with active osteoclasts separating the tumor from the bone and the connective tissue layer separating the tumor/bone [6].

Marginal resection is considered as the best treatment option if the carcinoma reaches close to the bone without any invasion or with mild invasion [5]. Marginal resection involves the removal of 1 cm of margins from all sides [7]. Nomura et al. in 2005 reported that in case of oral squamous cell carcinoma, the tumor extended to the periosteum in 33%, to the cortical bone in 23%, and to the bone marrow in 9% of the patients who underwent mandibular resection. The remaining 35% of the patients had no evidence of mandibular invasion. The area of bone resorption on preoperative clinical and radiographic examinations often disagreed with the extent of mandibular invasion on histopathologic examination [8].

The clinical presentation of oral squamous cell carcinoma can range from a white plaque to an ulcerated lesion [9]. Malignant lesions in the gingiva may resemble

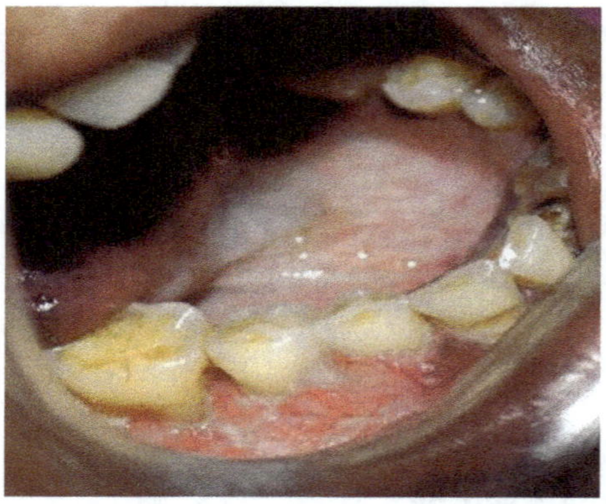

FIGURE 1: Desquamative changes in relation to the 43, 44, 45, and 46 regions.

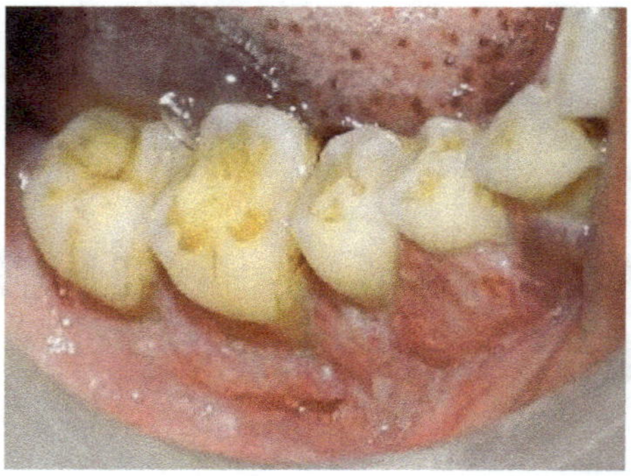

FIGURE 2: Ulceroproliferative lesion extending from the 44 to 47 regions.

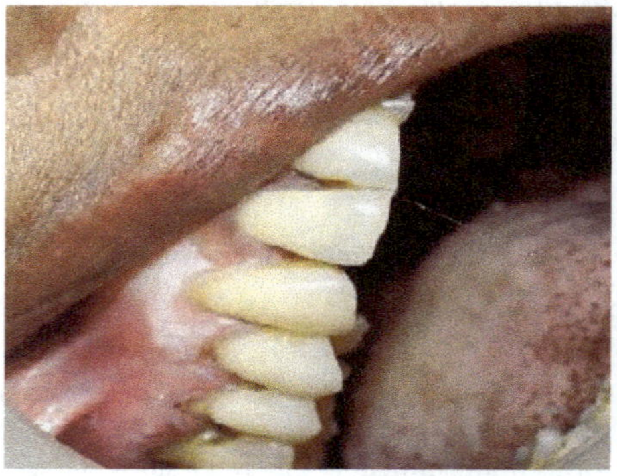

FIGURE 3: Desquamative lesion noted in relation to 13 extending to the 15 regions.

frequently seen inflammatory lesions of the gingiva. Oral carcinomas can often be misdiagnosed as other inflammatory lesions in the oral cavity leading to delay in delivering prompt treatment. Thus, the early diagnosis and treatment of oral carcinoma by health care providers is mandatory for optimum treatment outcome [10]. Treatment of squamous cell carcinoma is mainly a surgical excision and a radical neck dissection in the case of lymph node metastasis. Radiotherapy is considered as adjunct postoperative treatment along with chemotherapy and is a definite treatment of choice in case of advanced stages of cancer.

Oral carcinoma has emerged as a major health problem in India mainly because of the high prevalence of smokeless tobacco use. Oral SCC metastases to regional lymph nodes in the neck and distant metastases are seen in the later stages as diseases progress [11]. Here, we are reporting a nontobacco-related case of SCC of the lower alveolus with atypical presentation of desquamative gingival lesions and often more chance to misdiagnose the case.

2. Case Report

A 48-year-old female patient presented to the Department of Periodontics with the chief complaint of acute pain in relation to the lower right back teeth region for the past 2 months. The patient gave a history of antibiotic and analgesic medication for one week after consulting with a nearby hospital. Pain was the throbbing type and continuous in nature, and it aggravates on opening the mouth, during mastication, and while brushing teeth.

General clinical examination revealed normal mouth opening. Multiple tender lymph nodes were noted on the right side of the face and neck region. On palpation, submandibular and cervical lymph nodes were tender and palpable (2 cm in diameter) and were firm and fixed to the skin.

The intraoral examination revealed desquamative changes in relation to the 43, 44, 45, and 46 regions (Figure 1). Grade 2 mobility in relation to the 44, 46, and 47 regions and grade 3 mobility in relation to 45. No associated paraesthesia was reported. An ulceroproliferative lesion extending from the 44 to 47 regions with mixed keratotic and erythematous area with granular appearance was noted (Figure 2). On palpation, the lesion was tender with mild induration. Desquamative lesion was noted in relation to 13 extending to 15 regions (Figure 3). Periodontal probing resulted in profuse bleeding in relation to 45 and 46 regions. Deep pockets (>6 mm) in relation to the 16, 17, 26, 27, 44, 45, 46, and 47 regions.

Hard tissue examination revealed an end-on-end occlusion. A comprehensive periodontal examination was done which revealed heavy deposits of calculus on the lingual surface of mandibular posteriors. Generalized cervical abrasion and attrition were present. The oral hygiene maintenance was compromised due to severe pain while brushing interfering with proper plaque removal.

2.1. Radiographic Evaluation. OPG revealed generalized horizontal bone loss with severe bone loss in relation to the 45 and 46 regions with widening of PDL space and furcation radiolucency in relation to 46. Impacted 18 and 28 were noted (Figure 4). Diffused poorly defined radiolucency was noted in relation to 45 and 46 extending up to the superior border of the mandibular canal (Figure 5).

Based on clinical and radiographic examination, a provisional diagnosis of chronic generalized periodontitis and carcinoma alveolus was made. Differential diagnosis is erosive lichen planus.

Staging of oral squamous cell carcinoma is done based on the American Joint Committee on Cancer. cTNM is the stage given after the clinical examination of the patient, while

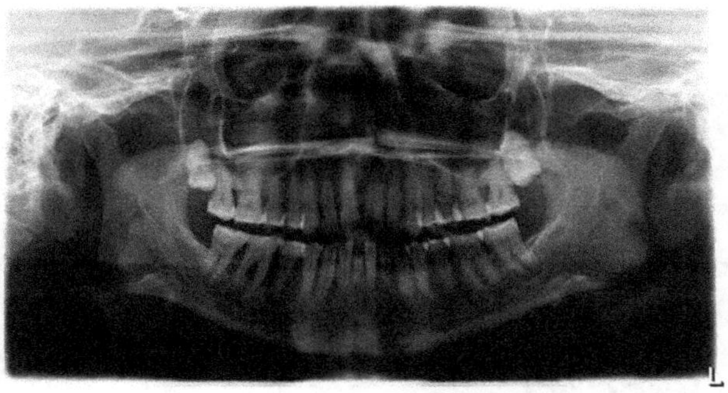

FIGURE 4: Generalized horizontal bone loss with severe bone loss in relation to the 45 and 46 regions with widening of the PDL space and furcation involvement in relation to 46. Impacted 18 and 28.

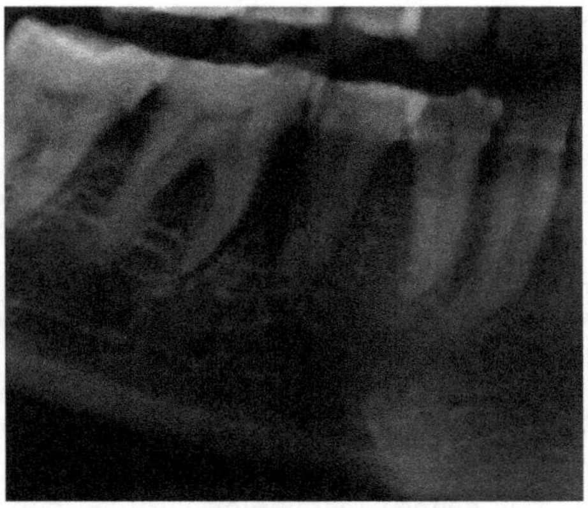

FIGURE 5: Diffused poorly defined radiolucency was noted in relation to 45 and 46 extending up to the superior border of the mandibular canal.

pTNM is the stage after the histopathological examination of the surgical specimen. Based on the American Joint Committee on Cancer January 2018, the cTNM cancer staging of this case is AJCC Stage IVA and stage grouping T4aN1M0 as there is involvement to the jaw bone and presence of a palpable lymph node of size 2 cm.

2.2. Treatment. Initially, nonsurgical periodontal therapy including scaling and root planing was performed. Incisional biopsy of the oral lesion extending from the marginal gingiva of 44 to 46 to the mucogingival junction (measuring about $1.4 * 1.3 * 0.6$ cm in size) was performed under LA (Figure 6). The excised tissue was sent for histopathological examination (Figure 7). 3-0 vicryl sutures placed and a surgical pack given (Figure 8). The patient was kept under antibiotic and anti-inflammatory therapy for one week.

2.3. Histopathological Examination. Histopathological examination of the given soft tissue section revealed islands and sheets of malignant squamous epithelial cells infiltrating into the connective tissue (Figures 9(a) and 9(b)). The neoplastic cells exhibit numerous keratin pearl formation, nuclear and cellular pleomorphism, and mitotic figures (Figure 9(c) (c1, c2) 40x). Areas of severely atrophic epithelium with few saw toothed rete pegs and basal cell degeneration are also seen. Based on clinical, radiographic, and histopathological examinations, the case is diagnosed as squamous cell carcinoma (SCC). The patient was referred to the Regional Cancer Centre (RCC), Thiruvananthapuram, for further treatments. We tried to contact the patient for further follow up but was in vain.

3. Discussion

Squamous cell carcinoma is considered as the most common malignant neoplasm of the oral cavity. The tongue, oropharynx, and floor of the mouth are the most common sites, and SCC of the gingiva and lips is rarely seen. SCC of the mandibular gingiva is more common than the maxillary gingiva [12].

Most of the cases of oral carcinoma are associated with tobacco chewing habit and usually appear as a premalignant lesion like leukoplakia before progressing to the malignant stage, but rare cases have also been reported with nontobacco-associated squamous cell carcinoma. The case reported here is one without the history of tobacco chewing habit.

Carcinoma of the gingival region often mimics desquamative lesions of the gingiva and other inflammatory gingival lesions. The gingiva is one of the most common sites for chronic inflammation as it is often associated with irritants like calculus and abundant microbial flora. Attached gingiva is more involved than free gingiva [4]. Misdiagnosis is often encountered in the absence of detailed clinical examination and radiographic investigation.

Mandibular alveolus is the second most common site for oral carcinoma. Oral squamous cell carcinoma is more frequently seen among men compared to women as men are often exposed to high risk habits such as smoking and tobacco chewing (Liviu Feller et al. 2012). Age is another critical factor for oral SCC; as age advances, pronounced genetic and epigenetic changes take place. The case presented here is a female patient of age 48 years with a lesion mimicking desquamative lesion in relation to the lower right back teeth region. Another desquamative lesion was noted in the maxillary region in relation to 13, 14, and 15 without the clinical presentation of SCC.

Regional lymph node metastasis is another feature of squamous cell carcinoma. Cervical lymph nodes of the submandibular triangle and upper jugular regions have stronger predilection of regional lymph node metastasis in the case of SCC of the lower alveolus [13]. Tender and palpable submandibular and cervical lymph nodes (which are firm and fixed to the skin) of about 2 cm in diameter were detected in the present case. Prognosis is better in early oral SCC, especially those that are well-differentiated and without metastasis, but the worst part is that most cases of OSCC are not diagnosed at the earlier stage of the disease. The prognosis can vary based on a number of factors that are related to the tumor or treatment or to the patient.

Squamous cell carcinoma was found to enter the medullary cavity through the upper border of the mandible, either through the occlusal ridge alone or in combination with

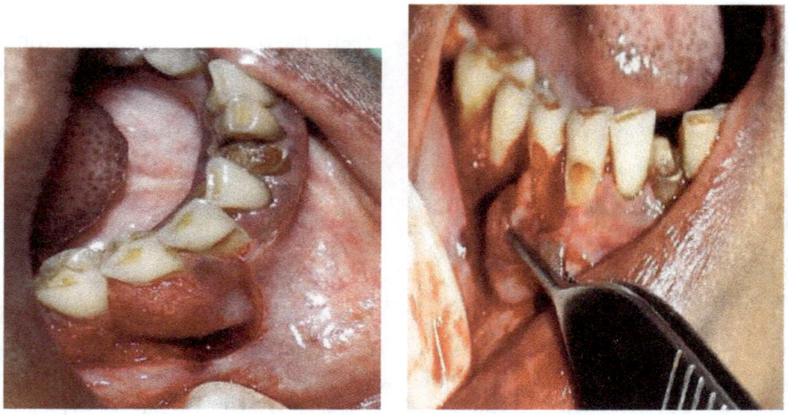

(a) (b)

Figure 6: (a, b) Incisional biopsy.

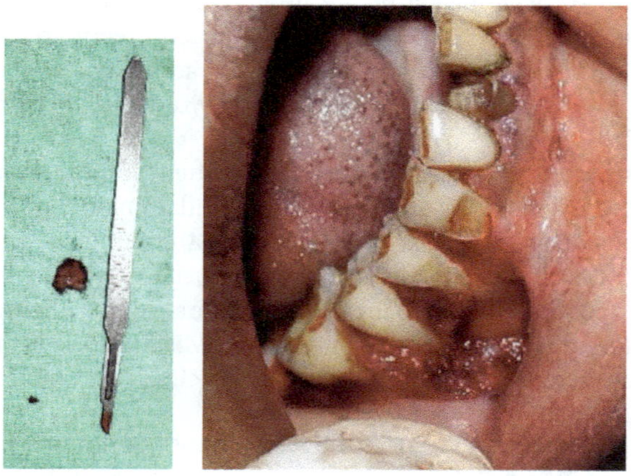

(a) (b)

Figure 7: (a, b) Excised tissue and surgical site after excision.

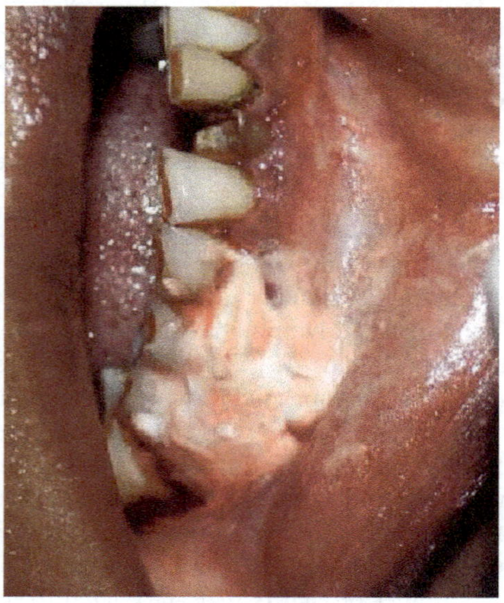

Figure 8: Surgical pack.

penetration of either the buccal or lingual plates. The spread through the foramina is another important route of entry. When the carcinoma is not that deep, that is, if it does not reach the alveolar canal, then there is no spread along the alveolar canal and little or no insinuation of the cancer cells beyond the tumor front [7].

The radiologically detected bone defects in squamous cell carcinoma were classified as follows: (a) erosive—well-defined margins of the absorbed bone and (b) moth eaten—irregular, ill-defined margins of absorbed bone. Histopathologic patterns of bone involvement were classified as follows: (a) expansive—outline of the eroded bone appears smooth or slightly concave and (b) infiltrative—tumors will infiltrate the mandible through spaces or aggressively by destroying the bone. The extent of radiologically detected bone defects and the histological pattern of bone involvement can be graded as follows: (a) grade 1—bone defects limited to the alveolar bone, (b) grade 2—bone defects exceeded the alveolar bone but did not extent beyond the mandibular canal or the temporary line between right and left mental foramen, and (c) grade 3—bone defects extend beyond the mandibular canal or the temporary line between the right and the left mental foramen [14]. The case presented here shows diffuse, ill-defined radiolucency in relation to 45 and 46 extending up to the superior border of the mandibular canal.

Treatment of squamous cell carcinoma is primarily a surgical excision followed by radiation therapy and chemotherapy as postoperative adjunct treatment modalities. Radical neck dissection is often required in case of lymph node metastasis. Marginal resection is considered as a treatment option when the bone defects did not extend beyond the mandibular canal and segmental resection if it extends beyond the mandibular canal. The 5-year cumulative survival rate for the mandibular marginal resection group is about 78.1% and 72.8% in the segmental resection group [14]. Other innovations in the field of cancer therapy were laser-based technology (photodynamic therapy), immunotherapy, and gene therapy to treat oral squamous cell carcinoma at a much earlier stage [15].

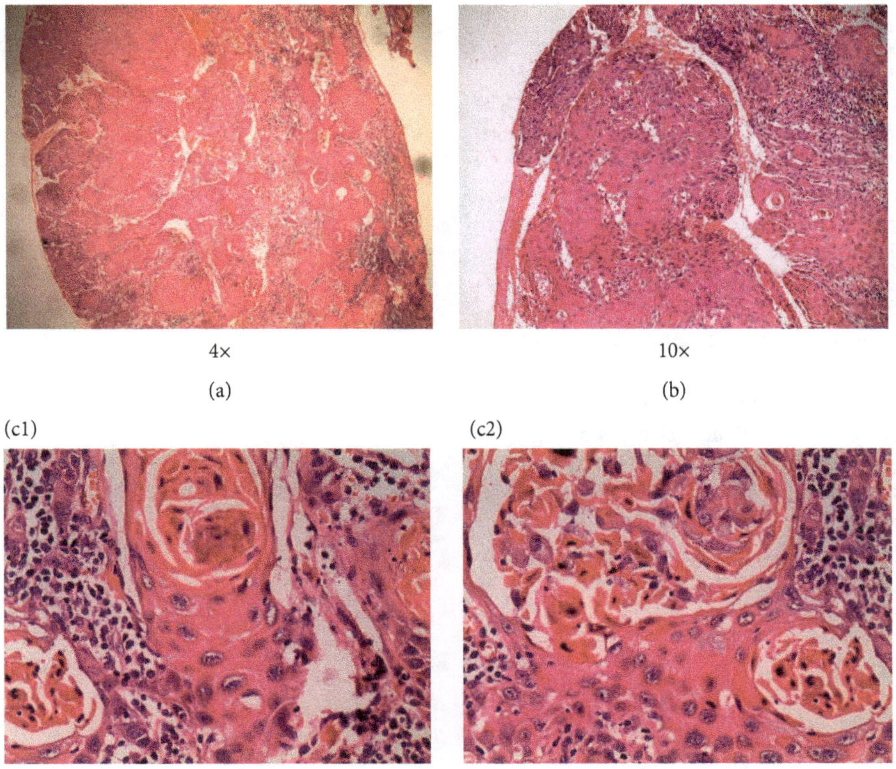

4× (a)

10× (b)

(c1) 40×

(c2) 40×

(c)

Figure 9: (a) 4x and (b) 10x: histopathologic view of the lesion showing islands and sheets of malignant squamous epithelial cells infiltrating into the connective tissue. Areas showing severely atrophic epithelium with few saw toothed rete pegs and basal cell degeneration are also seen. (c1, c2) 40x: higher magnification showing neoplastic cells with numerous keratin pearl formations, nuclear and cellular pleomorphisms, and mitotic figures. Few dilated blood vessels were also noted.

4. Conclusion

Squamous cell carcinoma is the most common malignant epithelial neoplasm with varied oral presentations. Therefore, the dentist should be aware of the characteristics of the disease. The most fatal complication is the distant metastasis as the disease progresses. Hence, correct and timely diagnosis is of utmost importance and there are more chances for misdiagnosis as the clinical presentation of oral squamous cell carcinoma can mimic inflammatory gingival lesions.

References

[1] J. Ferlay, H. R. Shin, F. Bray, D. Forman, C. Mathers, and D. M. Parkin, *GLOBOCAN 2008 v2.0, Cancer Incidence and Mortality Worldwide: IARC Cancer Base No. 10*, International Agency for Research on Cancer, Lyon, France, 2010.

[2] M. L. Wallace and B. W. Neville, "Squamous cell carcinoma of the gingiva with an atypical appearance," *Journal of Periodontology*, vol. 67, no. 11, pp. 1245–1248, 1996.

[3] S. Warnakulasuriya, "Global epidemiology of oral and oropharyngeal cancer," *Oral Oncology*, vol. 45, no. 4-5, pp. 309–316, 2009.

[4] S. T. Ildstad, M. E. Bigelow, and J. P. Remensnyder, "Squamous cell carcinoma of the alveolar ridge and palate. A 15-year survey," *Annals of Surgery*, vol. 199, no. 4, pp. 445–453, 1984.

[5] J. C. de Vicente, O. R. Recio, S. L. Pendás, and J. S. López-Arranz, "Oral squamous cell carcinoma of the mandibular region: a survival study," *Head & Neck*, vol. 23, no. 7, pp. 536–543, 2001.

[6] R. L. Carter, S. W. Tsao, J. F. Burman, M. R. Pittam, P. Clifford, and H. J. Shaw, "Patterns and mechanisms of bone invasion by squamous carcinomas of the head and neck," *American Journal of Surgery*, vol. 146, no. 4, pp. 451–455, 1983.

[7] K. H. Lam, L. K. Lam, C. M. Ho, and W. L. Wei, "Mandibular invasion in carcinoma of the lower alveolus," *American Journal of Otolaryngology*, vol. 20, no. 5, pp. 267–272, 1999.

[8] T. Nomura, T. Shibahara, N.-H. Cui, and H. Noma, "Patterns of Mandibular Invasion by Gingival Squamous Cell Carcinoma," *Journal of Oral and Maxillofacial Surgery*, vol. 63, no. 10, pp. 1489–1493, 2005.

[9] T. Y. Yoon, I. Bhattacharyya, J. Katz, H. J. Towle, and M. N. Islam, "Squamous cell carcinoma of the gingiva presenting as localized periodontal disease," *Quintessence Int*, vol. 38, no. 2, pp. 97–102, 2007.

[10] P. A. Levi Jr., D. M. Kim, S. L. Harsfield, and E. R. Jacobson,

"Squamous Cell Carcinoma Presenting as an Endodontic-Periodontic Lesion," *Journal of Periodontology*, vol. 76, no. 10, pp. 1798–1804, 2005.

[11] J. G. Buckley, A. Ferlito, A. R. Shaha, and A. Rinaldo, "The treatment of distant metastases in head and neck cancer–present and future," *ORL*, vol. 63, no. 4, pp. 259–264, 2001.

[12] O. A. Effiom, W. L. Adeyemo, O. G. Omitola, O. F. Ajayi, M. M. Emmanuel, and O. M. Gbotolorun, "Oral squamous cell carcinoma: a clinicopathologic review of 233 cases in Lagos, Nigeria," *Journal of Oral and Maxillofacial Surgery*, vol. 66, no. 8, pp. 1595–1599, 2008.

[13] J. P. Shah, N. W. Johnson, and J. G. Batsakis, *Textbook of Oral Cancer*, Martin Dunitz, London, 2003.

[14] K. Tei, Y. Totsuka, T. Iizuka, and K. Ohmori, "Marginal resection for carcinoma of the mandibular alveolus and gingiva where radiologically detected bone defects do not extend beyond the mandibular canal," *Journal of Oral and Maxillofacial Surgery*, vol. 62, no. 7, pp. 834–839, 2004.

[15] S. M. Balaji, "Oral squamous cell carcinoma: advances in management," *Indian Journal of Dental Research*, vol. 26, no. 6, p. 559, 2015.

16

A Rare Case of Orthograde Retrieval of Extruded Instrument following Periapical Tissue Healing

Ahmed Elhakim[1,2] **and Tarek Mohamed Abd El-Wahab**[1]

[1]*Department of Endodontics, Faculty of Dentistry, Mansoura University, Mansoura, Egypt*
[2]*Department of Conservative Dentistry, Yonsei University College of Dentistry, Seoul, Republic of Korea*

Correspondence should be addressed to Tarek Mohamed Abd El-Wahab; tarek.abdelwahab@mans.edu.eg

Academic Editor: Sukumaran Anil

The ideal retrieval protocol of separated instruments reverts the case to the initial situation prior to the fracture incidence while preserving the tooth hard tissue and the integrity of the supporting structures. When a patient presented for emergency treatment of tooth #37 diagnosed with acute suppurative apical periodontitis, radiographic examination revealed a fractured instrument extruded into the periapex. The treatment options for retrieval were limited to replantation. The initial emergency treatment which consisted of orthograde pus drain, radicular disinfection, and intracanal calcium hydroxide dressing completely resolved patient's symptoms. The follow-up radiographs revealed an interesting finding: gradual shift in the separated fragment position into the radicular space allowing a successful nonsurgical removal of the broken instrument. In conclusion, the reaction of periodontal tissues to an extruded instrument fragment remaining in situ may be favourable; thus, a risk and benefit analysis approach is essential to fractured instrument retrieval.

1. Introduction

The reported rates of endodontic instrument separation during treatment range from 0.4% to 7.4% [1]. This considerable variation in fracture prevalence reflects its complex and multifarious nature. Canal geometry, instrument properties, mode of action, and operator skill are identified as the main determining factors of separation risk [2]. Nevertheless, it is well-acknowledged among practicing specialist that endodontic files frequently separate even with meticulous adherence to the proper parameters of use.

Depending on its location and its relation to the curvature if present and the ability to visualize it by straight line access, management of separated endodontic instruments includes nonsurgical retrieval, bypassing, follow-up, and surgical treatment [3, 4]. Higher rates of treatment failure are associated with unretrieved instruments impeded in canals with preexisting preapical lesions, especially when separations occur earlier in the treatment [5–7]. This is attributed to the residual bacterial biofilms harbored in the artificial isthmus created by the instrument and beyond the point of impedance [3]. When the separated fragment extends beyond the apex due to an improper working length control at the moment of fracture or being pushed during a failed attempt of retrieval, additional complications may arise including injury to vital structures, persistent infection, and foreign body reaction [8].

Fractured instruments extending beyond the apical foramen have a significantly reduced probability of retrieval which explains the noticeable paucity of reports on these cases [3, 4]. The available literature is comprised of single case reports discussing management of partially extruded instrument fragments only, mainly by apical surgery or replantation with few reports describing successful orthograde retrieval [9–13]

To the best of our knowledge, this is the first report describing the unusual periodontal tissue reaction to and the successful nonsurgical retrieval of a fractured endodontic instrument completely extruded outside the root canal.

2. Case Report

A 30-year-old healthy female patient presented with pain and swelling in the lower left side of the mandible. The pain was severe, disturbed her sleep, and was not relived by medication. She reported a recurrent mild swelling (2 or 3 times annually) in the same area for the past three years.

The patient had facial asymmetry caused by cellulitis. Intraoral examination revealed a fluctuant swelling on the buccal mucosa adjacent to grossly decayed tooth #36 and filled tooth #37 which was exceptionally sensitive to palpation. The gingival probing depths were normal. Radiographic examination revealed that tooth 37 had a single, poorly obturated canal and a periapical radiolucency with a separated instrument located 3 mm away from the apex (Figure 1).

Tooth 37 was diagnosed as the causative tooth with acute suppurative apical periodontists. After anesthesia and endodontic access, loosely packed root filling was removed the by H-Files (Mani Inc, Tochigi, Japan). Yellow purulent discharge drained through the access cavity and was encouraged by a sterile saline flushed using side vent needle (EndoTop, Cerkamed, Stalowa Wola, Poland). Following working length determination, apical diameter was gauged to reveal a #80 sized wide apical foramen. The canal walls were planned without enlargement using H-files while being irrigated with 2% sodium hypochlorite solution (Chloraxid, Cerkamed, Stalowa Wola, Poland) that was activated ultrasonically using irrisafe-20 (Acteon Satelec, Merignac, France). The canal was then dried and medicated with calcium hydroxide (Metapaste, Meta Biomed, Chungbuk, Korea), and the access was sealed by Cavit (3 M, MN, USA). The unrestorable tooth 36 was extracted, and amoxicillin/clavulanic acid 1 gm tab every 12 hours and Ibuprofen 600 mg tab every 8 hours were prescribed.

After three days, the patient experienced sudden pain exacerbation. The canal was re accessed and purulent discharges exuded once again from the canal. After copious irrigation with sodium hypochlorite and ultrasonic activation, the canal was dried, remedicated with Metapaste, and sealed.

The patient missed the obturation appointment and returned eight months later for an unrelated complaint. She reported complete absence of pain and normal functionality of the treated tooth since the last treatment. Clinical examination revealed an intact temporary restoration, healthy periapical mucosa with normal responses to percussion, and periapical palpation tests. Radiographic examination demonstrated partial bone healing and a shift in the separated fragment position towards the tooth apex (Figure 2).

The treatment plan changed to a follow-up approach with long-term calcium hydroxide dressing before obturation, to observe the possibility of further movement of the separated fragment. Annual follow-up radiographs demonstrated gradual movement of the broken fragment towards and into the radicular space (Figure 3). Thirty-two months after the initial visit, the entire segment settled inside the root canal, and retrieval attempt using ultrasonically activated irrigant was successful. The canal was dried and obturated with guttapercha and resin sealer (Adseal, Meta Biomed, Chungbuk, Korea) by continuous wave of compaction technique, and the coronal structure was restored using resin composite (Filtek Z350, 3 M ESPE, USA) (Figure 4).

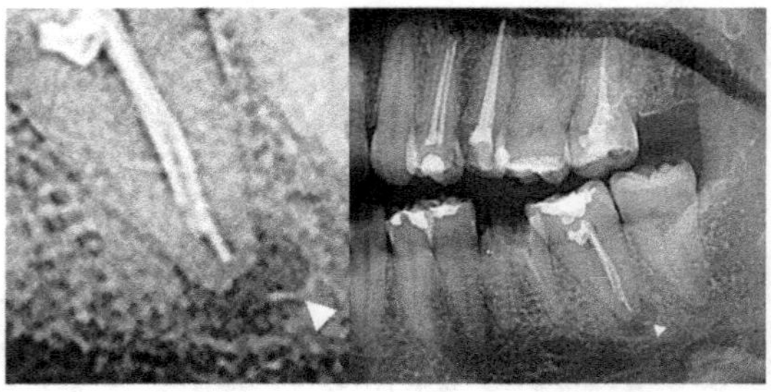

Figure 1: Emergency visit. The patient had severe pain and cellulitis with a fractured instrument beyond the apex (arrowhead). The patient was treated with systemic antibiotic with orthograde pus discharge followed by radicular disinfection and intracanal calcium hydroxide dressing.

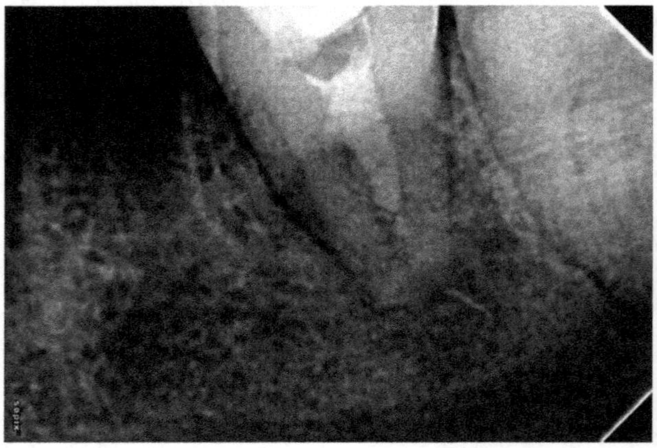

Figure 2: First recall after 8 months. Due to the change in orientation of the broken instrument and the wide apical foramen, a decision was taken to remedicate the canal and follow-up the case as the tooth was functional, and the patient was asymptomatic.

3. Discussion

The main goal of managing a separated instrument is to eliminate or minimize its impact on long-term prognosis. Proper and complete disinfection of the radicular spaces after the incidence of instrument separation neutralize its deleterious effect regardless of the outcome of management protocol. Thus, analysis of the risk and benefit and decision-making are integral to separated instrument retrieval [14]. In certain cases, bypassing or follow-up may be preferred over instrument retrieval where excessive removal of dentin to gain access to and free the impeded fragment may compromise the biomechanical integrity of the tooth and lead to perforations [15, 16]. This statement is especially true in cases involving strategic teeth where

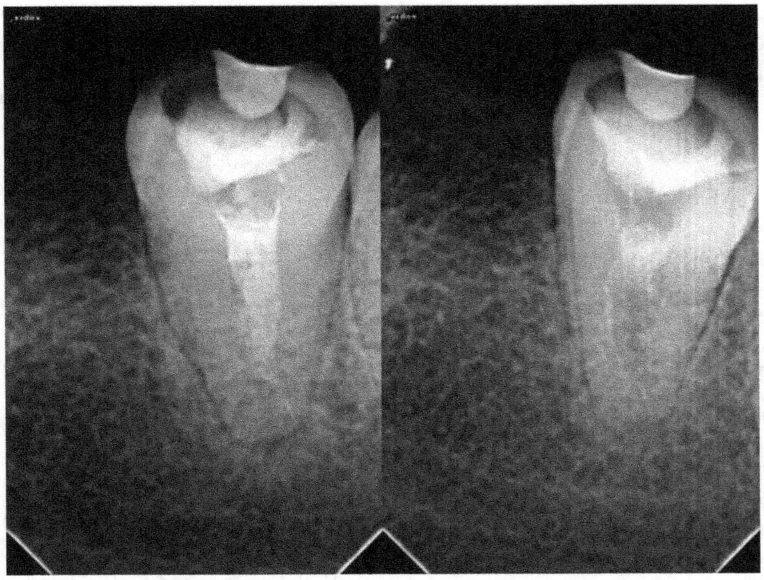

FIGURE 3: Annual follow-up radiographs demonstrating movement of the fractured segment into the root canal.

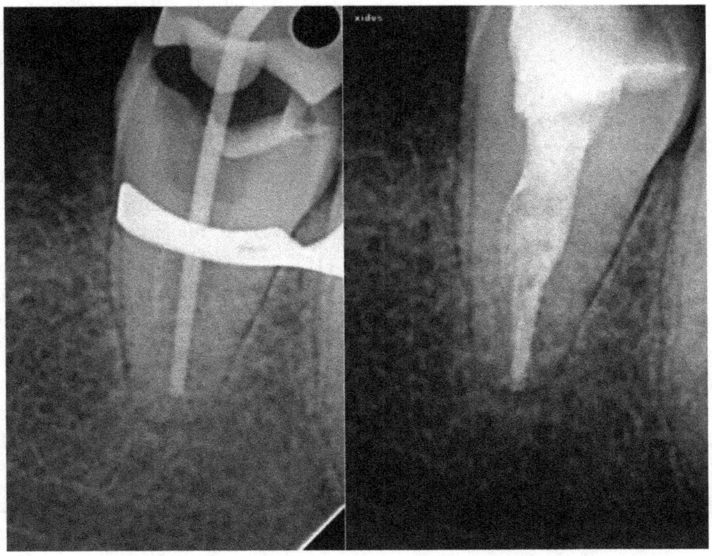

FIGURE 4: Retrieval of the fractured segment and obturation 32 months after the initial treatment. Patient remains asymptomatic.

uncertain prognosis may halt the treatment or lead to undesirable consequences.

Similarly in our case, tooth 37 was initially planned for replantation to curette the periapical area and remove the extruded file segment since apical surgery was not feasible due to the thick buccal bone ridge. However, the inherent risk of replantation-associated resorption could lead to undesirable outcomes including tooth loss and necessity of a later complex prosthodontic restoration. When the periapical lesion demonstrated signs of healing after the emergency visits, the treatment changed from an active intervention to a passive follow-up.

Stainless steel files are corrosion resistant and biologically inert, while NiTi metal alloys are well tolerated by human tissues [17, 18]. Although we cannot determine whether the lesion developed prior to or after the incident of fracture, it is clear that the abscess drainage and radicular disinfection were crucial to initiation of healing and that the remaining fragment did not retard the process of healing. Consequently, an endodontic instrument extruded into the periapex alone may not constitute a sufficient reason of treatment failure [19, 20].

Previous studies concluded that either an inflammatory or isolative reaction (granulation or calcification) takes place around foreign bodies extruded beyond the tooth apex [19, 21]. Smith's observations on the sequestration of fractured roots and bone fragments have conclude that an intermediate layer of inflammatory exudates surrounding the fragment is necessary to facilitate sequestration which may be retreaded in its absence [22]. In the current case, the initial active inflammation and suppuration might have prevented encapsulation of the extruded fragment by granulation tissue and tipped the periradicular tissue reaction towards sequestration, while the wide apical foramen mostly caused by over instrumentation and the unfilled radicular space may have facilitated tissue drainage and file repositioning into the root canal.

4. Conclusion

We described the spontaneous retrieval of an instrument fragment extruded into the periapex of tooth 37. Within the limitation of this single study, the findings from this case support the available evidence from the literature of a risk and benefit analysis approach when managing a fractured endodontic instrument. If the source of infection within the radicular spaces has been addressed, the periodontal reaction to an extruded endodontic instrument may be favorable even with maintenance of the fragment in situ. As single observations do not permit any more than a speculation as to the nature of this phenomena and because our understanding of the periodontal tissue reaction to foreign bodies is based on limited classical observations, further studies are needed to elude its governing dynamics and the underlying mechanisms.

Authors' Contributions

All authors have contributed significantly in this case report and are in agreement with the manuscript.

References

[1] M. B. McGuigan, C. Louca, and H. F. Duncan, "Endodontic instrument fracture: causes and prevention," *British Dental Journal*, vol. 214, no. 7, pp. 341–348, 2013.

[2] M. B. McGuigan, C. Louca, and H. F. Duncan, "Clinical decision-making after endodontic instrument fracture," *British Dental Journal*, vol. 214, no. 8, pp. 395–400, 2013.

[3] B. Suter, A. Lussi, and P. Sequeira, "Probability of removing fractured instruments from root canals," *International Endodontic Journal*, vol. 38, no. 2, pp. 112–123, 2005.

[4] M. Hülsmann and I. Schinkel, "Influence of several factors on the success or failure of removal of fractured instruments from the root canal," *Endodontics & Dental Traumatology*, vol. 15, no. 6, pp. 252–258, 1999.

[5] M. B. McGuigan, C. Louca, and H. F. Duncan, "The impact of fractured endodontic instruments on treatment outcome," *British Dental Journal*, vol. 214, no. 6, pp. 285–289, 2013.

[6] P. Panitvisai, P. Parunnit, C. Sathorn, and H. H. Messer, "Impact of a retained instrument on treatment outcome: a systematic review and meta-analysis," *Journal of Endodontia*, vol. 36, no. 5, pp. 775–780, 2010.

[7] P. Spili, P. Parashos, and H. H. Messer, "The impact of instrument fracture on outcome of endodontic treatment," *Journal of Endodontia*, vol. 31, no. 12, pp. 845–850, 2005.

[8] R. H. Kaddoura and A. A. Madarati, "Management of an over-extruded fragment in a C-shaped root canal configuration: a case report and literature review," *Journal of Taibah University Medical Sciences*, vol. 15, no. 5, pp. 431–436, 2020.

[9] R. Fujii, K. Morinaga, T. Asai et al., "Intentional replantation to treat apical periodontitis of maxillary first molar with foreign body located outside apical foramen using CBCT: a case report," *The Bulletin of Tokyo Dental College*, vol. 61, no. 2, pp. 127–133, 2020.

[10] S. L. Satheesh, S. Jain, A. C. Bhuyan, and L. S. Devi, "Surgical management of a separated endodontic instrument using second generation platelet concentrate and hydroxyapatite," *Journal of Clinical and Diagnostic Research*, vol. 11, no. 6, pp. ZD01–ZD03, 2017.

[11] A. Heydari, M. Rahmani, and M. Heydari, "Removal of a broken instrument from a tooth with apical periodontitis using a novel approach," *Iranian Endodontic Journal*, vol. 11, no. 3, pp. 237–240, 2016.

[12] H. Plascencia, A. Cruz, R. Solís, M. Díaz, and J. Vázquez, "Iatrogenic displacement of a foreign body into the periapical tissues," *Case Reports in Dentistry*, vol. 2014, Article ID 698538, 2014.

[13] N. Srivastava and N. Vineeta, "Foreign body in the periradicular area," *Journal of Endodontics*, vol. 27, no. 9, pp. 593-594, 2001.

[14] P. Parashos and H. H. Messer, "Rotary NiTi instrument fracture and its consequences," *Journal of Endodontics*, vol. 32, no. 11, pp. 1031–1043, 2006.

[15] Y. Gao, Y. Shen, X. Zhou, and M. Haapasalo, "Remaining root dentin thickness in mesiobuccal canals of maxillary first molars after attempted removal of broken instrument fragments," *Australian Endodontic Journal*, vol. 41, no. 3, pp. 122–127, 2015.

[16] A. A. Madarati, A. J. Qualtrough, and D. C. Watts, "Vertical fracture resistance of roots after ultrasonic removal of fractured instruments," *International Endodontic Journal*, vol. 43, no. 5, pp. 424–429, 2010.

[17] P. D. Eleazer, "Lack of corrosion of stainless steel instruments in vivo by scanning electron microscope and microprobe analysis," *Journal of Endodontics*, vol. 17, no. 7, pp. 346–349, 1991.

[18] J. Ryhänen, M. Kallioinen, J. Tuukkanen et al., "In vivo biocompatibility evaluation of nickel-titanium shape memory metal alloy: muscle and perineural tissue responses and encapsule membrane thickness," *Journal of Biomedical Materials Research*, vol. 41, no. 3, pp. 481–488, 1998.

[19] H. Yusuf, "The significance of the presence of foreign material periapically as a cause of failure of root treatment," *Oral Surgery, Oral Medicine, and Oral Pathology*, vol. 54, no. 5, pp. 566–574, 1982.

[20] P. N. Ramachandran Nair, "Non-microbial etiology: foreign body reaction maintaining post-treatment apical periodontitis," *Endodontic Topics*, vol. 6, no. 1, pp. 114–134, 2003.

[21] M. G. Khabbaz and P. D. Papadopoulos, "Deposition of calcified tissue around an overextended gutta-percha cone: case report," *International Endodontic Journal*, vol. 32, no. 3, pp. 232–235, 1999.

[22] R. L. Smith, "The role of epithelium in the healing of experimental extraction wounds," *Journal of Dental Research*, vol. 37, no. 2, pp. 187–194, 1958.

17

Management of Edentulous Microstomia Patient: A Case Report and Classification System

Maria S. Abbasi,[1] Naseer Ahmed,[1,2] Adil Bin Irfan,[1] Samar Al-Saleh,[3] Tariq Abduljabbar,[3] and Fahim Vohra[3]

[1]*Department of Prosthodontics, Altamash Institute of Dental Medicine, Karachi 75500, Pakistan*
[2]*PhD Scholar Prosthodontics Unit University Sains Malaysia, School of Dental Sciences, Health Campus, 16150 Kubang Kerian, Kelantan, Malaysia*
[3]*Department of Prosthetic Dental Science, College of Dentistry, King Saud University, 60169, Riyadh 11545, Saudi Arabia*

Correspondence should be addressed to Fahim Vohra; fvohra@ksu.edu.sa

Academic Editor: Kevin Seymour

Microstomia is an abnormally reduced oral aperture. In the literature, it is not classified by any particular size criteria, rather defined by its effects on function and esthetics. Prosthodontic management of edentulous patients with microstomia is a challenging task. Use of conventional methods for recording an impression and fabricating prosthesis is not effective in such patients. To fabricate well-fitting prosthesis, accuracy of impression recording important anatomic landmarks is essential. Formation of an exacting custom tray and diagnostic cast is critical for final impression accuracy. Provision of a well-fitting prosthesis in microstomia patient will restore esthetics, comfort, and function with oral and systemic patient wellbeing. This paper presents a case report of managing an edentulous microstomia patient with sectional removable prosthesis. Furthermore, it proposes a novel classification system for microstomia patients according to severity of the condition.

1. Introduction

Microstomia is a congenital, developmental, and acquired condition, which presents with reduced oral aperture resulting in esthetics and functional impairment [1, 2]. It is usually associated with congenital syndromes and autoimmune diseases that cause connective tissue disorder [3]. It is majorly reported as a result of scarring following surgeries and trauma (accidental, thermal, chemical, and electric burns) around the perioral tissues, facial burn injuries, and head and neck irradiation [3]. In a study by Patil et al., 38.2% of the reported microstomia cases were due to postsurgical complications and 41.1% cases were due to systemic sclerosis [4]. Mostly microstomia is associated congenitally with Freeman-Sheldon, Treacher Collins, and Pierre Robin syndromes [5]. The occurrence of microstomia congenitally has also been reported with an unknown cause [6].

Microstomia patients may present with clinical problems including severe facial scarring, reduced width and mobility of lips, and loss of elasticity and altered anatomy of the oral tissues, particularly thickening of the labial and buccal tissues and contraction of the tissues around the mouth [4]. These features affect oral health-related quality of life, i.e., compromised chewing, speech difficulty, and appearance. Furthermore, a diminished intraoral access will affect oral hygiene maintenance and manual dexterity. Additionally, it makes the provision of dental prostheses quite challenging [5], especially among edentulous patients, in which oral function, esthetic, comfort, and self-esteem are at its lowest [6].

Therefore, treating such cases of edentulism and microstomia is pivotal not only from a functional standpoint but also from a psychological perspective. The goals of prosthodontic treatment are to restore masticatory function, improve esthetics, restore vertical dimension, establish lip

Table 1: Classification systems based on diagnosis and management for microstomia patients.

Class	IOA severity	Vertical mouth opening	Accessibility/visibility	Treatment options	Prosthetic fabrication difficulty	Manual dexterity
DM-1	Mild	Minimally compromised: 31-35 mm	(i) Denture-bearing areas of the mouth are fully accessible and visible (ii) Impressions and JRR can be recorded easily	(i) Conventional removable dentures (ii) Implant-supported prosthesis (iii) Flexible dentures	Not technique sensitive	Adequate
DM-2	Moderate	Moderately compromised: 21-30 mm	(i) Denture-bearing areas of the mouth have moderately compromised accessibility and visibility (ii) Moderately difficult to record impressions and JRR (modification of the tray/ technique is required*)	(i) Surgical correction (ii) Prosthodontic mx: (1) Implants supported/retained prosthesis (2) Flangeless prosthesis (3) Sectional complete removable dental prostheses—various cross pins, bolts, attachments, buttons, and Lego pieces can be used for the locking mechanism (4) Swing lock denture with cobalt-chromium framework	Moderately technique-sensitive design, moderately skilled lab/technician required	Fair
DM-3	Severe	Substantially compromised: 10-20 mm	(i) All the denture-bearing areas of the mouth have substantially compromised accessibility and visibility (ii) Extremely difficult to record impressions and JRR	(i) Surgical correction (ii) Prosthodontic mx: Sectional collapsible complete removable dental prosthesis	Highly technique-sensitive designs, highly skilled lab/ technician required	Poor
DM-4	Extreme	Severely compromised: <10	(i) Denture-bearing areas hardly visible (ii) Impressions and JRR are not possible	Prosthetic rehabilitation not possible	—	—

DM = diagnosis and management; IOA = index of oral access; mx = management; JRR = jaw relation record; *flexible trays = sectional impression trays using die pins, sectional trays with interlocking-type handle or manually dispensing silicone putty.

support and competency, reduce drooling, and improve articulation [7]. The need for a classification based on diagnosis and overall patient management is lacking. The existing classification on microstomia which is the "index of oral access[1]" (IOA) does not address vertical mouth opening, difficulty in prosthesis fabrication, manual dexterity of the patient, and treatment options.

Proposed strategies for microstomia patients include use of sectional or flexible trays for primary impressions [8]. Sectional custom trays for maxillary and mandibular final impression, flexible dentures, and sectional complete removable dental prostheses using various cross pins, bolts, and attachments are proposed by clinical experts for hard and soft tissue replacement [9, 10],11. However, management strategies for edentulous microstomia patients are limited and challenging, with lack of defined standards. Therefore, in this report, the authors propose a classification system according to the severity of microstomia (Table 1), to guide practitioners in formulating diagnosis and treatment options according to the complexity of microstomia. We also present a case report of an edentulous microstomia patient managed successfully with a sectional complete denture.

2. Case Report

A 62-year-old, male, edentulous patient reported to the prosthodontic department with functional inadequacy. On examination, he had reduced oral aperture, 20 mm interridge distance and 32 mm intercommissural width, along with inelastic buccal and labial tissues as a result of scarring and fibrosis following surgery around the corner of the mouth (Figure 1(a)). The patient had type 2 diabetes mellitus and was on oral hypoglycemic drugs. He displayed adequate manual dexterity and psychological status and belonged to class IV assessment of Prosthodontic Diagnostic Index [12] and DM-3 class (Table 1), based on the severity of microstomia. After consideration of all options, a plan to provide a sectional collapsible complete denture was suggested.

The primary impression for the maxilla was recorded in three sections. Firstly, the right and left ridge impressions were recorded separately with impression compound (Compound Red Cakes, Kerr Dental, CA, USA), trimmed 4-5 mm from the midline, and irregular notches were made at the mesial surface. Additional material was then added over the two halves to index the impression and complete the

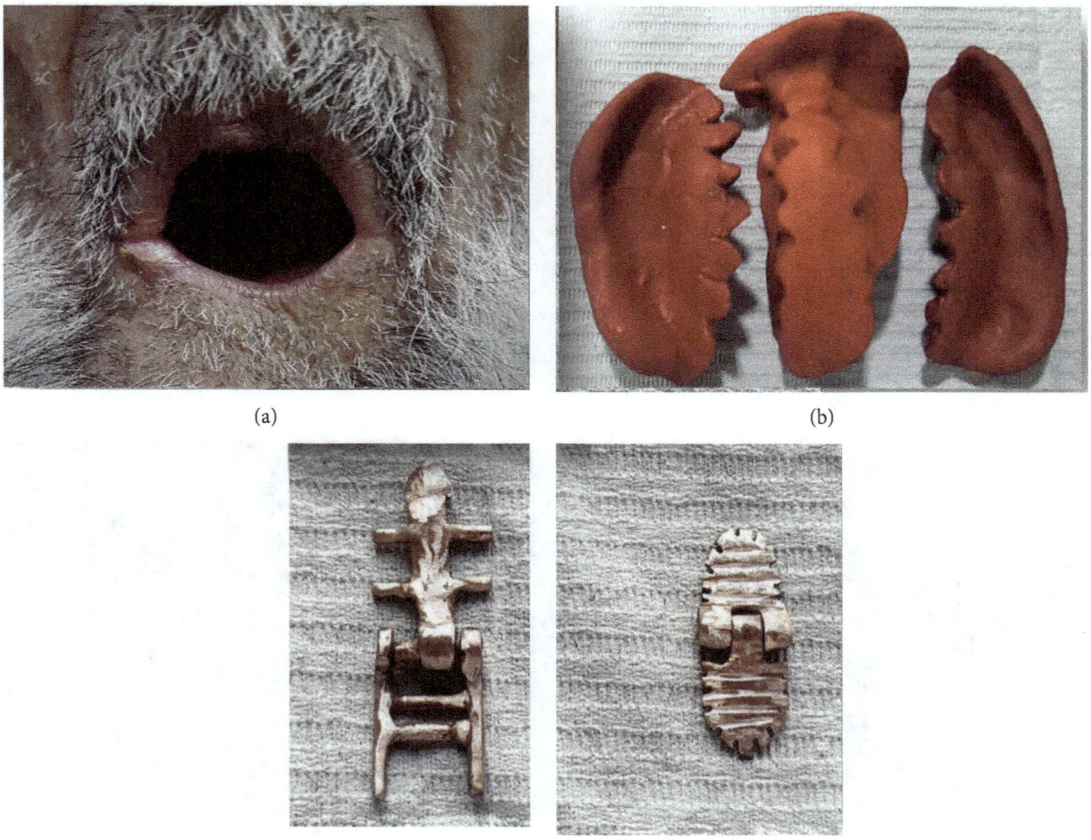

FIGURE 1: (a) Reduced oral access, 20 mm height and 32 mm intercommissural width. (b) Maxillary sectional primary impression. (c) Maxillary custom-made hinge. (d) Mandibular custom-made hinge.

maxillary impression record (Figure 1(b)). The mandibular impression was recorded with impression compound in one piece. Sectional custom trays were fabricated from the preliminary cast with a stepped butt joint along the midline. Border molding was carried out with green stick impression compound (Compound Green Sticks, Kerr Dental, CA, USA) with right and left sectional trays in the maxilla and mandible. Following border molding, definitive impressions of both segments were recorded simultaneously with medium body polyvinylsiloxane (PVS) (Aquasil, Monophase, Dentsply Sirona, PA, USA) along with an index over the 2 segments for stabilization of the trays.

Maxillary final record base was fabricated in two segments (Nature-Cryl® HI-20ET-GC America, CA, USA), anterior and posterior; a custom-made Co-Cr hinge was fabricated following the design guidelines presented by Conroy and Reitzik [13] (Figure 1(c)). This hinge was incorporated in the midline as far back as possible in the posterior segment making it collapsible in the horizontal plane. For stability and bracing of the posterior segment, an anterior segment was placed over it. Similarly, a mandibular record base (Nature-Cryl® HI-20ET-GC America, CA, USA) incorporating a custom-made Co-Cr hinge (Heraenium EH, Kulzer, Zaragoza, Spain) anterolingually in the midline was fabricated in one piece making the base collapsible in the horizontal plane (Figure 1(d)). Maxillomandibular relationship in centric relation was recorded using sectional resin base with wax rims (Figures 2(a) and 2(b)) and was transferred to the articulator. Semianatomic artificial teeth were arranged in bilateral balanced occlusion. Two ball attachments (Clix-Ball attachment, Preat Corp., ON, Canada) were incorporated in the posterior segment of the maxillary denture base in order to retain the anterior segment to the posterior segment. A dental surveyor was used to obtain parallel paths of insertion on both sides (Figure 2(c)). Two ball abutment housings (female component) (Clix-Ball attachment, Preat Corp., ON, Canada) on the tissue surface of the anterior denture segment were incorporated with autopolymerized acrylic resin (GC Pattern Resin-LS, GC America, CA, USA) (Figures 2(c) and 2(d)). The resistance provided by the slopes of the residual ridges and the tongue pressure was used to stabilize the collapsible-hinged mandibular complete denture.

At the denture insertion, overextension of borders and sharp edges were removed by relieving the intaglio surface using disclosing paste (Pressure Indicating Paste, Keystone, Singen, Germany) and carbide acrylic bur (Patterson Dental, MN, USA) on a slow-speed motor. Occlusion was adjusted to achieve equilibration in static and functional position of the mandible. The patient was instructed and trained for denture assembly and removal. He was provided postinsertion instructions on hygiene, safe storage, maintenance,

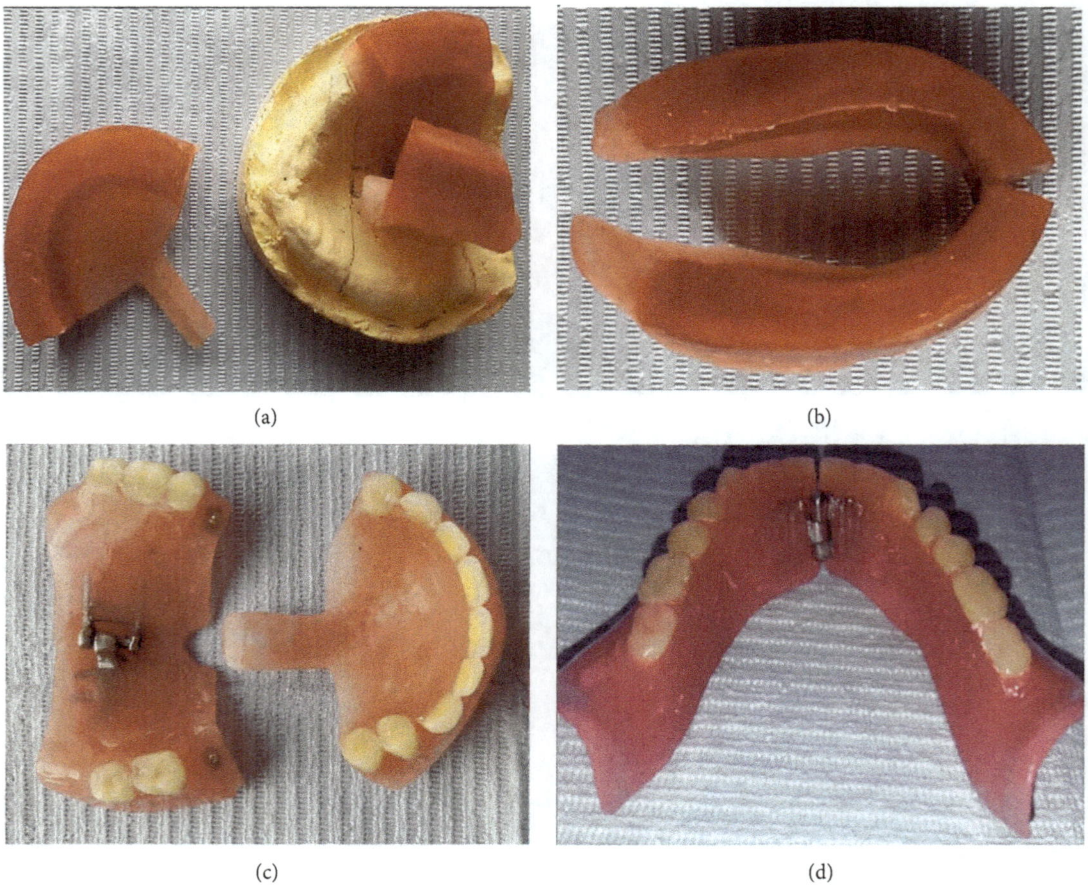

FIGURE 2: (a) Maxillary trial denture base and occlusion rim with custom-made hinge at midline of posterior segment. (b) Mandibular trial denture base and occlusion rim. (c) Sectioned maxillary prosthesis. (d) Sectioned mandibular prosthesis.

and regular follow-up to avoid mucosal ulcers and tissue inflammation, denture loss, and treatment failure.

3. Discussion

A planned and sequential approach is essential in treating microstomia cases. As the outcome is dependent on the clinical complexity of the case, along with the use of recommended materials and armamentarium, therefore, diagnosis and treatment planning are an essential component in the management [14]. A sectional complete denture prosthesis was provided based on the patient's treatment motivation, oral hygiene, extent of tissue loss, economic status, and available treatment duration. Sectional tray primary impression was recorded using impression compound with carved indexing in the center to assemble it extraorally. It allowed for staged process to overcome minimal access and maintained accuracy of the anatomic record [15]. The impression compound used for primary impression also acts as a flexible impression tray, in case the impression requires retake and improvements. The PVS medium body final impression was made for increased accuracy, dimensional stability, and elastic recovery [16].

The presented technique involved the fabrication of a sectional maxillary denture (anterior and posterior) and a combined incorporation of CoCr hinge in the center and ball abutments at the periphery of the posterior segment. This allowed for two-part insertion and enhanced stability due to the engagement of ball abutments and central hinge [17]. It is pertinent to mention that the success of prosthodontic treatment provided is multifactorial and improvement in mouth opening, soft and hard tissue health, and discontinuation of habits, good oral hygiene, and regular maintenance of prosthesis are critical for good treatment prognosis. As the management of microstomia is multifaceted, a holistic management plan is difficult to execute in the absence of a comprehensive classification system.

The present paper also presents a diagnosis and management (DM) classification system developed by considering the index of oral access (IOA) as baseline [1], as the latter does not address vertical mouth opening, difficulty in prosthesis fabrication, manual dexterity of the patient, and treatment options. This DM classification will assist in diagnosis, monitoring disease progression, interoperator communication, and record keeping in relation to microstomia. The patients could be treated with a variety of prosthetic options from a range of fixed and removable prosthesis keeping in mind adequate patient comfort and acceptance. Additionally, patients with microstomia suffering with chronic oral manifestation could be treated reliably, if this strategy is adopted on a large scale.

In spite of all, in the current era of digital development, it is believed that microstomia management will become more convenient and efficient. Intraoral scanning, computer-aided design and manufacturing (CAD-CAM), and 3D rapid prototyping can be utilized to produce precise sectional dentures. The hassle of recording manual impression, dental cast replication, and designing can be replaced with a digital workflow. Nevertheless, the use of dental implant-supported fixed prosthesis can add up to improve oral function and patient satisfaction.

4. Conclusions

The DM classification presented will assist in diagnosis and management of microstomia patients. The use of sectional removable dentures in the rehabilitation of edentulous patients with microstomia is effective; however, treatment prognosis is dependent on patient motivation and adaptation, case complexity, prosthodontic technique, technical skill, and maintenance.

Consent

The patient signed a written ethical consent showing agreement for documentation and presentation of the completed microstomia case.

References

[1] E. King and J. Owens, "Flexible and sectional complete dentures with magnetic retention for a patient with microstomia–a case report," *Dental update.*, vol. 43, no. 3, pp. 212-213, 2016.

[2] I. Tulunoglu, M. H. Lee, M. L. Taifur, and O. Tulunoglu, "Restoring masticatory function in a patient with severe microstomia using rapid prototyped mesh and a custom-made hinge and swing-lock prosthesis," *The Journal of Prosthetic Dentistry*, vol. 119, no. 6, pp. 887–892, 2018.

[3] M. J. Garnett, F. S. Nohl, and S. C. Barclay, "Management of patients with reduced oral aperture and mandibular hypomobility (trismus) and implications for operative dentistry," *British Dental Journal*, vol. 204, no. 3, pp. 125–131, 2008.

[4] P. Sinavarat and C. Anunmana, "Sectional collapsible complete removable dental prosthesis for a patient with microstomia," *The Journal of Prosthetic Dentistry*, vol. 114, no. 5, pp. 627–632, 2015.

[5] H. Malkawi and M. Tarawneh, "The whistling face syndrome, or craniocarpotarsal dysplasia. Report of two cases in a father and son and review of the literature," *Journal of Pediatric Orthopaedics*, vol. 3, no. 3, pp. 364–369, 1983.

[6] K. N. Nguyen, I. Semenov, B. Blasiole, J. G. Robison, and D. H. Chi, "Congenital microstomia in a neonate with impending respiratory compromise," *Case reports in Anesthesiology*, vol. 2014, Article ID 739463, 3 pages, 2014.

[7] D. A. Givan, W. A. AuClair, J. C. Seidenfaden CDT, and J. Paiva, "Sectional impressions and simplified folding complete denture for severe microstomia," *Journal of Prosthodontics*, vol. 19, no. 4, pp. 299–302, 2010.

[8] A. Satpathy and A. K. Gujjari, "Complete denture in a microstomia patient," *Journal of Clinical and Diagnostic Research: JCDR*, vol. 9, no. 5, 2015.

[9] P. Malik and M. Rathee, "Restricted mouth opening- impressions making," *Scholars Journal of Dental Sciences*, vol. 2, pp. 24–29, 2015.

[10] A. S. Fernandes, K. Mascarenhas, and M. A. Aras, "Custom sectional impression trays with interlocking type handle for microstomia patients," *Indian Journal of Dental Research*, vol. 20, pp. 370–373, 2009.

[11] S. S. Colvenkar, "Sectional impression tray and sectional denture for a microstomia patient," *Journal of Prosthodontics*, vol. 19, no. 2, pp. 161–165, 2010.

[12] T. J. McGarry, A. Nimmo, J. F. Skiba, R. H. Ahlstrom, C. R. Smith, and J. H. Koumjian, "Classification system for complete edentulism," *Journal of Prosthodontics*, vol. 8, no. 1, pp. 27–39, 1999.

[13] B. Conroy and M. Reitzik, "Prosthetic restoration in microstomia," *The Journal of Prosthetic Dentistry*, vol. 26, no. 3, pp. 324-327, 1971.

[14] J. F. McCord, G. H. Moody, and A. S. Blinkhorn, "An overview of dental treatment of patients with microstomia," *Quintessence International*, vol. 21, no. 11, 1990.

[15] J. G. Egan and S. A. Swindells, "A novel prosthodontic alternative for patients who are edentulous and have microstomia: a case report," *Special Care in Dentistry*, vol. 32, no. 4, pp. 160–164, 2012.

[16] F. Vohra, F. Altokhais, A. B. Thafrah et al., "Effect of contemporary retraction agents and cleaning with hydrogen peroxide on the polymerization of elastomeric impression materials," *Journal of Applied Biomaterials & Functional Materials*, vol. 18, 2020.

[17] B. Öwall, "Precision attachment-retained removable partial dentures: part 2. Long-term study of ball attachments," *International Journal of Prosthodontics*, vol. 8, no. 1, 1995.

18

Piezosurgery-Assisted Surgical Treatment in Impacted Canine Transmigration

Matheus Francisco Barros Rodrigues,[1] **Layla Louise de Amorim Rocha,**[1] **Rodrigo da Franca Acioly,**[2] **Cristofe Coelho Lopes da Rocha,**[3] **and Daniel do Carmo Carvalho**[2]

[1]*Dentistry Course, Faculdade Cathedral, Boa Vista 69307-053, Brazil*
[2]*Department of Oral and Maxillofacial Surgery and Traumatology, Hospital Geral de Roraima, Boa Vista 69305-455, Brazil*
[3]*Infrastructure Department, Instituto Federal, Boa Vista 69303-340, Brazil*

Correspondence should be addressed to Matheus Francisco Barros Rodrigues; matheusfbr18@gmail.com

Academic Editor: Kevin Seymour

Delayed eruption of a canine tooth may represent a possible impaction. If this is the case, a slight elevation in the palatal or vestibular mucosa is often observed. Cases of transmigration, where the unerupted tooth crosses the midline, are less frequent. This article reports on the piezosurgery-assisted surgical treatment of a transmigrated canine in the mentonian region. Treatment for this condition varies depending on the clinical characteristics, symptoms, and location of the dental element. The surgical treatment established for this case was satisfactory, and full recovery of the patient was achieved without complications such as an intense postoperative inflammatory response.

1. Introduction

In human dentition, mandibular and maxillary canines are teeth that have relevance both in aesthetics and occlusion [1–5]. A small manifestation such as a cyst or root fragment or mandibular trauma at an early age can cause dental deviation that may lead to impaction [3, 6]. Common precipitating factors are neighboring tooth lesions, infection, ectopic eruption, and interference with prosthesis [2].

Most impacted canines are clinically asymptomatic and do not cause pain or discomfort [3, 6, 7]. A high index of suspicion should exist for canine impaction in the case of delayed eruption and a slight elevation in the palatal or vestibular mucosa [7]. Vestibular positioning of impacted canines is usually associated with spatial problems, while palatal positioning of impacted canines is associated with path abnormalities [8].

Transmigration cases, where the unerupted tooth migrates and crosses the midline, are less frequent [5, 6, 9]. Studies show that the canines are the only teeth in the dental arch able to cross the midline [3]. This form of impaction occasionally occurs in the maxillary region; however, canine transmigration is more common in the mandible [10, 11]. In most cases, periapical radiographs are not sufficient to detect transmigrated canines, making a panoramic radiograph essential [6].

This article is aimed at reporting on the piezosurgery-assisted surgical treatment of a transmigrated canine in the mentonian region, showing the clinical and radiographic aspects as well as the established treatment. In addition, it reviews the main concepts of management and demonstrates a comparative and indicative analysis of the proposed treatments.

2. Case Report

A 33-year-old man presented to the dental office with the complaint of an absent lower canine on the left side. The patient had no other symptoms and was classified as ASA I. The clinical examination revealed the absence of dental

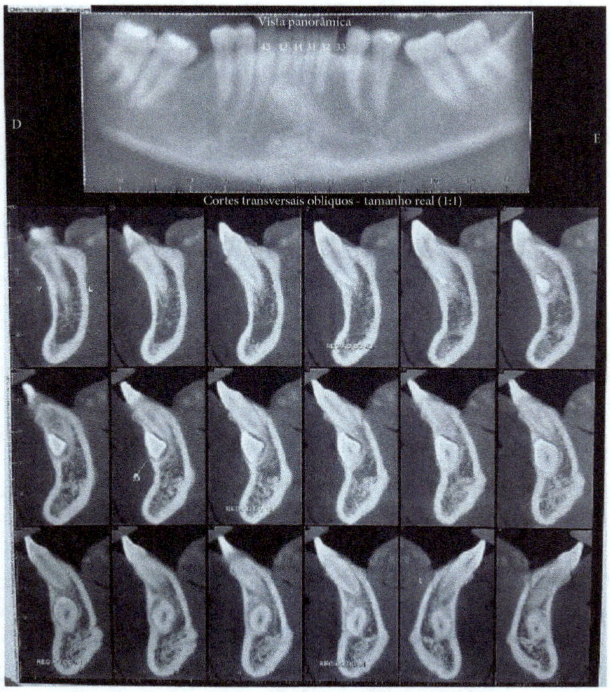

Figure 1: Computed tomography (CT) scan (panoramic view and oblique cross-sections).

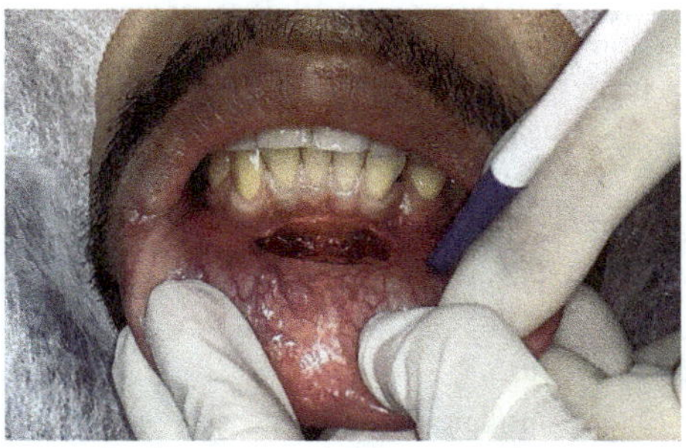

Figure 2: Horizontal incision 5 mm below the mucogingival line from canine to canine.

element 33. In light of the above, a computed tomography (CT) scan was requested, and transmigration of the left lower canine in the midline in the mentonian region, in the horizontal and vestibular position, was diagnosed, as shown in Figure 1.

Due to the unfavorable position of the dental element, orthodontic treatment was contraindicated, establishing surgical extraction as the preferred mode of treatment [1, 7]. The patient underwent surgery under local anesthesia (articaine 4% 1 : 100,000) with bilateral blocks of the lower alveolar nerve, complemented by a vestibular canine-to-canine infiltration terminal. During surgery, a horizontal incision was made 5 mm below the mucogingival line extending from canine to canine, as shown in Figure 2. The tissue was then detached, allowing partial visualization of the impacted tooth.

The surrounding tissue was then separated from the tooth and odontosection was carried out using a piezoelectric apparatus in order to minimize the trauma, as can be seen in Figure 3.

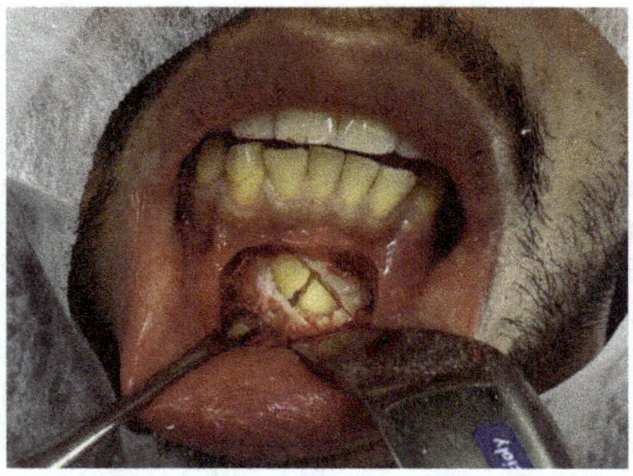

Figure 3: Osteotomy followed by piezosurgery-assisted odontosection.

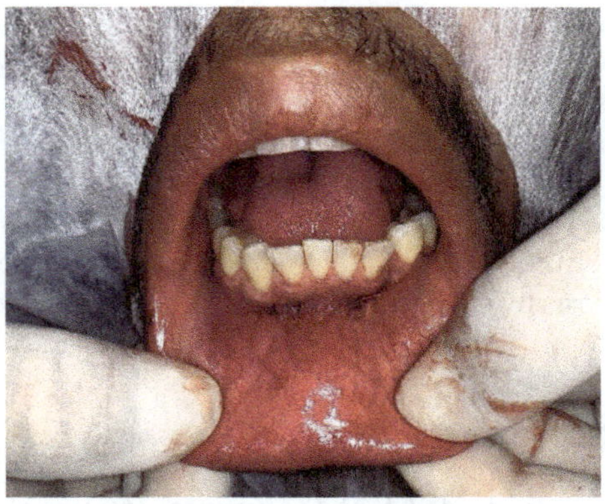

Figure 4: Suture in the deep and superficial plane.

After extracting the tooth, curettage and synthesis maneuver were performed in the internal musculature and in the superficial plane, both using an absorbable suture thread (Monocryl 5.0) as shown in Figure 4.

At the end of the surgical procedure, the patient received counselling regarding postoperative care. Antibiotic was prescribed (Amoxicillin 500 mg every 8 hours for 7 days) with an anti-inflammatory (Meloxicam 7.5 mg every 12 hours) and analgesic (Dipyrone Sodium 500 mg every 6 hours for three days). The patient underwent 5 laser therapy sessions during the recovery period and returned after 7 days to remove the sutures. At this presentation, there was no complaint of pain or paresthesia and no evidence of infectious symptoms.

3. Discussion

The teeth most affected by impaction are the third molars and permanent canines [12]. Surgeons should pay attention to the characteristics of impaction and select the appropriate treatment technique to appropriately manage each case on an individual basis [2].

Orthodontic traction and self-transplants were found in the literature as treatment options for impacted canines [6]. However, these are time-consuming and expensive treatments [2]. Important factors to consider when planning traction are patient age, root formation stage, tooth proximity to the site, tooth angulation between 0 and 15°, and the absence of root dilaceration [7].

Orthodontic traction of transmigrated teeth can be mechanically complex and may be contraindicated, depending on the angulation of these teeth [1, 7]. Following unsuccessful orthodontic treatment, surgical extraction is performed as a prophylactic measure against the formation of pathological lesions [1, 2].

Treatment success through the use of transplants depends on the degree of tooth development, as this procedure is more effective in cases where the impacted tooth has incomplete rhizogenesis. In addition, for the transplant to be viable, extensive ostectomy is necessary for full extraction of the impacted tooth and subsequent transplant placement in the dental arch [2].

Surgical treatment of an impacted element requires osteotomy and odontosection techniques that may damage the surrounding tissue [13]. However, piezosurgery-assisted surgery is useful in minimizing trauma [14], because the use of ordinary saws or high-speed drills applies pressure and a certain degree of heating to both the bone and the adjacent soft tissue. Use of the piezoelectric equipment results in comparatively minimum heating, therefore decreasing the risk of osteonecrosis by ensuring the vitality of the osteocytes [15].

4. Conclusions

It can been concluded that the surgical treatment strategy established for this case of transmigration and canine impaction was satisfactory and resulted in resolution of symptoms and a good clinical outcome. There was no intense inflammatory response or infectious condition in the postoperative period. The aid of piezosurgery assisted in minimizing trauma to soft and hard tissues and, therefore, reduced the risk of osteonecrosis in this case. Extraction of the dental element resulted in the prevention of future pathologies such as root resorptions and infections.

References

[1] N. M. S. P. Assis, F. W. Alves, and F. N. Carvalho, "Transmigracao de caninos mandibulares: relato de dois casos clínicos," *Revista Brasileira de Odontologia*, vol. 66, no. 1, 2009.

[2] J. O. P. Hyppolito, M. B. Paies, R. D. O. Veras Filho, F. Florian, and E. H. Vieira, "Tratamento cirúrgico de canino incluso em mento: relato de caso," *Revista de Odontologia da UNESP*, pp. 42–46, 2011, https://repositorio.unesp.br/handle/11449/125602.

[3] J. D. S. F. Filho, S. R. França, L. K. Araújo, J. J. de Negreiros Pereira, I. F. C. Belchior, and M. B. da Silva Sampieri, "Intervenção cirúrgica de um canino incluso em sínfise mandibular: relato de caso," *Revista da Faculdade de Odontologia - UPF*, vol. 23, no. 3, pp. 329–332, 2018.

[4] R. Pérez, L. Angélica, and M. JGE, "Transmigración del canino mandibular. Reporte de un caso clínico y revisión de la literatura," *Revista ADM*, vol. 70, no. 4, pp. 202–208, 2013.

[5] A. Auluck, A. Nagpal, S. Setty, K. M. Pai, and J. Sunny, "Transmigration of impacted mandibular canines—report of 4 cases," *Journal of the Canadian Dental Association*, vol. 72, no. 3, pp. 249–252, 2006.

[6] P. Mesquita and H. Salgado, "Transmigrant mandibular canine - Case report," *Revista Portuguesa de Estomatologia, Medicina Dentária e Cirurgia Maxilofacial*, vol. 56, no. 1, pp. 63–67, 2015.

[7] G. T. M. Candeiro and R. N. Tavares, "Tratamento cirúrgico em transmigração de canino inferior impactado-relato de caso," *Revista da Faculdade de Odontologia de Porto Alegre*, vol. 50, no. 3, pp. 39–41, 2011.

[8] M. A. Pérez Flores, P. Pérez Flores, and C. Fierro Monti, "Alteraciones en la erupción de caninos permanentes," *International Journal of Morphology*, vol. 27, no. 1, pp. 139–143, 2009.

[9] N. Umashree, A. Kumar, and T. Nagaraj, "Transmigration of mandibular canines," *Case Reports in Dentistry*, vol. 2013, 7 pages, 2013.

[10] I. F. Qaradaghi, "Bilateral transmigration of impacted mandibular canines: report of two cases and review," *Archives of Oral Research*, vol. 6, no. 3, 2010.

[11] S. Olate, J. P. Alister Herdener, J. L. Muñante-Cárdenas, L. Pozzer, and J. R. Albergaria-Barbosa, "Tratamiento quirúrgico de caninos mandibulares bilaterales transmigrados," *International journal of odontostomatology*, vol. 4, no. 3, pp. 285–290, 2010.

[12] E. P. Alves, A. F. Montagner, S. P. Antonizazzi, and L. F. D. Oliveira, "Prevalência e posição de caninos superiores impactados e sua relação com reabsorção radicular," *Revista da Faculdade de Odontologia-UPF*, vol. 19, no. 2, 2014.

[13] A. L. M. Miranda, *Piezocirurgia no consultório de Medicina Dentária*, Tese de Doutorado, 2016.

[14] M. P. S. Kumar, "Newer methods of extraction of teeth," *International Journal of Pharma and Bio Sciences*, vol. 6, no. 3, pp. 679–685, 2015.

[15] M. F. M. O. Consolaro, E. Sant' Ana, and G. Moura Neto, "Cirurgia piezelétrica ou piezocirurgia em odontologia: o sonho de todo cirurgião," *Revista Dental Press de Ortodontia e Ortopedia Facial*, vol. 12, no. 6, pp. 17–20, 2007.

19

Esthetic Rehabilitation using Magnet-Retained Cheek Plumper Prosthesis

Alisha Rewari,[1] Nupur Dabas,[2] Reshu Sanan,[2] Shefali Phogat,[2] Sumit Singh Phukela,[2] and Monika Vigarniya[3]

[1]*Department of Prosthodontics, SGT University, India*
[2]*Department of Prosthodontics, Faculty of Dental Sciences, SGT University, India*
[3]*Shaheed Hasan Khan Mewati Government Medical College, India*

Correspondence should be addressed to Alisha Rewari; alisha.rewari@gmail.com

Academic Editor: Mine Dündar

Summary. Prosthetic rehabilitation of a completely edentulous patient is no more confined to replacement of missing teeth. Long span of edentulism and ageing leads to loss of support of the facial musculature, which is of great concern in treating completely edentulous patients. Flaccid facial musculature eventually leads to sunken cheeks and unesthetic appearance, causing a negative impact on psychological well-being of the patient. The use of conventional complete dentures can restore the loss to some extent, but in some cases, additional support is required. The present clinical report exemplifies the use of magnet-retained detachable maxillary cheek plumper prosthesis in a completely edentulous patient with sunken cheeks.

1. Introduction

Ageing has an impact on facial esthetics due to loss of alveolar process and teeth, loss of muscle tonicity, loss of elasticity of the skin, and impairment of function [1]. Prosthetic rehabilitation of a completely edentulous patient is no more confined to replacement of missing teeth. Any and every prosthesis should replace both function and esthetics. Conventional complete dentures with appropriate flange extensions customarily support the overlying lips and cheeks.

But, certain factors like early loss of posterior teeth, thinning of the tissues, and weight loss may cause concavities below the malar bone or slumped cheeks, which affects esthetics making the patient look much older than their age [2]. This also has a negative impact on their social and professional lives leading to a detrimental psychological effect on the patient. Thus, to support the sunken cheeks, a prosthesis known as cheek plumper can be used. A conventional cheek plumper, which is a single unit prosthesis that adds on to the weight of the denture, increases the mesiodistal width of the prosthesis, thereby making its insertion difficult in patients with limited mouth opening [3]. Moreover, its long-term use can cause muscle fatigue. Thus, to combat this situation, a detachable cheek plumper can be fabricated.

The present clinical report exemplifies the use of magnets to support a detachable cheek plumper prosthesis in a completely edentulous patient with sunken cheeks.

2. Case Report

A 42-year-old male patient reported to the Department of Prosthodontics, Faculty of Dental Sciences, SGT University, with the chief complaint of missing teeth and poor esthetics since 3 years. He lost some of his teeth due to a road accident while some due to poor periodontal health. On intraoral examination, the patient had completely edentulous, low, well-rounded maxillary and mandibular arch. Extraoral examination revealed wrinkling of the skin and unsupported musculature leading to sunken cheeks. The patient was very conscious of his appearance and desired a prosthesis which would make his face look fuller and healthier. Keeping the patient's demand in mind, fabrication of maxillary and mandibular complete dentures with intraoral magnet-retained, detachable cheek plumpers attached to the maxillary denture was planned (Figure 1). The steps of fabrication were as follows.

(1) Primary impressions of maxillary and mandibular arches were made using modelling plastic impression compound (DPI pinnacle®), and custom trays were fabricated using autopolymerizing acrylic resin

(2) Border moulding was done using green stick modelling plastic impression compound, and definitive impressions were made using zinc oxide eugenol impression paste

(3) Jaw relations were recorded; teeth setting followed by try-in was done to check for occlusion, esthetics, and phonetics

(4) Following try-in, cheek plumpers were made using green stick and impression compound in the ratio of 7 : 3 and were attached over the buccal flange of the waxed up maxillary denture in the premolar-molar region using magnetic attachments on either side for trial in the same appointment. The adapted plumpers were inspected extraorally for adequacy of cheek support and contour and interference with functional movements

(5) Significant change in facial esthetics was seen after attaching cheek plumpers and was readily accepted by the patient

(6) Magnets were removed from the cheek plumpers, and both the plumpers were processed using heat cure acrylic resin by reverse flasking (Figure 2)

(7) After deflasking, cured denture and cheek plumpers were retrieved, trimmed, finished, and polished

(8) Two 2 mm deep and 5 mm diameter holes on either side were made on the buccal flanges of the maxillary denture and corresponding area of cheek plumpers (Figures 3 and 4)

(9) Magnets (Magfit™ DX600) (Table 1) were incorporated in the denture as well as cheek plumpers with autopolymerizing acrylic resin, and complete polymerization was ensured by placing it in a pressure pot. Magnet specifications are shown in Figure 5

(10) After inserting the complete denture, plumpers were attached to the maxillary denture (Figure 6) and adequate clearance from the occlusal table was verified (Figure 6)

(11) Attachment and removal of cheek plumper were demonstrated, and necessary instructions were given to the patient. He was asked to visit for regular follow-ups (Figure 7)

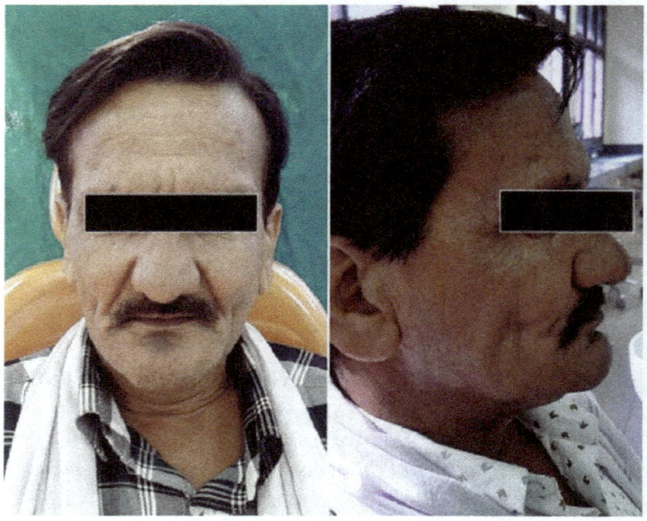

Figure 1: Straight profile and side profile of the edentulous patient showing sunken cheeks.

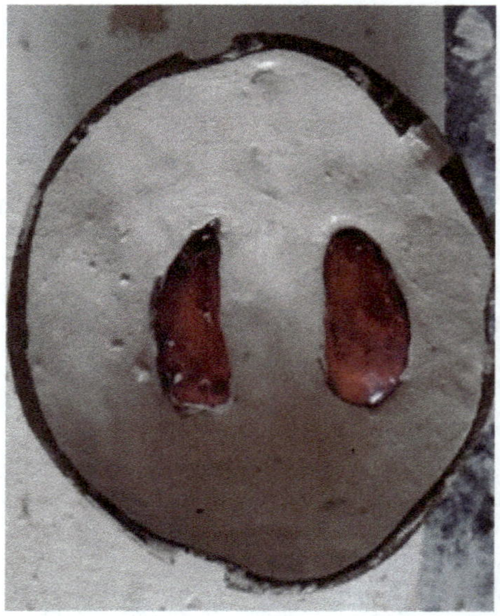

Figure 2: Investment of cheek plumper (wax pattern).

3. Discussion

The contour of the jaw bones, underlying teeth, and the soft tissues along with muscles around the teeth strongly influence the appearance of the lower half of the face [4]. Loss of teeth causes resorption of the alveolar ridge and loss of muscle tonicity. The apparent loss of subcutaneous fat, buccal pad of fat, and elasticity of connective tissue produces sunken cheeks. Rectification of drooping of cheeks can be done by different methods like reconstructive plastic surgery, injecting botulinum toxin (BOTOX) in the facial muscles, and various types of prosthesis [5]. Plastic surgery may be contraindicated in patients with a systemic disease. Moreover, it is a traumatic procedure and leaves behind a postsurgical scar.

Conventional cheek plumpers are single-unit prosthesis with extensions on either side of the posterior flange of denture base. Its continuous use leads to muscle fatigue and decreased retention of the prosthesis [6]. Muscle fatigue can be prevented if the patient has the option of removing cheek plumpers when experiencing discomfort. Therefore, in the present case, a detachable plumper prosthesis was planned

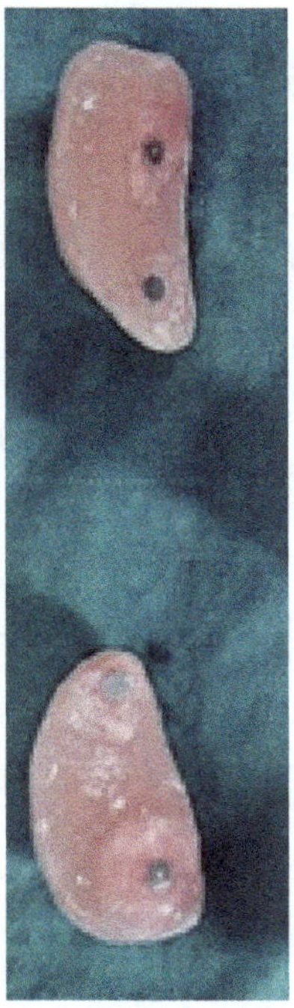

FIGURE 3: Cheek plumpers showing magnetic attachments.

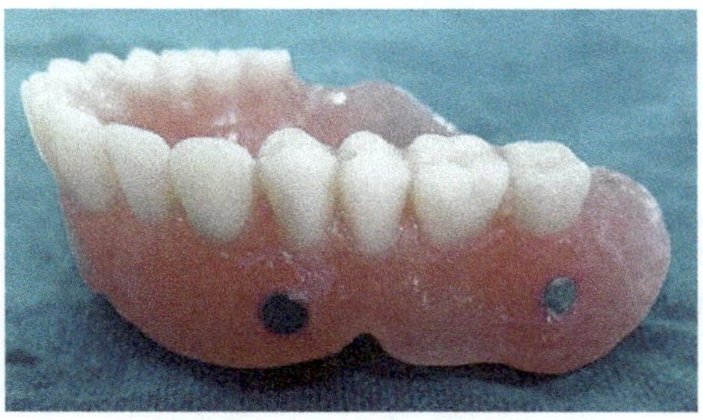

FIGURE 4: Buccal flange of maxillary denture showing magnetic attachments.

TABLE 1: Magfit DX is a new thin-type, uncoated magnetic attachment with improved wear resistance. The ellipsoidal outer lip of the magnetic assembly assures firm fixation to the denture base.

		Fe	Nd	Cr	Ni	Others
Magnetic assembly	Magnet	65%	29%	—	—	6%
	Yoke/disc	79%	—	19%	—	2%
	Nonmagnetic part	68%	—	16%	12%	4%
Keeper unit	Keeper	79%	—	19%	—	2%
	Surface	68%	—	30%	—	2%
	Holder	68%	—	16%	12%	4%

to reduce weight of the prosthesis and facilitate easy placement and removal. Various attachments like magnets, press stud fasteners, orthodontic elastic modules, stud attachments, and wires can be used to attach cheek plumpers with the denture [7, 8]. Magnets facilitate automatic reseating because of the magnetic force and easy detachment of plumper prosthesis making it easy to clean. It can provide a constant amount of retentive force even after a number of

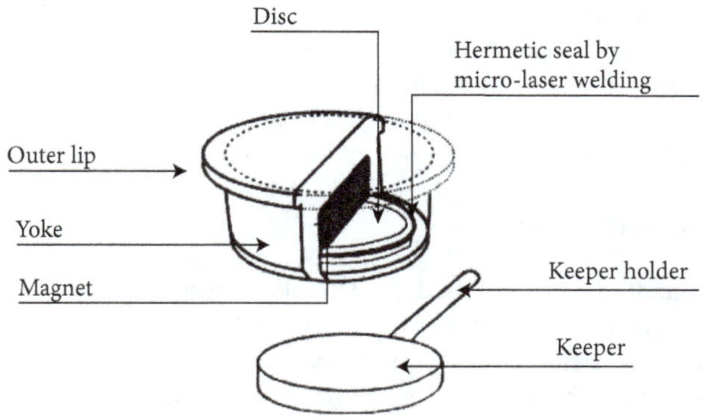

FIGURE 5: Magfit™ DX600.

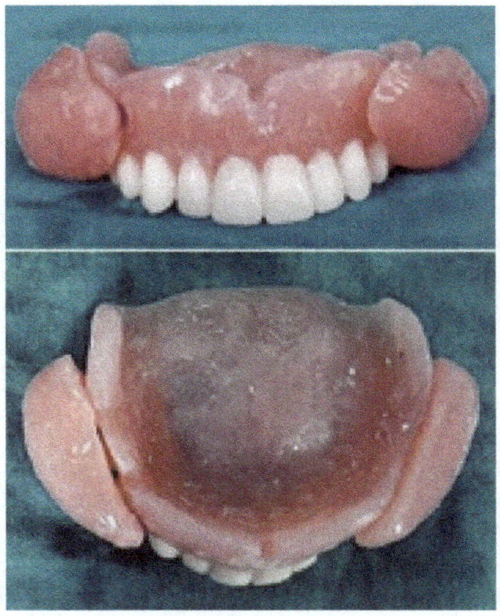

FIGURE 6: Maxillary denture with cheek plumper prosthesis (frontal view and intaglio surface).

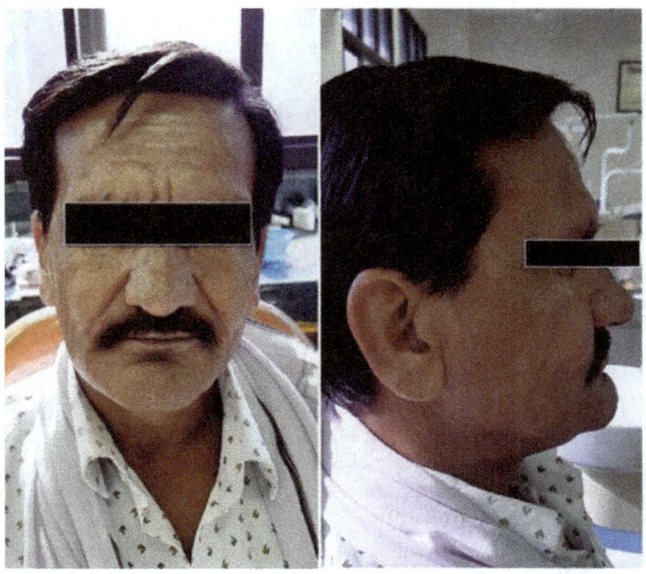

FIGURE 7: Straight profile and side profile of the patient with maxillary denture and cheek plumper prosthesis.

insertion and removal cycles of the prosthesis. Its disadvantage is having poor corrosion resistance with oral fluids and so may require encapsulation with relatively inert alloy. Periodic patient recall is essential to evaluate the attachments and their replacement, when required.

4. Limitations

Magnets cannot be used in patients allergic to metal. The patients need to be apprised regarding the fact that the magnetic field used in MRI tests damages the magnetic assembly. The patients need to remove dentures for MRI tests. The magnetic assembly should be kept away from high temperatures of more than 150°C.

5. Conclusion

Cheek plumpers are simple to fabricate and provide a noninvasive and cost-effective treatment option to enhance facial esthetics in patients with sunken cheeks, thereby improving the patient's psychological well-being. Magnet-retained detachable cheek plumper is a modification of the conventional technique of supporting the slumped tissues due to ageing.

References

[1] J. W. Bains and J. P. Elia, "The role of facial skeletal augmentation and dental restoration in facial rejuvenation," *Aesthetic Plastic Surgery*, vol. 18, no. 3, pp. 243–246, 1994.

[2] N. Verma, V. Chitre, and M. Aras, "Enhancing appearance incomplete dentures using magnetic retained cheek plumpers," *Journal Of Indian Prosthodontic Society*, vol. 4, no. 2, pp. 35–38, 2004.

[3] M. K. Marwah, K. Harshakumar, R. Ravichandran, and S. Lylajam, "Detachable magnet retained cheek plumpers to enhance complete denture esthetics - a case report," *International Journal of Health Sciences and Research*, vol. 6, no. 7, pp. 389–393, 2016.

[4] N. Javid, "The use of magnets in a maxillofacial prosthesis," *The Journal of Prosthetic Dentistry*, vol. 25, no. 3, pp. 334–341, 1971.

[5] S. R. Venkatachalapathy, G. N. Chander, and P. Gnanam, "A magnetically retained cheek plumper in a maxillary single complete denture: a clinical report," *Journal of Interdisciplinary Dentistry*, vol. 9, no. 1, pp. 25–30, 2019.

[6] V. Punia, R. Mishra, M. Khandelwal, N. Verma, and M. Handa, "Magnet retained detachable cheek plumper: innovation personified-a case report," *The Journal of Indian Prosthodontic Society*, vol. 4, pp. 16–20, 2013.

[7] J. S. Rupal, T. C. Anandmayee, G. P. Hardik, G. M. Farheen, J. D. Bhavyata, and A. K. Preeti, "Enhancement of patient aesthetics using detachable cheek plumpers incomplete dentures: case series," *Scholars Journal of Medical Case Reports*, vol. 2, no. 9, pp. 615–617, 2014.

[8] M. A. Riley, A. D. Walmsley, and I. R. Harris, "Magnets in prosthetic dentistry," *The Journal of Prosthetic Dentistry*, vol. 86, no. 2, pp. 137–142, 2001.

20

New Approach in the Management of Vertical Root Fracture with the Help of Biodentine and CBCT

H. C. Baranwal, Nidhi Singh, Neeraj Kumar, Riya Garg, Jyoti Yadav, and Richik Tripathi

Faculty of Dental Sciences, IMS, BHU, Varanasi, India

Correspondence should be addressed to Nidhi Singh; drnidhiconsendo@gmail.com

Academic Editor: Anut Itthagarun

Introduction. Vertical root fracture is a big challenge to dentists for its diagnosis and treatment. As the tooth presents poor prognosis, the most common treatment modality is extraction. One can save the tooth from extraction by the reconstruction of fracture fragments followed by intentional reimplantation. New treatment options have arrived for healing of the fracture site by hard tissue barrier formation with the help of bioceramic materials. *Case Report.* The present case report describes successful management of complete vertical root fracture of a maxillary left central incisor by trauma in a 35-year-old male with the help of Biodentine, a bonding agent, a fiber post, and dual-cure resin cement without tooth extraction, followed by all ceramic crowns. Up to two years of follow-up, there is no problem in the tooth, and radiographically, there is no radiolucency along the fracture line. Periodontal status and probing depth were within a normal physiological limit. *Conclusion.* Functional and aesthetic outcomes are achieved by combined therapy in the present case report.

1. Introduction

Vertical root fracture is defined as a longitudinally oriented fracture of the root, extending from the root canal to the periodontium [1]. Vertical root fracture is one of the most common causes of extraction [2]. Prevalence of vertical root fracture in permanent teeth was 3 to 5% in retrospective studies with etiology being multifactorial [3, 4]. The incidence of VRF is more commonly associated with endodontically than nonendodontically treated teeth [5]. In the vital tooth, physical trauma is the most common reason for tooth/root fracture. In anterior teeth, the line of spread of fracture is in the buccolingual direction [6]. VRF presents male predilection due to their stronger masticatory forces, high attrition, habitual hard food chewing, and less pliable supporting bone [7]. VRF repair using MTA has been already approved [8–11]. But it is difficult to handle; has long setting time, discoloration, and lower compressive and flexural strength than a dentine; and is high-cost [12–15]. Due to this, over the last years, several calcium silicate cements comparable to MTA have been presented, in which Biodentine (Septodont) is one of them. It is a calcium silicate-based cement which was used primarily as a substitute of dentine below resin composite filling material [16]. In contrast to MTA, Biodentine exhibits short setting time of about 15 min [15, 17] and appreciable mechanical features. It is a material which can set off periodontal regeneration and/or restoration. It has beneficial properties in the periodontium regarding biologic reaction of the cells. It is also called “bioactive cement” [18] because of the upregulating action on the activity of osteoblasts and periodontal cells.

Unfortunately, until today, no valid treatment option can be recommended to preserve teeth with VRF. In spite of that, the present case report used Biodentine as a new treatment option for a maxillary incisor with VRF. Using this material in the fractured tooth could be kept in situ for an observation period of two years, and the subject is free of any complaints until now.

2. Case Presentation

A 35-year-old male patient came to the Department of Conservative Dentistry and Endodontics, IMS, BHU, complaining of a fracture and pain along with cold and heat sensation in the upper left front tooth 8 days back. The patient had a history of trauma due to falling down at home 8 days back. On clinical intraoral examination, a horizontal fracture line was seen in

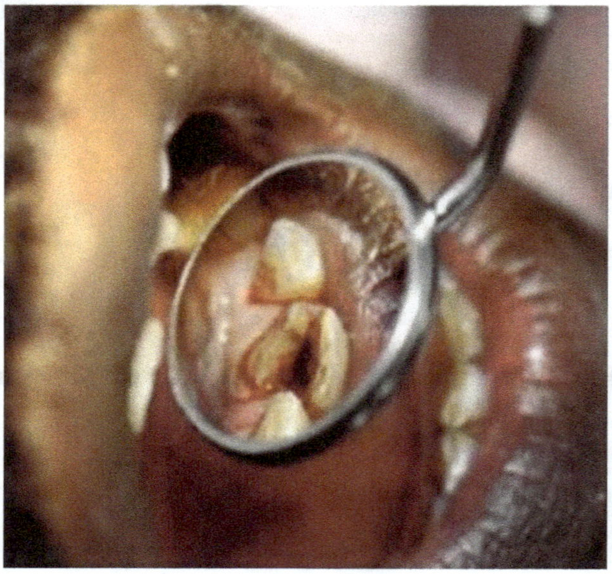

Figure 1: Preop photograph.

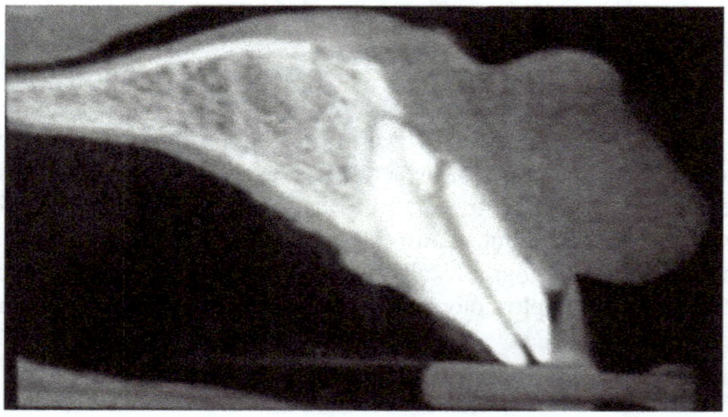

Figure 2: Preop CBCT.

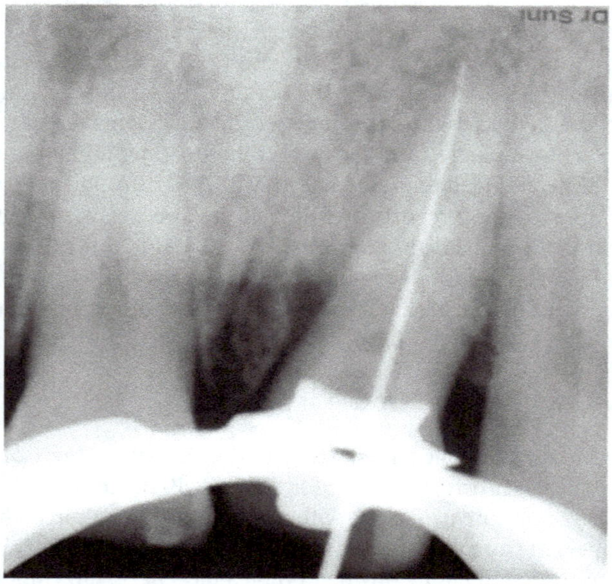

Figure 3: Working length determined.

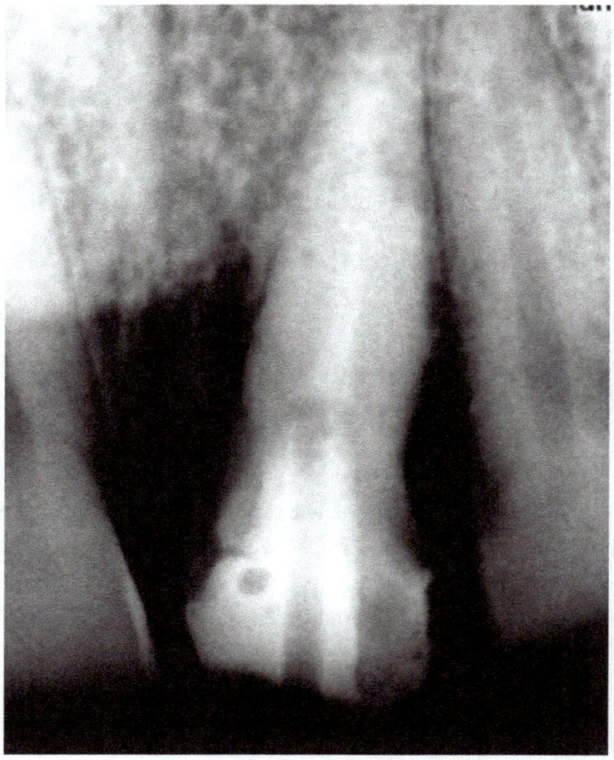

Figure 4: After postcementation.

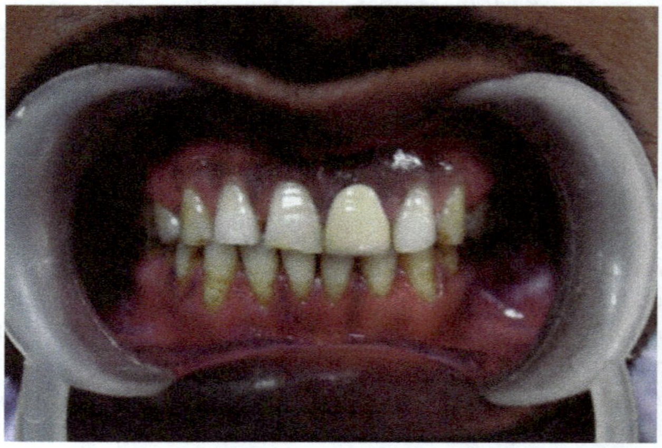

Figure 5: Postop photograph.

tooth no. 21 (Figure 1). Fractured tooth no. 21 was tender on percussion with a normal pocket depth. A pulp sensitivity test showed exaggerated response to a cold and heat test. On examination by CBCT, a vertical fracture line was shown mesiodistally along the root canal space to the apical third of the root directed labially (Figure 2). In a literature review, the treatment of complete vertical root fracture is the extraction of the tooth followed by dental prosthesis or implant or joining the separated fragments by different types of bonding system, laser or bioceramic cements, and reimplantation with a good success rate. None of these treatment options was accepted by the patient (because of fear of tooth extraction). To save the tooth, a new approach was planned to join the fragments without extraction of the tooth. Written informed

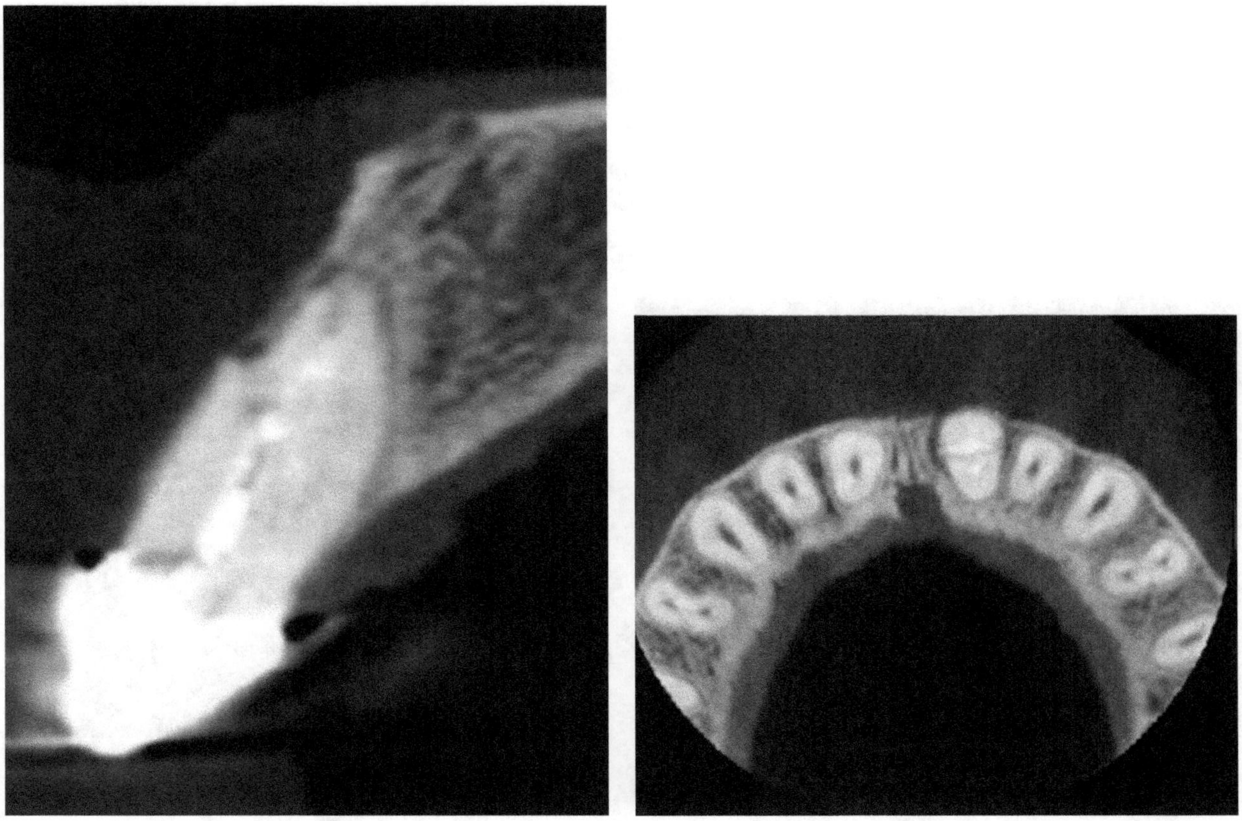

(a) (b)

Figure 6: (a) After 6 months of follow-up on CBCT (axial view). (b) After 6 months on CBCT (sagittal view).

consent was obtained, and the patient was scheduled for treatment on the next day after explaining all treatment plans. Before starting the root canal treatment, both separated fragments in the clinical crown region was bonded with a universal dentin bonding (Scotchbond Universal Adhesive 3M ESPE) agent and cured for 20 seconds, and then, flowable composite resin was used (Filtek Z 350xt 3M ESPE) and lightly cured. Firstly, isolation was done with a rubber dam (Hygenic dental dam) with local anesthesia administration (lignocaine, 1 : 150000) before starting the procedure. A proper access opening was done with endoaccess bur. Working length was established with a no. 15 k-file and confirmed by IOPA X-ray (Figure 3). Chemomechanical preparation was done using an up to no. 40 k-file as a master apical file. Irrigation was done by using normal saline and 0.5% NaOCl (Septodont Parcan) during CMP, and the final irrigation was done by using 5 ml 3% NaOCl and 5 ml 17% EDTA (Maarc Endo-L) followed by normal saline. After drying the root canal with a paper point, Biodentine (Septodont) was placed with the help of a Lentulo spiral in the apical part of the root canal, all fracture parts of the line and root canal space up to the intraosseous region. After 24 hours, postpreparation was done by using corresponding drill no. 2 (Tenax fiber post drill) and applying a bonding agent, and dual-cure resin cement (Kerr Maxcem Elite self-adhesive resin cement) was filled in the prepared post space; a no. 2 glass fiber post (Tenax fiber post, Coltene) was inserted and lightly cured for 40 seconds (Figure 4). After core buildup and reduction, impression was taken and the model was prepared. The cast was sent to the dental lab for all ceramic crowns on the same appointment. The crown was luted with the help of resin cement on the next visit (Figure 5). The patient was fully satisfied and happy with treatments even though slight pain and tenderness persist up to 30 days. After 30 days, all clinical signs and symptoms disappeared. The patient was recalled for a follow-up after 6 months (Figures 6(a) and 6(b)), 12 months (Figures 7(a)–7(c)), and 2 years (Figure 8) to check the progress of hard tissue formation on the fracture line by CBCT and X-ray. All periodontal conditions were within a normal limit after 24 months (Figure 9).

3. Discussion

Most of the vertical root fractures occur in the root canal-treated tooth and due to traumatic injury. There are very few choices of treatment for complete VRF in the anterior teeth due to traumatic injuries, due to the fact that complication naturally leads to extraction in most of cases. In the past, various successful treatment modalities in the anterior teeth have been suggested by uniting the fracture line by different adhesive techniques like dual-cure resin cement [19], 4 META/MMA/TBB [20], CO_2 laser, Nd:YAG laser [21], MTA [22], and Biodentine [23] followed by reimplantation of the tooth.

The main factors which lead to extraction are bacterial infection in the fracture line and the resorption of a nearby

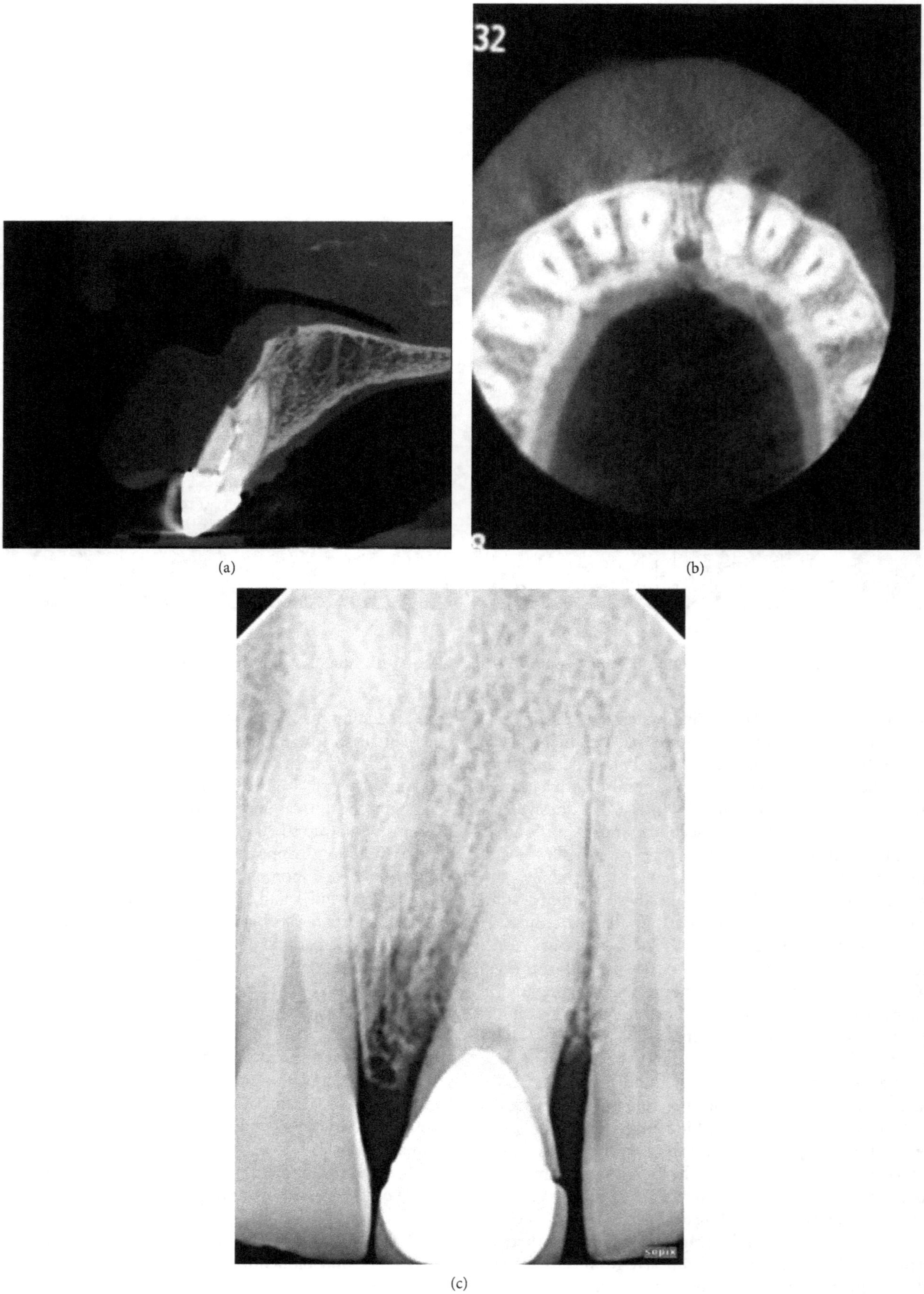

FIGURE 7: (a) After 1 year of follow-up (axial view). (b) One year of follow-up (sagittal view). (c) One year of follow-up on IOPAR.

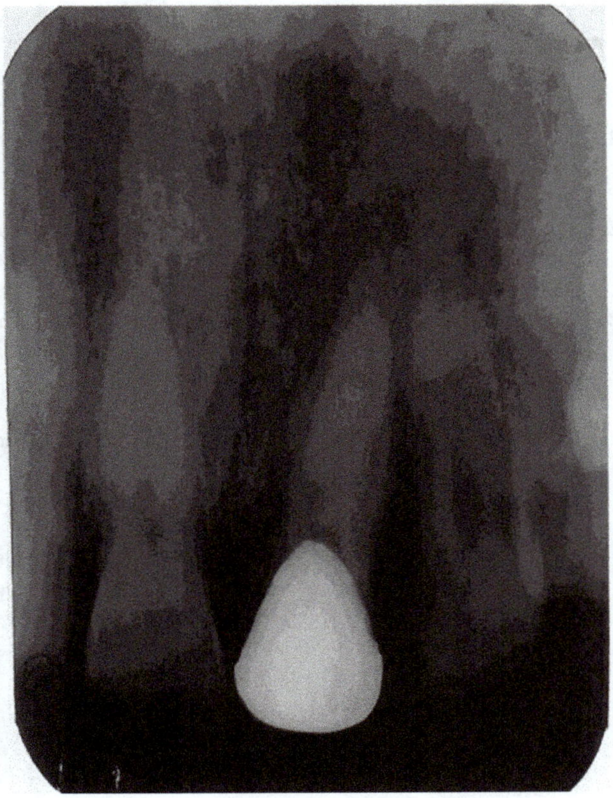

FIGURE 8: Two years of follow-up.

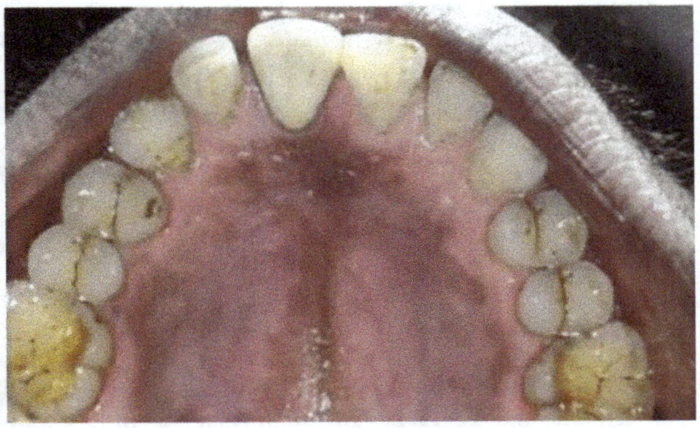

FIGURE 9: Palatal view photograph after 2 years.

alveolar bone [24]. So, especially in a vital tooth where there is no alveolar resorption and bacterial infection, a bioceramic material acts as an antibacterial and prevents the alveolar resorption and induces hard tissue deposition. The distance between separated fragments and the position and the extent of the fracture are also important features to determine the treatment modality. Erdem et al. [25] and Kusgoz et al. [26] in 2009 reported that MTA has the ability to seal the repair of horizontal root fracture.

Like MTA, Biodentine is also established for the management of horizontal root fracture, perforation repair, and external root resorption cases. Biodentine is biocompatible and has lesser setting time (15 minutes), and its Vickers hardness is 60 HV which was similar to that of dentin while the microhardness for ProRoot MTA was 40 HV [27]. Biodentine is available in the form of powder and liquid. In the powder form, it contains tricalcium silicate, dicalcium silicate, calcium carbonate, and zirconium dioxide. In the liquid form, it contains calcium chloride in aqueous solution with an admixture of polycarboxylate. Biodentine has greater resistance to hydrolysis during setting and does not dissolve in saliva [15, 17, 28]. Biodentine releases a higher amount of silicon and calcium in comparison to MTA. Silicon helps in bone calcification and stimulates bone growth and mineralization of the dentin [29]. Biodentine develops a calcium- or phosphate-rich hydroxyl apatite-like surface in the presence of body fluid. This surface helps in cell attachment and proliferation of the periodontal ligament [30, 31]. Biodentine might have great advantages when used as a canal obturation material because of its bioactive and physiochemical properties. Biodentine like MTA also provides an effective seal against dentin and cementum and promotes biological repair and regeneration of the periodontal ligament [32, 33]. So Biodentine may be a good choice for VRF without extraoral attachment of fragments and reimplantation. Biodentine was first used to fill the fracture line in prepared incomplete VRF in a maxillary central incisor extending through the buccal surface from the top of the coronal portion to the apex after careful removal and reimplantation, and after 24 months of follow-up, no pathosis was observed [23]. So, Biodentine was used in this case to fill in the prepared root canal for joining and healing the fracture fragments with good success up to two years of follow-up. A post and core may help in the prevention of coronal fracture, when the remaining coronal tooth structure is very thin after tooth preparation [5]. Root strength can also be improved by removing a smear layer. Chelating agents also induced an osteoinductive effect on hard tissue formation by releasing TGF beta1. CBCT can be valuable for the early detection of vertical root fracture in both endodontically and nonendodontically teeth.

4. Conclusion

Functional and aesthetic outcomes following treatment are achieved by a combined therapy in the present case report. A long regular follow-up is required to evaluate the success and to do the necessary alternation in the suggested treatment protocol if needed.

References

[1] D. L. Pitts and E. Natkin, "Diagnosis and treatment of vertical root fractures," *Journal of Endodontia*, vol. 9, no. 8, pp. 338–346, 1983.

[2] E. J. Nogueira Leal da Silva, G. Romão Dos Santos, R. Liess Krebs, and S. Coutinho-Filho Tde, "Surgical alternative for treatment of vertical root fracture: a case report," *Iranian Endodontic Journal*, vol. 7, no. 1, pp. 40–44, 2012.

[3] B. Bergman, P. Lundquist, U. Sjo¨gren, and G. Sundquist, "Restorative and endodontic results after treatment with cast

posts and cores," *The Journal of Prosthetic Dentistry*, vol. 61, no. 1, pp. 10–15, 1989.

[4] A. Torbjörner, S. Karlsson, O. Dr, and P. A. Ödman, "Survival rate and failure characteristics for two post designs," *The Journal of Prosthetic Dentistry*, vol. 73, no. 5, pp. 439–444, 1995.

[5] S. A. Khasnis, K. H. Kidiyoor, A. B. Patil, and S. B. Kenganal, "Vertical root fractures and their management," *Journal of Conservative Dentistry*, vol. 17, no. 2, pp. 103–110, 2014.

[6] J. Q. Holcomb, D. L. Pitts, and J. I. Nicholls, "Further investigation of spreader loads required to cause vertical root fracture during lateral condensation," *Journal of Endodontics*, vol. 13, no. 6, pp. 277–284, 1987.

[7] C. P. Chan, C. P. Lin, S. C. Tseng, and J. H. Jeng, "Vertical root fracture in endodontically versus nonendodontically treated teethA survey of 315 cases in Chinese patients," *Oral Surgery, Oral Medicine, Oral Pathology, Oral Radiology, and Endodontology*, vol. 87, no. 4, pp. 504–507, 1999.

[8] C. Bargholz, "Vertical tooth and root fractures," in *Problems in Endodontics: Etiology, Diagnosis, and Treatment*, M. Hülsmann and E. Schäfer, Eds., pp. 353–370, Quintessence, London, 2009.

[9] M. Torabinejad and N. Chivian, "Clinical applications of mineral trioxide aggregate," *Journal of Endodontia*, vol. 25, no. 3, pp. 197–205, 1999.

[10] S. Taschieri, A. Tamse, M. Del Fabbro, G. Rosano, and I. Tsesis, "A new surgical technique for preservation of endodontically treated teeth with coronally located vertical root fractures: a prospective case series," *Oral Surgery, Oral Medicine, Oral Pathology, Oral Radiology, and Endodontics*, vol. 110, no. 6, pp. e45–e52, 2010.

[11] S. Taschieri, M. Bortolin, T. Weinstein, and M. Del Fabbro, "Preservation of an injured vital tooth using ultrasonic device and mineral trioxide aggregate," *Minerva Stomatologica*, vol. 60, no. 9, pp. 467–477, 2011.

[12] B. Karabucak, D. Li, J. Lim, and M. Iqbal, "Vital pulp therapy with mineral trioxide aggregate," *Dental Traumatology*, vol. 21, no. 4, pp. 240–243, 2005.

[13] J. Stropko, "Micro-surgical endodontics," in *Endodontics*, A. Castellucci, Ed., vol. 3, pp. 1118–1125, Edizioni Odontoiatriche Il Tridente, Florence, 2009.

[14] I. Belobrov and P. Parashos, "Treatment of tooth discoloration after the use of white mineral trioxide aggregate," *Journal of Endodontia*, vol. 37, no. 7, pp. 1017–1020, 2011.

[15] T. Dammaschke, "Direct pulp capping," *Dentist*, vol. 27, no. 8, pp. 88–94, 2011.

[16] "Septodont Biodentine Active Biosilicate Technology scientific file," 2010.

[17] P. Laurent, J. Camps, M. De Meo, J. Dejou, and I. About, "Induction of specific cell responses to a Ca_3SiO_5-based posterior restorative material," *Dental Materials*, vol. 24, no. 11, pp. 1486–1494, 2008.

[18] S. Jung, J. Mielert, J. Kleinheinz, and T. Dammaschke, "Human oral cells' response to different endodontic restorative materials: an *in vitro* study," *Head & Face Medicine*, vol. 10, no. 1, p. 55, 2014.

[19] M. Öztürk and G. Çelik Ünal, "A successful treatment of vertical root fracture: a case report and 4-year follow-up," *Dental Traumatology*, vol. 24, no. 5, pp. e56–e60, 2008.

[20] N. Masaka, "Long-tenn observation of fractured tooth roots preserved by adhesion," *The Journal of Adhesive Dentistry*, vol. 3, pp. 156–171, 1995.

[21] S. Arakawa, C. M. Cobb, J. W. Rapley, W. J. Killoy, and P. Spencer, "Treatment of root fracture by CO_2 and Nd:YAG lasers: an in vitro study," *Journal of Endodontia*, vol. 22, no. 12, pp. 662–667, 1996.

[22] S. G. Floratos and S. I. Kratchman, "Surgical management of vertical root fractures for posterior teeth: report of four cases," *Journal of Endodontia*, vol. 38, no. 4, pp. 550–555, 2012.

[23] P. H. Hadrossek and T. Dammaschke, "New treatment option for an incomplete vertical root fracture–a preliminary case report," *Head & Face Medicine*, vol. 10, no. 1, 2014.

[24] N. Tani-Ishii, N. Mutoh, K. Muromachi, and J. Suzuki, "The clinical evaluation of vertical root fracture after endodontic treatment with mineral trioxide aggregate," *Integrative Molecular Medicine*, vol. 4, no. 3, pp. 1–5, 2017.

[25] A. P. Erdem, D. O. Ozdas, E. Dincol, E. Sepet, and G. Aren, "Case series: root healing with MTA after horizontal fracture," *European Archives of Paediatric Dentistry*, vol. 10, no. 2, pp. 110–113, 2009.

[26] A. Kusgoz, T. Yildirim, M. Tanriver, and C. Yesilyurt, "Treatment of horizontal root fractures using MTA as apical plug: report of 3 cases," *Oral Surgery, Oral Medicine, Oral Pathology, Oral Radiology, and Endodontics*, vol. 107, no. 5, pp. e68–e72, 2009.

[27] N. Pradelle-Plasse, X.-V. Tran, and P. Colon, "Physico-chemical properties," in *Biocompatibility or Cytotoxic Effects of Dental Composites*, M. Goldberg, Ed., pp. 184–194, Coxmoor, Oxford, 2009.

[28] G. Koubi, P. Colon, J.-C. Franquin et al., "Clinical evaluation of the performance and safety of a new dentine substitute, biodentine, in the restoration of posterior teeth - a prospective study," *Clinical Oral Investigations*, vol. 17, no. 1, pp. 243–249, 2013.

[29] T. Saito, H. Toyooka, S. Ito, and M. A. Crenshaw, "In vitro study of remineralization of dentin: effects of ions on mineral induction by decalcified dentin matrix," *Caries Research*, vol. 37, no. 6, pp. 445–449, 2003.

[30] L. Han and T. Okiji, "Uptake of calcium and silicon released from calcium silicate-based endodontic materials into root canal dentine," *International Endodontic Journal*, vol. 44, no. 12, pp. 1081–1087, 2011.

[31] M. G. Gandolfi, K. van Landuyt, P. Taddei, E. Modena, B. van Meerbeek, and C. Prati, "Environmental scanning electron microscopy connected with energy dispersive X-ray analysis and Raman techniques to study ProRoot mineral trioxide aggregate and calcium silicate cements in wet conditions and in real time," *Journal of Endodontia*, vol. 36, no. 5, pp. 851–857, 2010.

[32] M. Torabinejad, T. R. Pitt Ford, D. J. McKendry, H. R. Abedi, D. A. Miller, and S. P. Kariyawasam, "Histologic assessment of mineral trioxide aggregate as a root-end filling in monkeys," *Journal of Endodontics*, vol. 23, no. 4, pp. 225–228, 1997.

[33] E. L. Lamb, R. J. Loushine, R. N. Weller, W. F. Kimbrough, and D. H. Pashley, "Effect of root resection on the apical sealing ability of mineral trioxide aggregate," *Oral Surgery, Oral Medicine, Oral Pathology, Oral Radiology, and Endodontics*, vol. 95, no. 6, pp. 732–735, 2003.

21

Endodontic Management of Maxillary Second Molar Tooth with a Single Root and Single Canal

Neelam Mittal, Vijay Parashar, and Prasad Suresh Patel

Faculty of Dental Sciences, Institute of Medical Sciences, Banaras Hindu University, Varanasi, Up, India

Correspondence should be addressed to Prasad Suresh Patel; prasadpatel88@gmail.com

Academic Editor: Maria Beatriz Duarte Gavião

Comprehensive understanding of variations in the root canal morphology of a maxillary molar is useful for performing successful endodontic treatment in such cases. This case report describes endodontic management of a case with such aberrant root canal morphology of a maxillary second molar having a single root and single canal.

1. Introduction

The variations in root canal anatomy of multirooted teeth are a constant challenge for diagnosis and successful endodontic management [1]. Thus, it is necessary for a clinician to have thorough knowledge of variation in root canal anatomy of multirooted teeth. A maxillary second molar usually has three roots and three canals. The maxillary molar has been reported with various root canal anatomy having four roots [2], two roots [3, 4], and even a single root with a single canal [5]. The prevalence of a single canal in the maxillary molar is reported to be 0.5-0.6% [2, 5].

Fava et al. [6] have reported a study on morphologic variation in maxillary and mandibular molars. They have reported variations in the root canal system having a single root and single canal in maxillary and mandibular molars; however, it was reported to be most frequent with the mandibular molar. The majority of variations seen in the maxillary molar are seen with the maxillary first molar. Variations in root canal anatomy of the maxillary second molar are quite rare.

Kim et al. [7] in their study using CBCT found the incidence of a single-rooted maxillary second molar to be 10.7% in the Korean population, and Zhang et al. [8] found the incidence to be 10% in the Chinese population. However, study on the Indian population by Neelakantan et al. [10] reported 0.9% of maxillary second molars with a single root but none with a single root canal.

Use of multiple angled radiographs and advanced radiographic diagnostic methods such as cone beam computed tomography (CBCT) or use of magnifying loupes or operating microscope can lead to appropriate diagnosis and management of such complex root canal anatomy [8].

The aim of the present paper was to report an aberrant root canal anatomy with the maxillary second molar.

2. Case Report

A 32-year-old female reported to the Department of Operative Dentistry and Endodontics, Banaras Hindu University, Varanasi, India, with a chief complaint of pain in the upper left back tooth, which she reported was increasing while biting and taking cold or hot beverages. The patient's medical history was noncontributory. On clinical examination, there was deep proximal caries with the maxillary left second molar; thus, intraoral periapical radiograph (IOPA) of tooth 27 was advised. The tooth was nonmobile, and periodontal probing was also within the physiological limit. Radiographic examination revealed the carious exposure of tooth 27, and thus, root canal treatment of the teeth was advised. Radiographic examination also revealed some variation in root canal anatomy with tooth 27, and having a single root and single canal (Figure 1) was suspected.

The tooth was anesthetized with 1.8 mL (30 mg) 2% lignocaine containing 1 : 200,000 epinephrines (Xylocaine;

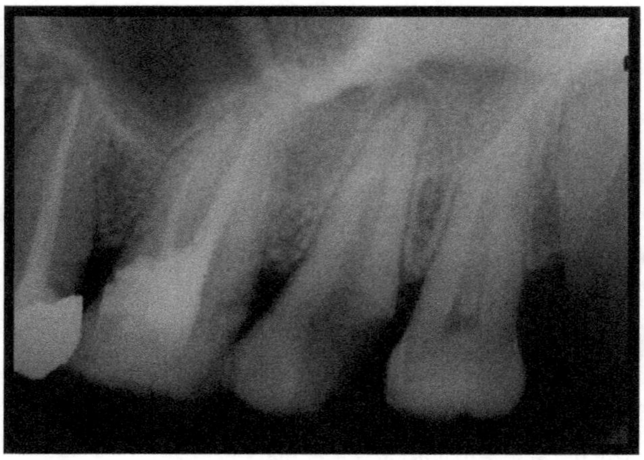

Figure 1: Preoperative IOPA.

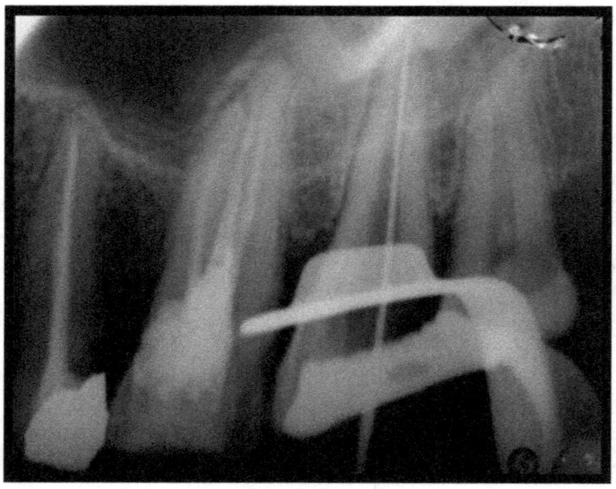

Figure 2: Working length IOPA.

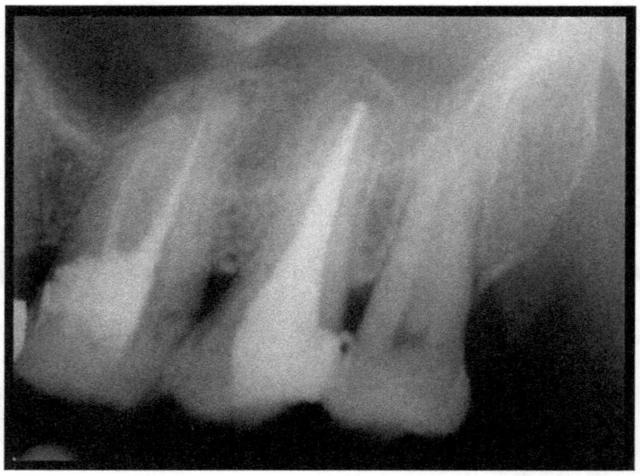

Figure 3: Post obturation IOPA.

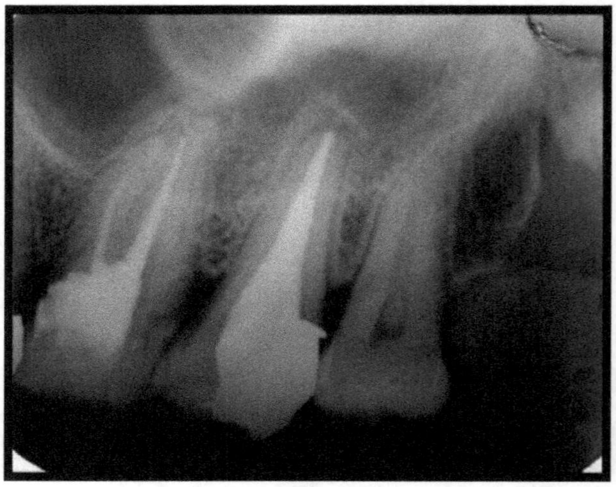

Figure 4: Final restoration IOPA.

AstraZeneca Pharma Ind Ltd., Bangalore, India.) followed by rubber dam isolation. Access opening with the aid of magnifying loupes (zumax 3.5X) of tooth 27 revealed a large single orifice and one single wide root buccolingually extending toward the root apex. Working length (WL) was determined with an apex locator (CanalPro Apex Locator, Coltene) and was confirmed with k-file (Figure 2). WL IOPA also confirmed the single-rooted maxillary second molar with a single canal. Root canal shaping was done with k-files using the conventional method of canal preparation and was irrigated with sodium hypochlorite (Sigma Aldrich, Germany). EDTA was used to remove the inorganic component of the root canal system, and a smear layer formed with filing the dentin. Saline was used as intermittent irrigation. Due to the wide nature of the canal, more attention was paid on chemical disinfection.

After canal preparation was done, IOPA was taken to confirm the fit of the master gutta percha cone. A lateral condensation technique of obturation with Apexit Plus as a sealer was used.

Post obturation, IOPA was taken to examine filling of the root canal system (Figure 3). Follow-up IOPA two weeks after (Figure 4) was taken, and final restoration with amalgam was done, and the patient was referred to the Department of Prosthodontics for further treatment.

3. Discussion

Such variation in the maxillary molar having a single root and single canal can be easily detected in routine radiograph. However, multiple preoperative radiographs can help us differentiate if two canals are present superimposing each other buccolingually. Use of an advanced diagnostic method such as CBCT can help rule out complex root canal anatomies where radiograph will be inconclusive.

Variation in root canal anatomy of the maxillary molar having a single root and single canal is reported less frequently. Literature review reported the incidence of the maxillary second molar having a single root and single canal to be 0.5-3.1% [2, 5, 9].

Study on the Indian population reported the incidence of 0.9% having a single root in the maxillary second molar, but none with a single root canal were reported [10].

The search for a missing canal can lead to common iatrogenic mishaps such as perforation or excessive tooth removal. Such error can be avoided if a clinician has general idea of variations present in the root canal system. This can be achieved with thorough preoperative evaluation of the root canal system with multiple angled root canals and use of CBCT when conflicting opinion presents about the complex root canal system. Use of magnifying loupes or a dental operative microscope can be very effective in such cases to perform ideal root canal treatment.

Various studies are reported in vivo and in vitro about the variations in root canal anatomy of the maxillary and mandibular molars.

Libfeld and Rotstein [2] in their study reported an incidence of 0.5% out of 200 radiographs of patients treated with endodontic treatment having maxillary second molars with a single root and a single canal in their in vivo study. Rwenyonyi et al. [11] also found a single root in a maxillary molar; however, the roots were found to be fused.

Wang *et al.* [12] in their study reported that the incidence of a maxillary second molar with a single root and a single canal is very rare. Ng et al. [13] and Alavi et al. [14] failed to find a case in their 77 maxillary second molars with a presence of a single root and a single canal.

Thus, these studies suggest that the incidence of a maxillary molar having a single root is not high. And so, it becomes important to recognize such cases while performing the endodontic treatment to avoid iatrogenic procedural errors.

4. Conclusion

Knowledge of variations in root canal anatomy guides in designing the therapy to be implemented in a particular case and can also affect the possibility of success with that therapy. Management of a maxillary second molar with a single root starts from proper diagnosis and modification in the treatment strategy accordingly. Therefore, practitioners need to be well equipped with knowledge of abnormalities in molar teeth and the prevalence of those abnormalities.

References

[1] V. Malagnino, L. Gallottini, and P. Passariello, "Some unusual clinical cases on root anatomy of permanent maxillary molars," *Journal of Endodontia*, vol. 23, no. 2, pp. 127-128, 1997.

[2] H. Libfeld and I. Rotstein, "Incidence of four-rooted maxillary second molars: Literature review and radiographic survey of 1,200 teeth," *Journal of Endodontia*, vol. 15, no. 3, pp. 129–131, 1989.

[3] J. V. Barbizam, R. G. Ribeiro, and F. M. Tanomaru, "Unusual anatomy of permanent maxillary molars," *Journal of Endodontia*, vol. 30, no. 9, pp. 668–671, 2004.

[4] E. Deveaux, "Maxillary second molar with two palatal roots," *Journal of Endodontia*, vol. 25, no. 8, pp. 571–573, 1999.

[5] G. Hartwell and R. Bellizi, "Clinical investigation of in vivo endodontically treated mandibular and maxillary molars," *Journal of Endodontics*, vol. 8, no. 12, pp. 555–557, 1982.

[6] L. R. G. Fava, I. Wienfeld, F. P. Fabri, and C. R. Pais, "Four second molars with single roots and single canals in the same patient," *International Endodontic Journal*, vol. 33, no. 2, pp. 138–142, 2000.

[7] Y. Kim, S. J. Lee, and J. Woo, "Morphology of maxillary first and second molars analyzed by cone-beam computed tomography in a Korean population: variations in the number of roots and canals and the incidence of fusion," *Journal of Endodontia*, vol. 38, no. 8, pp. 1063–1068, 2012.

[8] R. Zhang, H. Yang, X. Yu, H. Wang, T. Hu, and P. M. H. Dummer, "Use of CBCT to identify the morphology of maxillary permanent molar teeth in a Chinese subpopulation," *International Endodontic Journal*, vol. 44, no. 2, pp. 162–169, 2011.

[9] M. D. Peikoff, W. H. Christie, and H. M. Fogel, "The maxillary second molar: variations in the number of roots and canals," *International Endodontic Journal*, vol. 29, no. 6, pp. 365–369, 1996.

[10] P. Neelakantan, C. Subbarao, R. Ahuja, C. V. Subbarao, and J. L. Gutmann, "Cone-beam computed tomography study of root and canal morphology of maxillary first and second molars in an Indian population," *Journal of Endodontia*, vol. 36, no. 10, pp. 1622–1627, 2010.

[11] C. M. Rwenyonyi, A. M. Kutesa, L. M. Muvazi, and W. Buwembo, "Root and canal morphology of maxillary first and second permanent molar teeth in a Ugandan population," *International Endodontic Journal*, vol. 40, no. 9, pp. 679–683, 2007.

[12] Y. Wang, X. Hui, and D. M. Huang, "Maxillary second molar with curved single root and single canal: a case report," *Hua Xi Kou Qiang Yi Xue Za Zhi*, vol. 29, no. 1, pp. 104-105, 2011.

[13] Y. L. Ng, T. H. Aung, A. Alavi, and K. Gulabivala, "Root and canal morphology of Burmese maxillary molars," *International Endodontic Journal*, vol. 34, no. 8, pp. 620–630, 2001.

[14] A. M. Alavi, A. Opasanon, Y. L. Ng, and K. Gulabivala, "Root and canal morphology of Thai maxillary molars," *International Endodontic Journal*, vol. 35, no. 5, pp. 478–485, 2002.

22

Bilateral Atypical Facial Pain Caused by Eagle's Syndrome

V. Anuradha,[1,2] Ravi Sachidananda,[3] Satish Kumaran Pugazhendi,[2,4] Preeti Satish,[1,2] and Romir Navaneetham[5]

[1]*HOSMAT Hospital, Magrath Road, Richmond Road, Bangalore 560025, India*
[2]*Department of Oral and Maxillofacial Surgery, M R Ambedkar Dental College and Hospital, Bangalore, India*
[3]*People Tree Hospital, Tumkur Road, Goraguntepalya, Bangalore 560022, India*
[4]*Annasawmy Mudaliar General Hospital, Pulkeshi Nagar, Bangalore 560005, India*
[5]*Oral and Maxillofacial Surgery, Vydehi Dental College, EPIP Area, Whitefield, Bangalore 560066, India*

Correspondence should be addressed to Preeti Satish; preetiomfs@gmail.com

Academic Editor: Yuk-Kwan Chen

Recurrent throat pain, "foreign body" sensation, difficulty in swallowing, or vague facial pain is many times caused by the presence of an elongated styloid process. Many times, this condition is misdiagnosed and the patient is treated for facial neuralgia. But once Eagle's syndrome is confirmed by clinical and radiological examination, the treatment is always surgical resection. The approach maybe intraoral or extraoral. In this paper, we present a case of Eagle's syndrome caused by bilateral elongation of the styloid process and where surgical resection of the same gave instant permanent relief for the patient.

1. Introduction

One of the rarer conditions causing chronic craniofacial pain is Eagle's syndrome. This was first described by Watt W. Eagle in 1937 [1]. Many times the vague nature of presentation and quality of the pain serves to muddy the waters and leads to the patient being seen by many consultants like the neurosurgeon; the ear, nose, and throat surgeon; and many times even by a psychiatrist. Therefore, it is very common for these patients to be diagnosed with idiopathic nonspecific facial pain and to be treated without any positive result or relief from pain [2, 3].

The normal styloid process is a part of the temporal bone and usually measures about 25 mm in length. Clinically, discomfort is seen in patients where the elongated styloid processes are 40 mm or longer. Presenting symptoms include intermittent facial pain, sore-throat-like symptoms, ear pain, "foreign body" in throat sensation, or vague cervical pain [3, 4].

Eagle's syndrome is caused by a lengthened styloid process or by the links of the stylohyoid ligament getting ossified like a chain. Because of this, Eagle's syndrome is also sometimes called the stylohyoid syndrome [5]. This elongation of the styloid process maybe unilateral or bilateral. It is important to note that many times this abnormality is found only during routine radiographic examination without any presenting clinical symptoms [6]. In these patients, no active intervention is necessary and the presence of an elongated styloid process may be treated as an anatomical variation.

The normal styloid process is angulated downward, forward, and medially from the temporal bone. The tip of the process is situated between the internal and external carotid arteries and posterior to the tonsillar fossa and lateral to the wall of the pharynx. It is here that many times the tip can be felt intraorally. The muscular attachments of the styloid process is the stylopharyngeus, stylohyoid, and styloglossus. There are also two ligaments attached to the process, the stylohyoid and stylomandibular ligaments [7].

The pain is caused by (1) pressure on the glossopharyngeal nerve or trigeminal nerve or the chorda tympani branch of the facial nerve; (2) compression of adjacent structures; (3) compression of the sympathetic chain on the carotid sheath; (4) tendonitis of the stylohyoid muscle; (5) pressure on the mucosa covering the pharynx; (5) rarely, neuropraxia of cranial nerves 5, 7, 9, and 10 after tonsillectomy; (6) rarely, death due to vagus-mediated cardiac arrest; and (7) pressure

Table 1: Classification of the elongated styloid process.

Type I: a single-piece elongated process
Type II: a union of the stylohyoid ligament and stylohyoid process by a pseudoarticulation which is single
Type III: consists of multiple segments of the ossified stylohyoid ligament with multiple pseudoarticulations

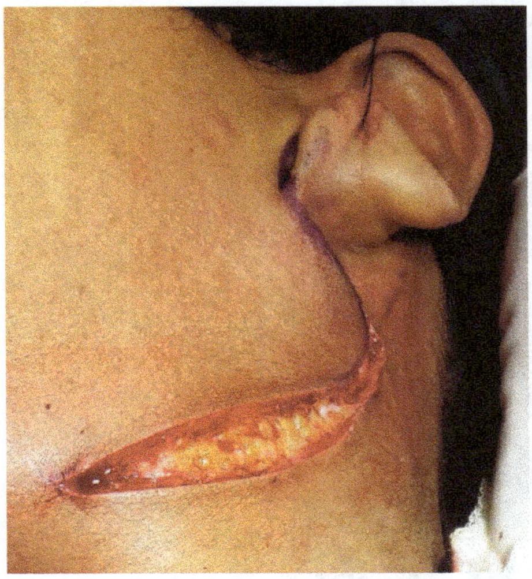

Figure 1: Incision.

on the internal carotid artery causing a transient ischemic attack [3, 8].

Commonly, routine orthopantamographs or computed tomography scans reveal the elongation of the styloid process. There is a classification that strives to describe the elongated styloid process radiographically [9] (Table 1).

The only accepted permanent treatment protocol for this anatomical abnormality is surgical removal of the elongated styloid process.

2. Case Presentation

A thirty-two-year-old female patient presented to the HOSMAT hospital with a complaint of bilateral neck pain which was exacerbated when the head was turned to either side and during swallowing since 4 years. She had been reviewed by many consultants over the past few years for the same without getting any relief. She was referred to us by the Ear, Nose, and Throat Team. There were no other clinical symptoms like headache, temporomandibular pain, or ear pain. There was no history of previous trauma or any surgical procedure. On palpation, the styloid process could be felt quite easily intraorally and extraorally. A course of oral amitriptyline was offered to the patient in an attempt to treat the condition conservatively, but this did not help the patient get relief from pain. Therefore, surgical excision via Risdon's incision (Figure 1) was planned for the bilaterally elongated styloid processes. The patient was offered surgical excision through an intraoral approach, but declined the same when advised of the need for elective tonsillectomy bilaterally.

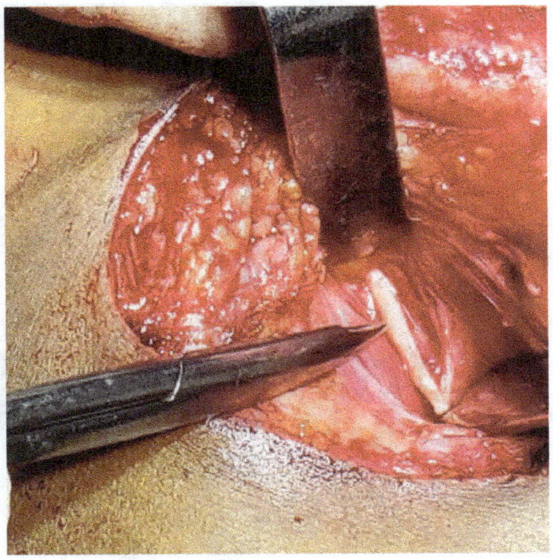

Figure 2: Right-side styloid process (Type II).

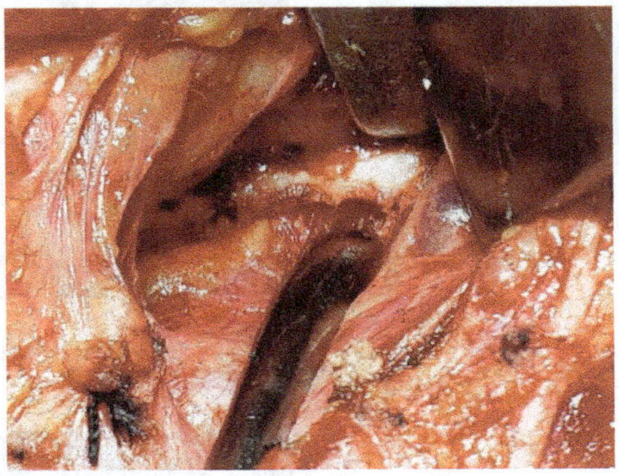

Figure 3: Left-side styloid process (Type I).

When the styloid process was evaluated radiographically, on the right side it was found to be a Type II variation and on the left side a Type I variation. This was confirmed during the intraoperative phase (Figures 2 and 3). Investigations performed included computed tomography scan with 3 dimensional reconstruction (Figures 4 and 5).

The resection of the elongated styloid process was done with general anesthesia with oral intubation. After Risdon's incision, a subplatysmal flap was elevated with care to preserve the marginal mandibular branch of the facial nerve. The posterior border to the sternocleidomatoid muscle and the posterior belly of the digastric muscle was identified carefully, and the dissection was done in the stylopharnygeal recess. The tip of the elongated styloid process was easily felt in this gap. The entire length was exposed with judicious use of monopolar and bipolar diathermy. The tissues underneath the styloid process were protected using retractors, and the dissection was carefully extended cranially to enable a lengthier resection. A 701 bur was used to cut the elongated styloid process (Figures 6 and 7). Plastic closure with drains in situ was employed (Figure 8). When the patient was reviewed after 24 hours, she was totally symptom-free. Now at one year after surgery, she continues to be symptom-free and is free of any medication.

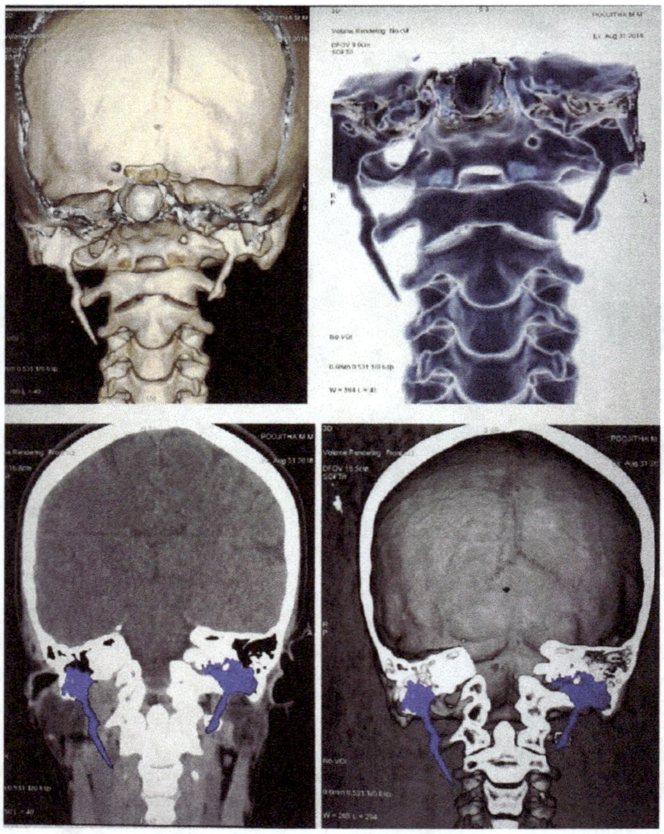

Figure 4: Computed tomography and 3D reconstruction.

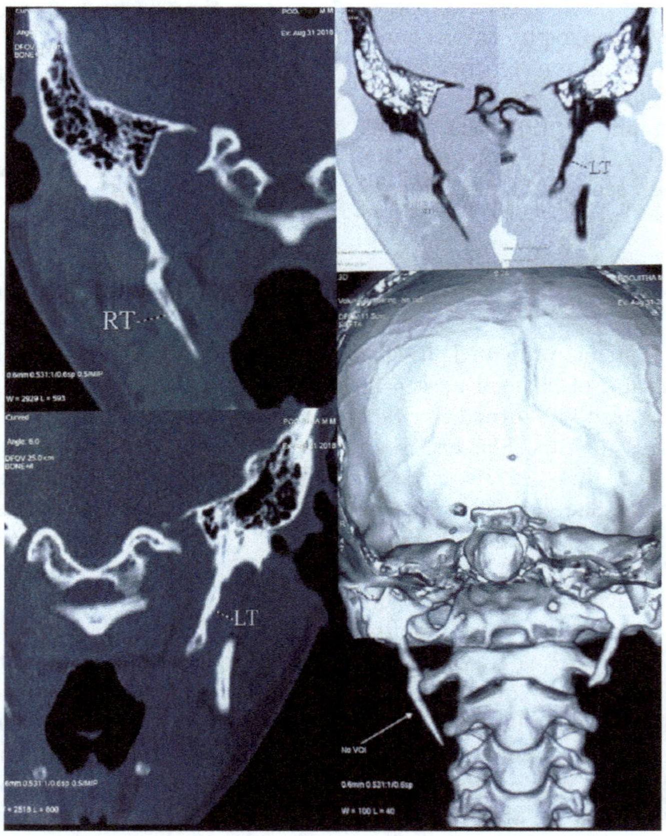

Figure 5: Computed tomography and 3D reconstruction.

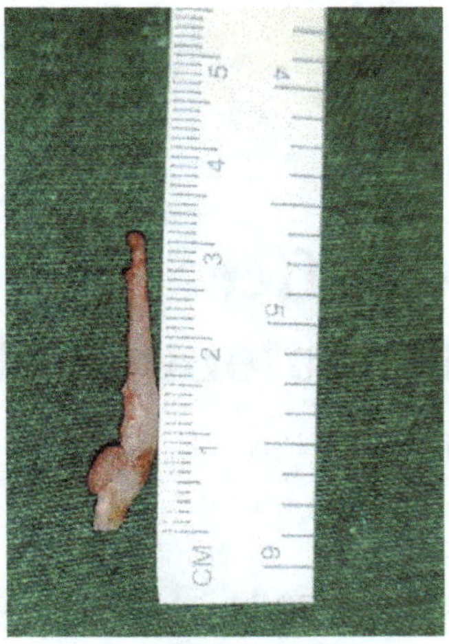

FIGURE 6: Excised right styloid process.

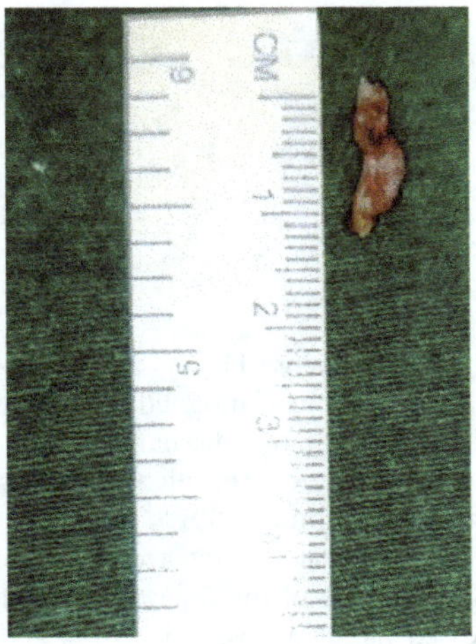

FIGURE 7: Excised left styloid process.

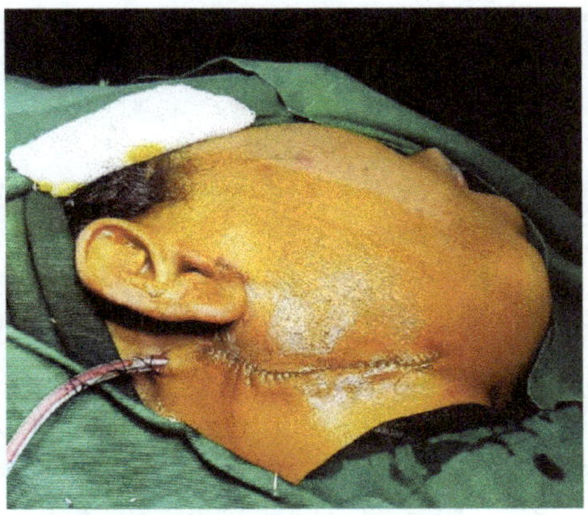

FIGURE 8: Closure.

3. Conclusion

A thorough knowledge of the pain symptoms caused by the elongated styloid process is very important for the oral and maxillofacial surgeon. Eagle's syndrome must always be considered in the differential diagnosis of patients with cervico-facial pain. Once the diagnosis is confirmed by clinical and regional imaging, resection of the styloid process is the treatment of choice. The immediate relief from pain and other symptoms of the patient is indeed a justification for the surgical resection of the elongated styloid process.

References

[1] M. Politi, C. Torro, and G. Tenani, "A rare cause for cervical pain: eagle's syndrome," *International Journal of Dentistry*, vol. 2009, Article ID 781297, 3 pages, 2009.

[2] J. W. Blackett, D. J. Ferraro, J. J. Stephens, J. L. Dowling, and J. J. Jaboin, "Trigeminal neuralgia post-styloidectomy in Eagle syndrome: a case report," *Journal of Medical Case Reports*, vol. 6, no. 1, p. 333, 2012.

[3] S. K. Swain, A. Jena, M. C. Sahu, and A. Banerjee, "Eagle's syndrome: our experiences in a tertiary care teaching hospital of Eastern India," *Journal of Head & Neck Physicians and Surgeons*, vol. 5, no. 2, pp. 66–70, 2017.

[4] K. C. Prasad, M. P. Kamath, K. J. M. Reddy, K. Raju, and S. Agarwal, "Elongated styloid process (Eagle's syndrome): a clinical study," *Journal of Oral and Maxillofacial Surgery*, vol. 60, no. 2, pp. 171–175, 2002.

[5] V. B. Feldman, "Eagle's syndrome: a case of symptomatic calcification of the stylohyoid ligaments," *The Journal of the Canadian Chiropractic Association*, vol. 57, pp. 21–27, 2003.

[6] V. Arora, A. Shetti, and V. Keluskar, "Eagle syndrome: a review of current diagnostic criteria and evaluation strategies," *Journal of Indian Academy of Oral Medicine and Radiology*, vol. 20, no. 1, pp. 1–5, 2008.

[7] G. Fini, G. Gasparini, F. Filippini, R. Becelli, and D. Marcotullio, "The long styloid process syndrome or Eagle's syndrome," *Journal of Cranio-Maxillofacial Surgery*, vol. 28, no. 2, pp. 123–127, 2000.

[8] J. H. Song, S. K. Ahn, and C. B. Cho, "Elongated styloid process as a cause of transient ischemic attacks," *JAMA Neurology*, vol. 70, no. 8, pp. 1072-1073, 2013.

[9] R. P. Langlais, D. A. Miles, and M. L. Van Dis, "Elongated and mineralized stylohyoid ligament complex: a proposed classification and report of a case of Eagle's syndrome," *Oral Surgery, Oral Medicine, and Oral Pathology*, vol. 61, no. 5, pp. 527–532, 1986.

23

Delayed Epistaxis which was Developed after Orthognathic Surgery with Le Fort I Osteotomy and Managed by Endoscopic Cauterization

Yuya Kurasawa,[1] Hitoshi Sato,[1] Ryogo Katada,[2] Takanobu Inada,[2] Tatsuo Shirota,[2] and Toshikazu Shimane[1]

[1]Department of Oral and Maxillofacial Surgery, Division of Oral Oncology, Showa University, School of Dentistry, Tokyo, Japan
[2]Department of Oral and Maxillofacial Surgery, Showa University, School of Dentistry, Tokyo, Japan

Correspondence should be addressed to Hitoshi Sato; h.sato@dent.showa-u.ac.jp

Academic Editor: Ozkan Ozgul

A case of delayed epistaxis from the mucosa behind the right side of the inferior nasal mucosa 11 days after orthognathic surgery by Le Fort I osteotomy is presented. The patient was a 31-year-old man who underwent orthognathic surgery under general anesthesia. No abnormal findings were found during or after the operation. The patient was discharged from the hospital 10 days postoperatively. However, bleeding from the right nasal cavity occurred suddenly on the night after discharge, and he presented to our hospital again. The epistaxis was stopped once by nasal packing containing 0.001% epinephrine and systemic infusion of carbazochrome sulfonic acid and tranexamic acid. However, when the nasal packing was removed the next day, right nasal epistaxis was observed again. Curvature of the nasal septum and thickening of the inferior turbinate mucosa were seen on inspection; although, no active bleeding point was identified. Decreased nasal mucosa thickening and bleeding were observed after nasal packing containing 0.02% epinephrine. When the inside of the nasal cavity was observed endoscopically, an approximately 2 mm laceration was found in the mucosa behind the side wall of the right inferior nasal mucosa, and bleeding from the same part was confirmed. After endoscopic cauterization for hemostasis of the nasal mucosa, no rebleeding was observed. Although delayed epistaxis after Le Fort I osteotomy are often performed CT angiography to confirm the bleeding site, endoscopic cauterization would be primarily useful because of less invasiveness.

1. Introduction

The Le Fort I osteotomy to correct maxillary deformities is a versatile technique that avoids complications. The osteotomy design has undergone modification to enhance the ability of the surgeon to accurately reposition the maxilla and to improve bony contact and thus the initial stability of the mobilized jaw [1, 2]. Even though it is a simple and reliable procedure after years of clinical use, it is not completely free of complications [3, 4]. Although most complications are fortunately nonfatal, major intraoperative and postoperative bleeding that is potentially life-threatening may occur. The authors present a case of delayed, massive epistaxis caused by a ruptured nasal mucosa as a postoperative complication of Le Fort I osteotomy.

2. Case Presentation

A 31-year-old Japanese man (height, 164.0 cm; weight, 63.5 kg) with a chief complaint of an occlusal abnormality began treatment in the orthodontic department of our institution in November 2017. His personal and family medical histories were unremarkable. The diagnosis was facial asymmetry with class III malocclusion accompanied by skeletal mandibular prognathism (Figure 1). The frontal cephalometric X-ray showed the left upper and lower first molars

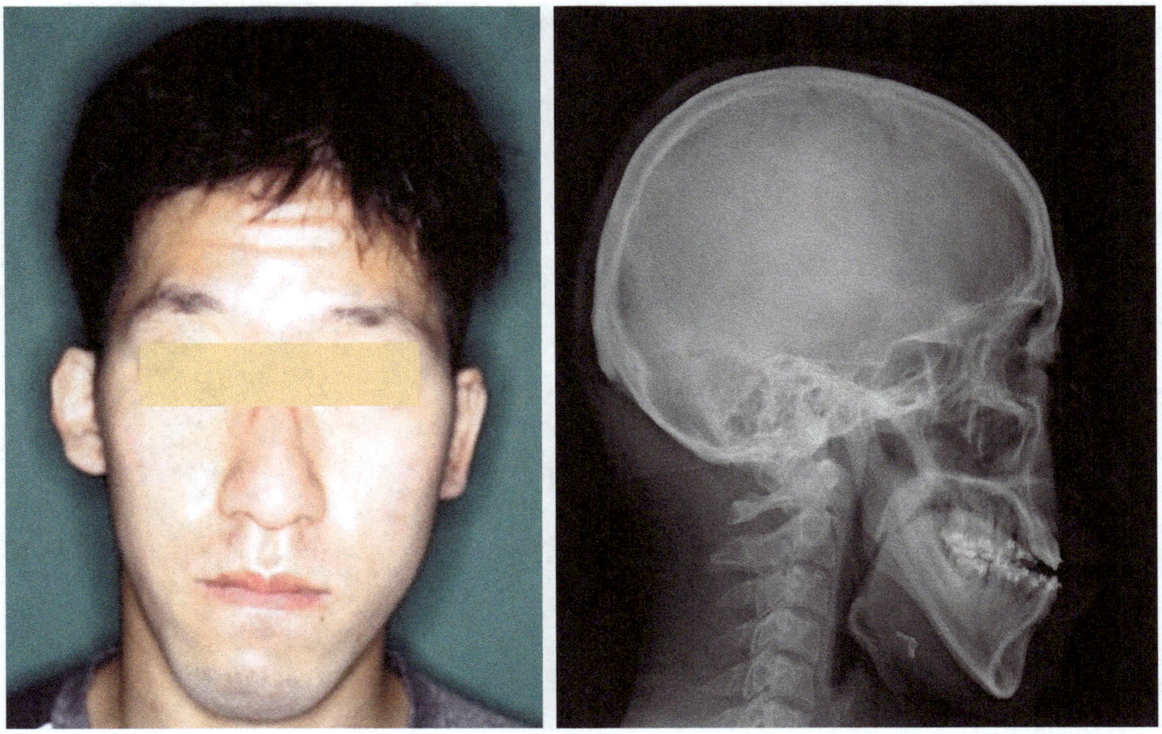

FIGURE 1: Preoperative facial photograph and lateral cephalometric radiograph. The mandible is deviated to the right, with anterior crossbite.

positioned about 2 mm lower than those on the right, and the occlusal plane inclined upwards, toward the right. Three-dimensional skeletal analysis showed the left upper first molar positioned about 1 mm more forward than the right upper first molar. Thus, orthognathic surgery, including Le Fort I osteotomy and bilateral sagittal split ramus osteotomy, was scheduled for August 2020 after the patient completed presurgical orthodontic treatment. His nutritional status was good, and laboratory findings three weeks before surgery showed no abnormalities. Le Fort I osteotomy and bilateral sagittal split ramus osteotomy proceeded under general anesthesia in August 2020. The left first molar region was elevated 2.5 mm, and the maxilla was rotated with the right first molar as the center. The mandible was repositioned posteriorly (right and left, 5.0 and 2.0 mm, respectively). Bilateral descending palatine arteries were exposed by removing interfering bone around them. The maxillary tuberosity was also carefully removed with an ultrasonic vibration cutting device. The volume of intraoperative blood loss was 155 mL, and surgical duration was 4 h and 54 min. Osteosynthesis was performed with bioabsorbable plates for the maxilla (Super Fixsorb, Teijin, Tokyo, Japan) and titanium plates for the mandible (MOJ system, Johnson & Johnson, Tokyo, Japan). The patient was free of adverse events and abnormalities and was discharged 10 days after surgery (Figure 2).

The night after discharge, he presented to our hospital again with epistaxis from the right side. The patient was hemodynamically stable. Laboratory investigations were normal, with a hemoglobin of 12 g/dl. After readmission to our hospital, bilateral anterior nasal packing containing 0.001% epinephrine was performed. In addition, systemic infusion of carbazochrome sulfonic acid and tranexamic acid was performed. The bleeding was controlled.

On the second day of readmission, continuous posterior nasal bleeding was noted when the nasal packing was removed. The complete blood count showed that the hemoglobin had decreased to 10.6 g/dl. Inspection of the right nasal cavity showed protrusion of the nasal septal cartilage and thickening of the inferior turbinate mucosa. However, the bleeding site could not be confirmed. Bleeding became weaker with insertion of nasal packing containing 0.02% for about 15 min, and a rigid endoscope (Olympus, Tokyo, Japan) could be inserted. On endoscopy, a laceration of about 2 mm was found in the mucosa behind the side wall of the right inferior nasal passage, and arterial bleeding from the same part was confirmed (Figure 3(a)). Therefore, cauterization was performed with a suction coagulator for hemostasis while visually observing the bleeding site under an endoscope, and an alginate wound dressing (Sorbsan®, ALCARE Co., Ltd., Tokyo, Japan) was inserted into the cauterization site to complete the hemostasis treatment (Figure 3(b)). Subsequently, there was no further epistaxis, and the patient was discharged on the day after the cauterization procedure for hemostasis. Seven days after the procedure, the scarred tissue on the bleeding site was seen endoscopically (Figure 4). Since then, regular follow-up has continued, with no remarkable adverse events, including no unstoppable epistaxis.

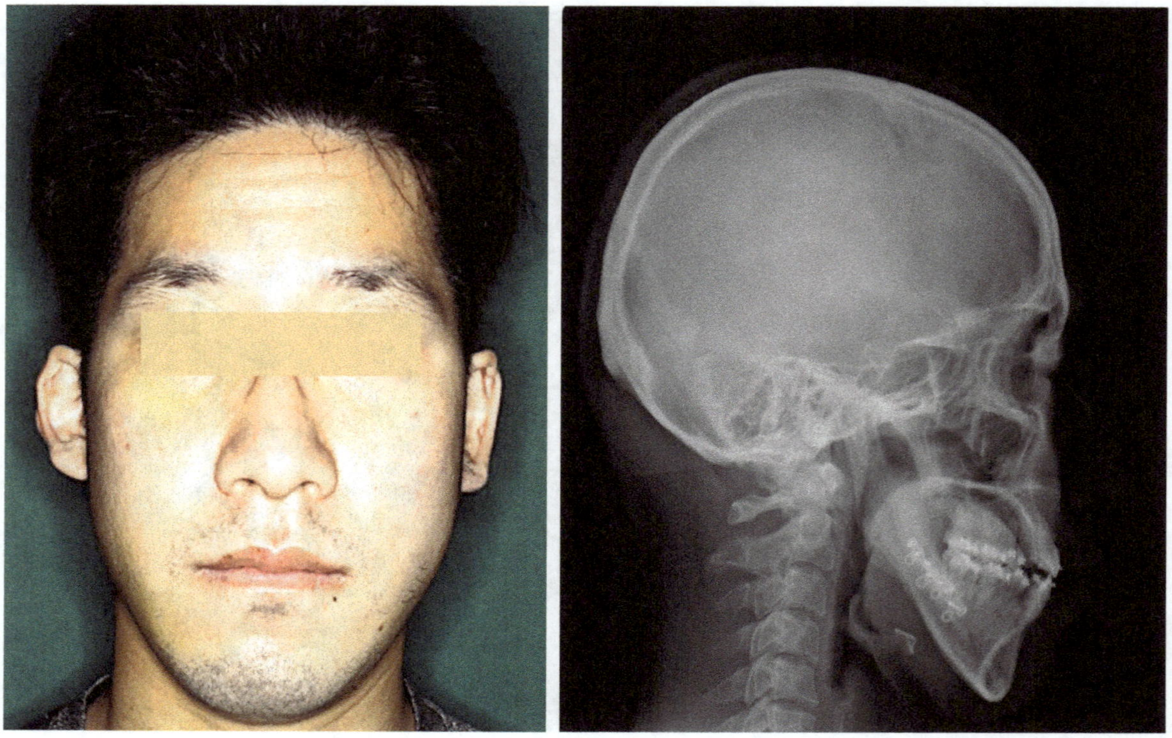

Figure 2: Postoperative facial photograph and lateral cephalometric radiograph. Mandibular deviation and occlusal relationships are improved.

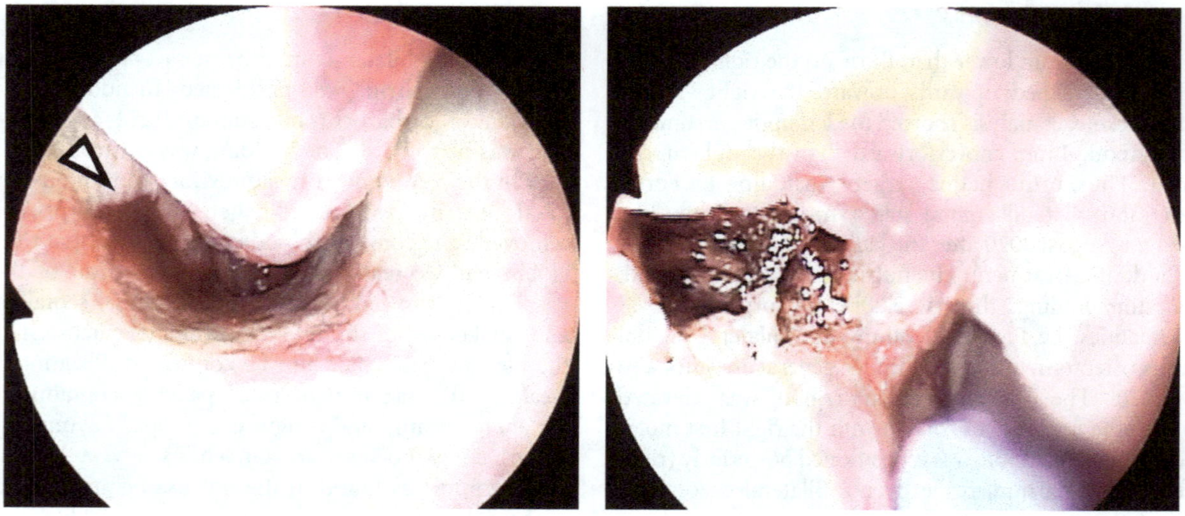

(a) (b)

Figure 3: Endoscopic image ((a) at the time of bleeding, (b) at the time of hemostasis). (a) A laceration is found on the side wall of the right inferior nasal passage, and arterial bleeding is observed (arrowhead). (a) Hemostasis is achieved by cauterization of the nasal mucosa.

3. Discussion

It has been reported that complications following Le Fort osteotomy are relatively rare compared to the number of procedures performed [5]. Fortunately, most of the complications are not severe and/or fatal. Politis noted that only two cases of life-threatening bleeding were reported following 750 Le Fort I osteotomies [6]. On the other hand, the article mentioned that such complications could be underestimated, since patients experiencing massive nasal bleeding are not necessarily treated in the same hospital or by the same surgeon.

During Le Fort I osteotomies, pterygomaxillary separation leads to damage to the descending palatine artery and pterygoid venous plexus. A tomodensitometric study to measure the position of the maxillary artery in relation to

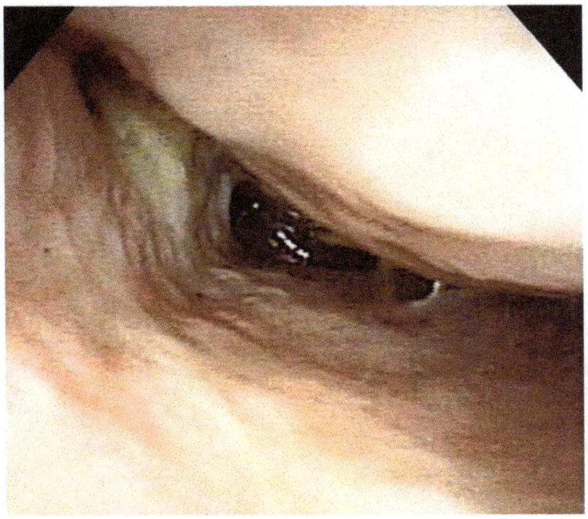

FIGURE 4: Endoscopic image (7 days after endoscopic cauterization hemostasis). Scarring of the nasal mucosa at the bleeding point is observed.

pterygomaxillary junction shows that there is a risk of injuring the artery around 20 mm above the inferior extremity of the pterygomaxillary junction [7]. Thus, to avoid bleeding complications during or after surgery, care is needed when performing pterygomaxillary separation. An ultrasonic bone curette is useful for a safe procedure when performing pterygomaxillary separation without damaging the surrounding tissues [8]. In the present case, an ultrasonic device was also used to perform procedures in the pterygomaxillary area to safely mobilize the pterygoid process, and the postoperative bleeding was not from this area. Recently, a large clinical trial for down fracture in Le Fort I osteotomy by digital pressure alone showed no severe complications [9]. Moreover, there are no strong evidences of the usefulness of osteotomes in pterygomaxillary disjunction or disjunction via the maxillary tuberosity [9]. Thus, pterygomaxillary separation without an osteotome such as a bone chisel should be considered to avoid bleeding complications.

In general, vessel injury causes acute bleeding that should be controllable intraoperatively. However, in a case with partial vessel injury, vulnerability of the vessel wall can lead to the formation of a pseudoaneurysm [10]. It has been reported that the cause of delayed epistaxis in Le Fort I osteotomy may be rupture of a pseudoaneurysm [10–14]. The epistaxis in the present case was managed by endoscopic cauterization, achieving hemostasis for a laceration of the nasal mucosa. Thus, the cause of the epistaxis might have been a pseudoaneurysm and/or postoperative traumatic injury to a small artery on the nasal mucosa. Although most patients with a pseudoaneurysm develop postoperative bleeding within 14 days postoperatively, longer delays of up to 3 months postoperatively have been reported [14]. The incidence of this complication is rare, and more cases need to be studied to determine the best approach for diagnosis and treatment. Angiography confirms the diagnosis, precisely locating the site of bleeding, and treatment can be provided immediately if necessary. Thus, it was used in many previous reports with delayed epistaxis after the Le Fort I osteotomy were used it. However, CT angiography would take time and have the risk of unnecessary radiation exposure. Endoscopically confirmation of the bleeding site should be primarily performed the delayed epistaxis after the orthognathic surgery, because of the convenience and noninvasive procedure of it. In the management of the present case, it was elected not to perform embolization because hemostasis was achieved with endoscopic cauterization.

4. Conclusion

We described a case with delayed epistaxis after Le Fort I osteotomy which was managed by endoscopic cauterization. Although CT angiography might be useful to confirm the bleeding site, careful endoscopic examination should be performed prior to that in order to avoid the unnecessary radiation exposure.

Acknowledgments

The authors would like to thank Kojiro Hirano, the otolaryngologist who performed the endoscopic cauterization hemostasis.

References

[1] S. M. Sullivan, "Le Fort I Osteotomy," *Atlas of the Oral and Maxillofacial Surgery Clinics of North America*, vol. 24, no. 1, pp. 1–13, 2016.

[2] B. O'Regan and G. Bharadwaj, "Prospective study of the incidence of serious posterior maxillary haemorrhage during a tuberosity osteotomy in low level Le Fort I operations," *The British Journal of Oral & Maxillofacial Surgery*, vol. 45, no. 7, pp. 538–542, 2007.

[3] O. H. Junior, R. Guijarro-Martínez, A. P. de Sousa Gil, L. da Silva Meirelles, R. B. de Oliveira, and F. Hernández-Alfaro, "Stability and surgical complications in segmental Le Fort I osteotomy: a systematic review," *International Journal of Oral and Maxillofacial Surgery*, vol. 46, no. 9, pp. 1071–1087, 2017.

[4] M. Eshghpour, V. Mianbandi, and S. Samieirad, "Intra- and postoperative complications of Le Fort I maxillary osteotomy," *The Journal of Craniofacial Surgery*, vol. 29, no. 8, pp. e797–e803, 2018.

[5] D. T. Lanigan, J. H. Hey, and R. A. West, "Major vascular complications of orthognathic surgery: false aneurysms and arteriovenous fistulas following orthognathic surgery," *Journal of Oral and Maxillofacial Surgery*, vol. 49, no. 6, pp. 571–577, 1991.

[6] C. Politis, "Life-threatening haemorrhage after 750 Le Fort I osteotomies and 376 SARPE procedures," *International Journal of Oral and Maxillofacial Surgery*, vol. 41, no. 6, pp. 702–708, 2012.

[7] R. Bendrihem and C. Vacher, "Radiologic anatomy of the maxillary artery in the pterygopalatine area applied to Le Fort 1 osteotomies," *Surgical and Radiologic Anatomy*, vol. 39, no. 1, pp. 23–27, 2017.

[8] K. Ueki, K. Nakagawa, K. Marukawa, and E. Yamamoto, "Le Fort I osteotomy using an ultrasonic bone curette to fracture

the pterygoid plates," *Journal of Cranio-Maxillo-Facial Surgery*, vol. 32, no. 6, pp. 381–386, 2004.

[9] J. Breeze, C. V. Linares, and P. Stockton, "Is an osteotome necessary for pterygomaxillary dysjunction or dysjunction through the tuberosity during Le Fort I osteotomy? A systematic review," *The British Journal of Oral & Maxillofacial Surgery*, vol. 54, no. 3, pp. 248–252, 2016.

[10] R. L. Avelar, J. G. Goelzer, O. E. Becker, R. B. de Oliveira, E. F. Raupp, and P. S. C. de Magalhães, "Embolization of pseudoaneurysm of the internal maxillary artery after orthognathic surgery," *The Journal of Craniofacial Surgery*, vol. 21, no. 6, pp. 1764–1768, 2010.

[11] V. S. Albernaz and T. A. Tomsick, "Embolization of arteriovenous fistulae of the maxillary artery after Le Fort I osteotomy: a report of two cases," *Journal of Oral and Maxillofacial Surgery*, vol. 53, no. 2, pp. 208–210, 1995.

[12] I. M. Smith, P. J. Anderson, M. J. Wilks, and D. J. David, "Traumatic arteriovenous malformation following maxillary Le Fort I osteotomy," *The Cleft Palate-Craniofacial Journal*, vol. 45, no. 3, pp. 329–331, 2008.

[13] L. Goffinet, B. Laure, T. Tayeb et al., "An arteriovenous fistula of the maxillary artery as a complication of Le Fort I osteotomy," *Journal of Cranio-Maxillo-Facial Surgery*, vol. 38, no. 4, pp. 251–254, 2010.

[14] M. R. Bykowski, A. Hill, C. Garland, W. Tobler, J. E. Losee, and J. A. Goldstein, "Ruptured pseudoaneurysm of the maxillary artery and its branches following Le Fort I Osteotomy," *The Journal of Craniofacial Surgery*, vol. 29, no. 4, pp. 998–1001, 2018.

24

Genetic Risk of Talon Cusp: Talon Cusp in Five Siblings

Nuha Abdel-Rahman Elmubarak

Department of Restorative Dentistry, National Ribat University, Khartoum, Sudan

Correspondence should be addressed to Nuha Abdel-Rahman Elmubarak; naina82000@yahoo.com

Academic Editor: H. Cem Güngör

Talon cusp is a rare dental anomaly that appears as a cusp-like projection on anterior teeth. Although numerous articles considering this anomaly have been published, this report has displayed a unique presentation of talon cusp. This case series is the first report in literature on which talon cusp has been presented in multiple siblings which highlights the genetic/familial component of the etiology. The report has also displayed unfamiliar morphological appearance (heart shape) of the talon cusp. Furthermore, talon cusp has shown an association with taurodontism in this report. Taurodontism has never been mentioned in the previous literature among the odontogenic variations that may associate talon cusp. A 25-year-old male has presented with talon cusps on the palatal surface of anterior teeth. Family history revealed four of his siblings had the same anomaly on anterior teeth. Talon cusps in the five cases cause clinical problems like occlusal interference, displacement and proclination of the anterior tooth, caries in the grooves delineating talon cusp, or pulp necrosis. Free dental treatment has been offered in the university clinic. However, they live in remote rural areas making it difficult to follow up with treatment.

1. Introduction

Talon cusp is a developmental dental anomaly in which an accessory cusp arises from the cingulum or cementoenamel junction of the anterior teeth in maxilla or mandible. It can affect deciduous or permanent teeth [1]. As all other cusps, talon cusp is composed of normal enamel underlined by dentin. It may or may not contain pulpal tissue [2]. However, large talon cusps, particularly those which stand away from the crown surface, more probably have pulp tissue [3].

Talon cusp was first reported in 1892 by Mitchell, who reported a maxillary central incisor with a horn-like bulge extending from the palatal surface [4]. It resembles an eagle's talon; hence, Mellor and Ripa give it the name talon cusp [5].

The etiology of talon cusp is not totally clear. Talon cusp arises during the morphodifferentiation stage of tooth development. It is proposed to be a normal consequence of outward bulging of the inner enamel epithelial cells (precursors of ameloblasts) and focal hyperplasia of the mesenchymal peripheral cells of dental papilla (precursors of odontoblasts) [2].

Clinically, some talon cusps possess sharp tips whereas others have smooth rounded tips. The tip of the cusp may stand away from the rest of the crown, or it may be fused with the tooth surface. Morphologically, talon cusps can be presented as horn-like, pyramidal, or conical shape [5–7].

On radiograph, talon cusp appears as a V-shaped radiopaque structure overlapping the affected crown with its apex directed incisally. Talon cusp on an unerupted tooth may be misinterpreted as mesiodens or compound odontoma. This misdiagnosis may lead to unnecessary surgical intervention in an attempt to remove it [2].

Based on histopathology, Danker et al. [8] and Uyeno and Lugo [9] described talon cusp as a form of dens evaginatus. Also, a previous literature review has considered talon cusp as a descriptive term of dens evaginatus on the lingual surface of anterior teeth [10]. However, depending upon the site, rate of incidence, and clinical appearance, dens evaginatus and talon cusp should be treated as separate anomalies [11]. The term dens evaginatus should be used for tubercles presented on the occlusal surfaces of premolars and molars [12].

Talon cusp usually occurs as an isolated anomaly rather than being part of any disorder [13]. Nevertheless, the anomaly has been reported in patients with Mohr syndrome [14],

Rubinstein-Taybi syndrome [15], Sturge-Weber syndrome [7], and Ellis-van Creveld syndrome [16].

Talon cusp is not an innocent anomaly as large talon cusp may lead to many clinical problems including traumatic occlusion; displacement of the affected and opposing teeth; compromised esthetics in cases of facial talon cusp; plaque retention and caries susceptibility in the developmental grooves that delineate the cusp; attrition of the opposing teeth; periodontal problems; hypersensitivity, pulpal necrosis, and periapical pathosis due to excessive attrition; accidental cusp fracture; irritation of the tongue during speech and mastication; interference with tongue space; speech disturbance; breast-feeding problems; and temporomandibular joint pain due to excessive occlusal forces [4, 17–19].

The present report describes five siblings with talon cusps in all upper anterior teeth.

2. Case Presentation

A 25-year-old Sudanese male came to Students' Dental Clinic in the Faculty of Dentistry, National Ribat University, Sudan, to treat his lower molar. During oral examination, large tubercles have been noticed in the palatal surface of all upper anterior teeth and diagnosed as talon cusps. On family history, he mentioned that four of his siblings had the same tubercles on anterior teeth. The siblings have been contacted and invited for dental examination.

2.1. Case 1. A 25-year-old male presented with talon cusps in all upper anterior teeth. Despite the name, talon cusps in both central incisors presented as heart-shaped tubercles rather than talon shape. However, lateral incisors and canines have the typical talon shape appearance (Figure 1).

Deep carious grooves separate the heart-shaped tubercles in both central incisors from the palatal surfaces of the teeth. Meanwhile, in the lateral incisors and canines, the grooves are not deep and not carious and the tubercles are in close proximity to the palatal surfaces. However, grooves in the lateral incisors are darkly stained.

All anterior teeth except the left central incisor have responded normally to the sensibility test. The left central incisor has no response to the sensibility test and shows discoloration (Figure 2).

The tubercles have been measured mesiodistally (MD) and incisogingivally (IG), and accordingly, talon cusps have been classified following Hattab et al.'s classification [2] (Table 1). Proclination of anterior teeth in this case occurs due to occlusal interference of the tubercles with the lower teeth. This proclination makes teeth at risk of trauma (Figures 2–4).

Dental variations like dens invaginatus in the upper left central incisor (Figure 5) and taurodontism in posterior molars (Figure 6) are associated with talon cusps.

On radiographic examination for the left central incisor, radiolucency around its open apex has been noticed. It has been diagnosed as chronic apical periodontitis. Pulp pathology on the left central incisor may be due to one of two reasons.

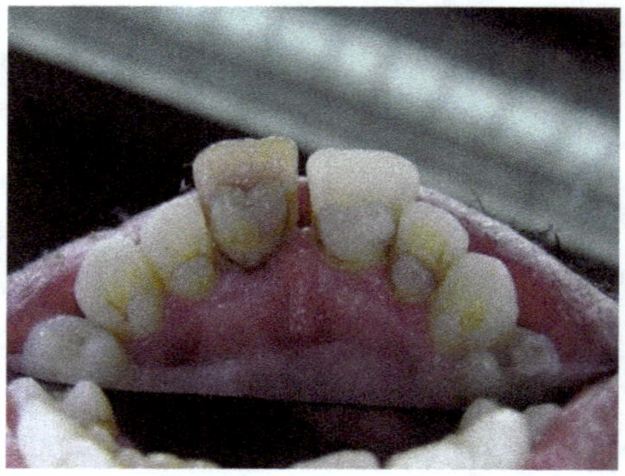

FIGURE 1: Case 1: heart-shape tubercles on both central incisors and typical talon-shape tubercles on both laterals and canines.

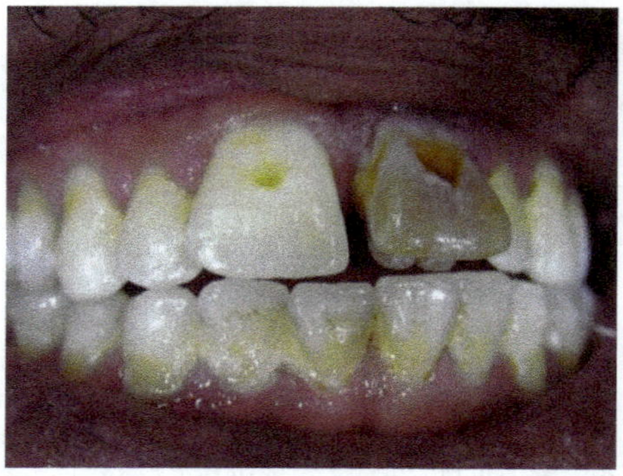

FIGURE 2: Case 1: discolored necrotic left central incisor (facial aspect).

(1) *Trauma.* As shown in Figures 3 and 4, tubercle interference with lower teeth leads to proclination of upper incisors and makes them at risk to trauma. Proclination of the left central incisor is greater than other incisors, and this make it at a higher risk to trauma leading to pulp necrosis. Measurements of the tubercles revealed that the larger tubercle is located on the left central incisor, and this justifies why the left central incisor is more proclined than other anterior teeth.

(2) *Dens Invaginatus.* Radiograph shows dens invaginatus on the left central incisor. Risk of pulp necrosis is well known in teeth with dens invaginatus if early precaution is not considered.

2.2. Case 2. A 21-year-old male, brother of case 1, also has talon cusps in the palatal aspect of all upper anterior teeth. Measurements of the tubercles have been presented in Table 1.

The right central incisor has been destructed by caries distally. So, MD dimension could not be measured. Talon cusps in both canines appear in a form of large bifid cingula (Figure 7).

According to Hattab et al.'s classification [2], both central incisors have been classified as Type 1 (talon), lateral incisors regarded as Type II (semitalon), and canines regarded as Type III (trace talon) (Table 1).

Table 1: Comparison between measurements of talon cusps of the five cases and Hattab et al.'s classification for each tubercle.

Tooth type	Case number Case 1	Case 2	Case 3	Case 4	Case 5
Right central incisor 11	IG = 6 mm MD = 6 mm Type 1 (talon)	IG = 5 mm MD = ?? Type 1 (talon)	IG = 5 mm MD = 4 mm Type 1 (talon)	IG = 4.5 mm MD = 4.5 mm Type 2 (semitalon)	No clinical examination (out of reach)
Right lateral incisor 12	IG = 4.5 mm MD = 4 mm Type 2 (semitalon)	IG = 4 mm MD = 3 mm Type 2 (semitalon)	IG = 3 mm MD = 3 mm Type 2 (semitalon)	IG = 3 mm MD = 3 mm Type 2 (semitalon)	No clinical examination (out of reach)
Right canine 13	IG = 4 mm MD = 3 mm Type 2 (semitalon)	Enlarged bifid cingulum Type 3 (trace talon)	IG = 3 mm MD = 2.5 mm Type 2 (semitalon)	Enlarged cingulum Type 3 (trace talon)	No clinical examination (out of reach)
Left central incisor 21	IG = 7 mm MD = 7 mm Type 1 (talon)	IG = 5.5 mm MD = 5 mm Type 1 (talon)	IG = 5 mm MD = 5 mm Type 1 (talon)	IG = 4.5 mm MD = 4 mm Type 2 (semitalon)	No clinical examination (out of reach)
Left lateral incisor 22	IG = 4 mm MD = 4 mm Type 2 (semitalon)	IG = 4 mm MD = 3 mm Type 2 (semitalon)	IG = 4 mm MD = 3.5 mm Type 2 (semitalon)	IG = 3 mm MD = 3 mm Type 2 (semitalon)	No clinical examination (out of reach)
Left canine 23	IG = 4 mm MD = 4 mm Type 2 (semitalon)	Enlarged bifid cingulum Type 3 (trace talon)	IG = 3 mm MD = 2.5 mm Type 2 (semitalon)	IG = 3 mm MD = 3 mm Type 2 (semitalon)	No clinical examination (out of reach)

MD: the mesiodistal dimension of the tubercle (in millimeters); IG: the incisogingival dimension of the tubercle (in millimeters); ??: the dimension could not be measured due to caries destruction.

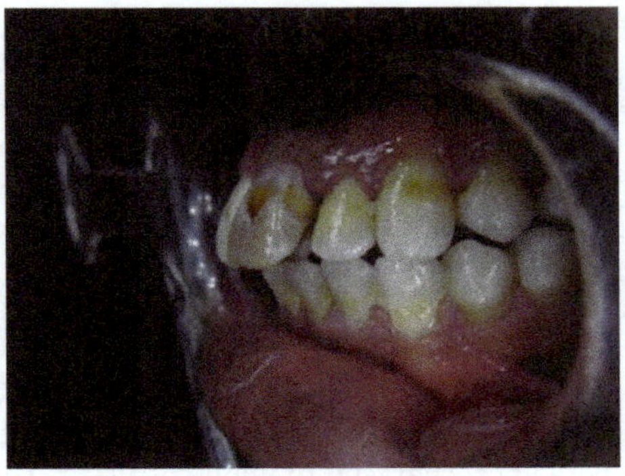

Figure 3: Case 1: proclination of upper teeth due to occlusal interference of the tubercles.

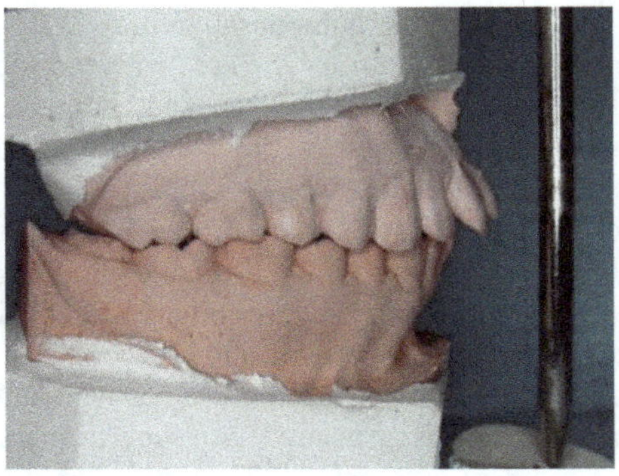

Figure 4: Case 1: study cast shows the large overjet of both central incisors.

The sensibility test has revealed that all anterior teeth are vital except the right central incisor which is nonvital and discolored and the distal half of its tubercle destructed by caries (Figure 7).

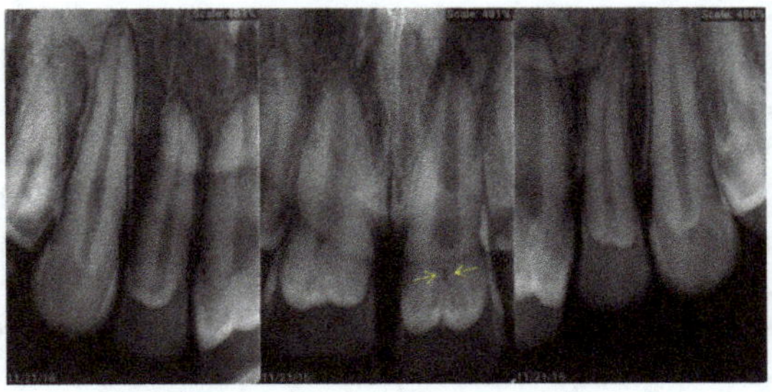

Figure 5: Case 1: periapical radiograph shows talon cusps in all upper anterior teeth. Notice the small radiolucent teardrop in the centre of the crown of the left central incisor (dens invaginatus).

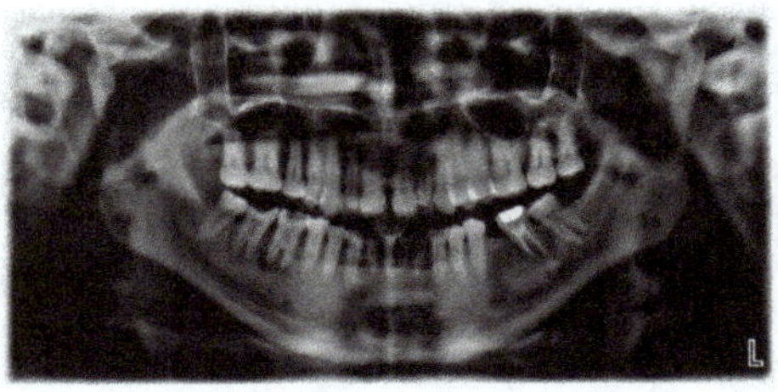

Figure 6: Case 1: dental panoramic tomography (DPT) shows taurodontism in molars.

Radiographic appearance of talon cusps has been shown in Figure 8.

Talon cusp in this patient is also associated with taurodontism in posterior teeth (Figure 9).

2.3. Case 3. A 19-year-old male, the second brother of case 1, has also presented with talon cusps in the palatal aspect of all upper anterior teeth (Figures 10–12).

Dimensions and classification of the tubercles according to Hattab et al. [2] have been shown in Table 1.

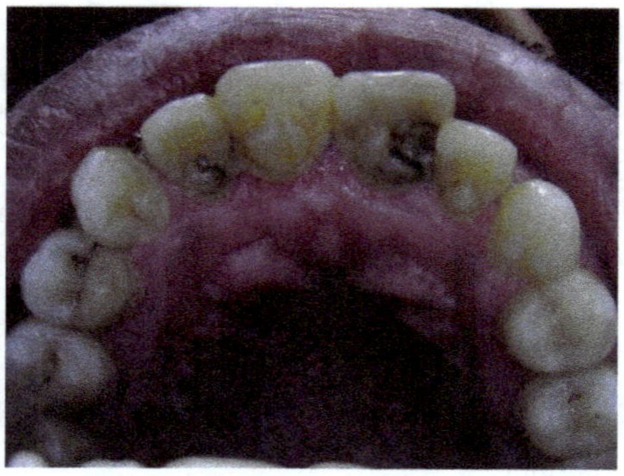

Figure 7: Case 2: talon cusps in all upper anterior teeth.

The tubercle on the right central incisor is detached from the tooth surface and separated with a deep groove, while in the left central incisor, the tubercle is merged with the tooth surface. The tubercles on lateral incisors are separated with shallow grooves, so are the canines (Figures 10 and 11).

Clinically, the teeth look generally smaller than normal size, which may be due to gingival enlargement or incomplete eruption. This can only be discovered after gingival treatment and oral hygiene improvement (Figures 13–15).

On clinical examination, shovel-shape appearance has been noticed on both mandibular canines (Figure 16) and both maxillary lateral incisors (Figure 10).

Taurodontism in molars was shown in dental panoramic tomography (DPT) (Figure 17).

2.4. Case 4. A 15-year-old female, the youngest sister of case 1, has also presented with talon cusps in all upper anterior teeth. All taloned teeth have responded normally to the sensibility test. On both central and lateral incisors, there are grooves separating talon cusps from the palatal surfaces of the teeth. The grooves are carious except that on the left central incisor (Figure 18).

As in the previous three cases, taurodontism in molars has appeared in DPT (Figure 19).

The usual V-shape radiographic appearance of talon cusps is clearly shown in the periapical view and DPT (Figures 19 and 20).

Table 1 shows dimensions of talon cusps of this case and its classification according to Hattab et al. [2].

Clinical examination has revealed a supernumerary tooth (paramolar) on the right upper posterior quadrant (Figure 21).

General examination of the teeth has revealed abnormally small teeth which may be due to incomplete eruption of teeth (Figure 22).

2.5. Case 5. A 27-year-old male, the oldest brother of case 1, like his siblings, has also talon cusps in all anterior maxillary teeth. Unfortunately, this patient works in a far rural area. He could not come for dental examination. Photos for this case have been sent by a medical officer who works there (Figure 23).

Talon cusps interfere with the occlusion of anterior teeth. This interference has resulted in a slight malalignment on anterior teeth (Figure 24).

Dental variations associated with talon cusp anomaly in this report have been summarized in Table 2.

3. Discussion

Talon cusp is an uncommon condition which affects primary and permanent teeth. Literature is not rich with data of talon cusp per se. Most of the papers concerning talon cusp have entitled and focused on dens evaginatus, as previous literature considers them as one entity.

Up to 2014, the total number of articles published on "talon cusp" is about 170 articles that described 407 teeth with talon cusp. Of the total 407 taloned teeth, 375 talon cusps were located on the palatal/lingual surface while 32 cusps were located on the facial surface. The same reviews reveal that 309 out of 407 taloned teeth were permanent whereas 98 were primary teeth [12].

The prevalence of talon cusp varies according to populations. Sedano et al. in a survey done in Mexico to determine dental anomalies in children found that this condition was present in only 0.06% [20]. Also, a smaller survey done on 536 patients in Malaysia showed that 5.2% of children had talon cusp in one of their incisors [21].

According to Hattab's review, the prevalence of talon cusp ranges from 0.06% to 7.7% and there is a racial variation for distribution of this anomaly. It occurs with a higher incidence in the Arab population than in Caucasians and Blacks [12]. This report has added to literature 30 taloned teeth in five cases that belong to the Arab population (Sudanese). Although prevalence of talon cusp in the Sudanese population has not been studied yet, according to the author's clinical experience, it is not very uncommon.

Literature reported familial evidence of talon cusp: the anomaly has been described affecting two siblings [16, 22], two sets of female twins [23], two family members [24], and three siblings [25]. Based on this data, the literature supports the hereditary character of talon cusp [13]. This report of five siblings with talon cusps adds to literature a firm evidence of a genetic background for this anomaly.

It has been noticed that sometimes talon cusp affected patients who had consanguineous parents [2, 24]. Hattab et al. mentioned that 8 out of 13 cases with talon cusp had first-cousin parents [1, 2]. This report is compatible with which had been mentioned in the literature, as parents of the five siblings are cousins.

Mader suggested that talon cusp may be associated with other somatic and odontogenic anomalies like peg-shaped lateral incisors and impacted mesiodens and canine [26]. Natkin et al. reported a case of talon cusp associated with complex odontoma and impaction [6]. Davies and Brook found that talon cusp is associated with supernumerary teeth, megadont, and dens evaginatus [27]. Hattab added a number of dental variations that may be associated with talon cusp. It includes ectopic canine, hypodontia, double teeth, dens invaginatus, shovel-shaped incisors, bifid cingula, and exaggerated Carabelli cusp [12]. Taurodontism has never been mentioned in literature to be associated with talon cusp. The present report is the first one that has mentioned taurodontism as one of the dental anomalies that may associate talon cusp.

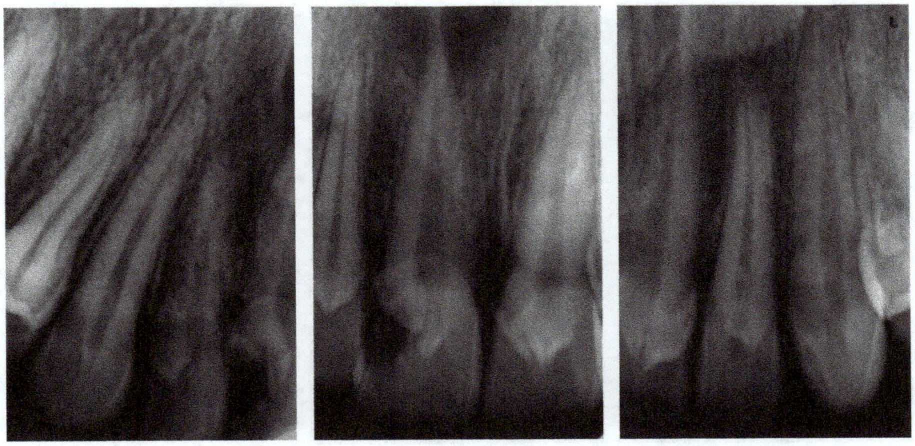

FIGURE 8: Case 2: periapical radiograph shows radiographic appearance of talon cusp.

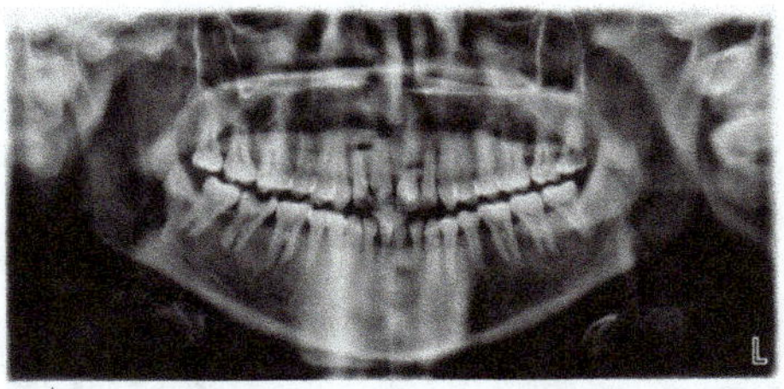

FIGURE 9: Case 2: dental panoramic tomography (DPT) shows taurodontism in molars.

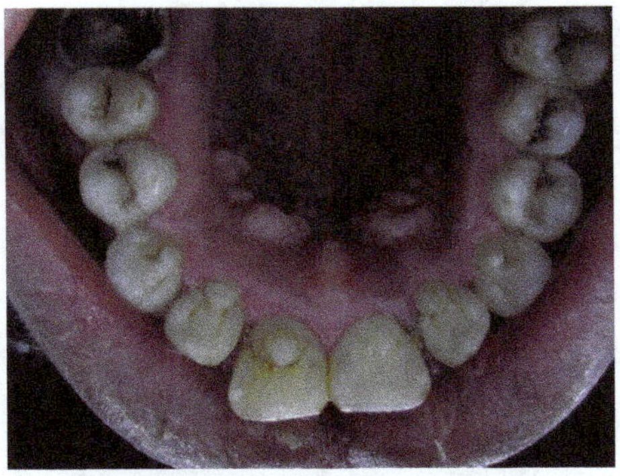

FIGURE 10: Case 3: palatal view shows talon cusps in all upper anterior teeth.

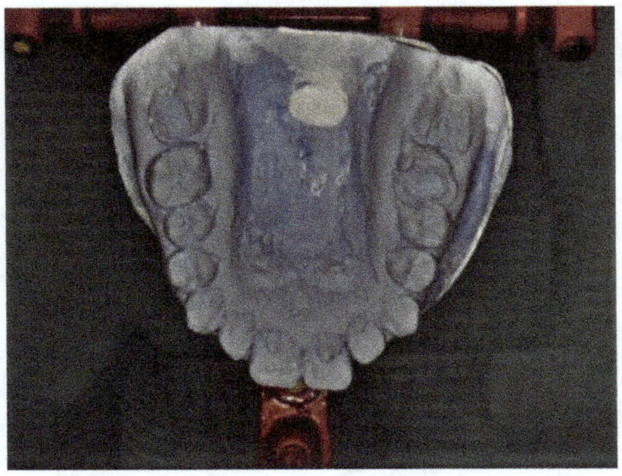

FIGURE 11: Case 3: talon cusps in all upper anterior teeth (study cast).

The treatment of talon cusp requires careful clinical and radiographic judgment. Each case should be assessed separately. Size of talon cusp plays an important role in the treatment plan. A small cusp which is asymptomatic needs no treatment while a large prominent cusp associated with functional and esthetic problems like case 1 requires definitive treatment.

The groove that separates talon cusp from the tooth surface requires especial considerations. If talon cusp blends with the tooth surface with no definite groove that delineates it like in the left central incisor in case 3, no preventive measure should be taken. However, a preventive measure should be taken if the groove is deep but noncarious: it should be cleaned from debris and plaque and prophylactically sealed with a fissure sealant. In case of carious grooves, then the lesion should be eradicated and the cavity filled with glass ionomer cement [2].

The anomalous cusp should be reduced in case of occlusal interference [2]. The amount of pulp extension within talon cusp is one of the challenges that may face the clinician when cusp reduction is required. Grinding of the palatal projection must be performed, with the possibility of exposure of the dentin-pulp complex, and consequently, pulp necrosis may be expected [28]. However, many grinding trials to remove occlusal interference of talon cusp did not end up with pulp exposure. Pitts and Hall reduce a talon cusp by 3 mm in one visit without pulp exposure [29]. Hattab et al. suggested to treat the ground surface with fluoride varnish (Duraphat) as a desensitizing agent to enhance reparative dentin formation [30]. One to 1.5 mm has been ground from six talon cusps in one visit also without exposing the pulp [2]. Dankner et al. have performed selective grinding for talon cusp in the lower mandibular incisor through sessions which continue for 12 months. Each grinding session was followed by application of Duraphat sodium fluoride gel. After 10 years of follow-up period, the tooth remains asymptomatic and vital [31]. Hattab and Hazza'A have tried to complete grinding of the cusp on two sessions at 6- to 8-week intervals without exposing the pulp [32].

Superimposition of talon cusp over the tooth crown makes it difficult to use ordinary radiographic evaluation like

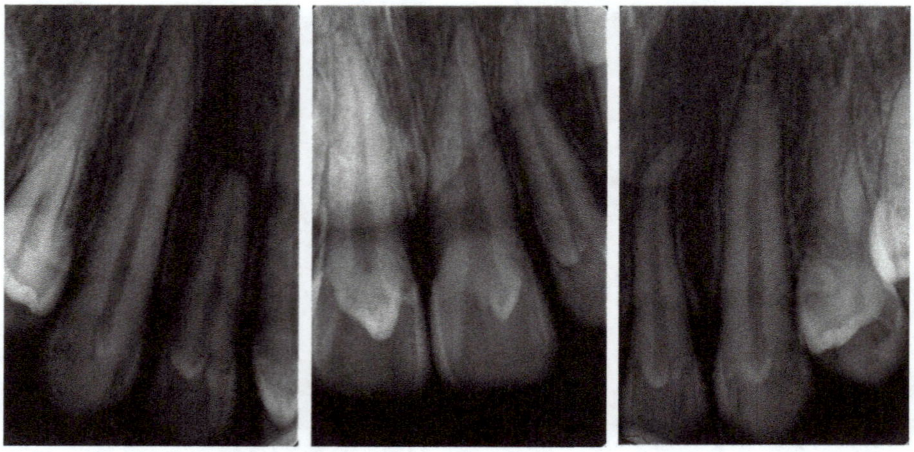

Figure 12: Case 3: periapical radiograph shows radiographic appearance of talon cusps.

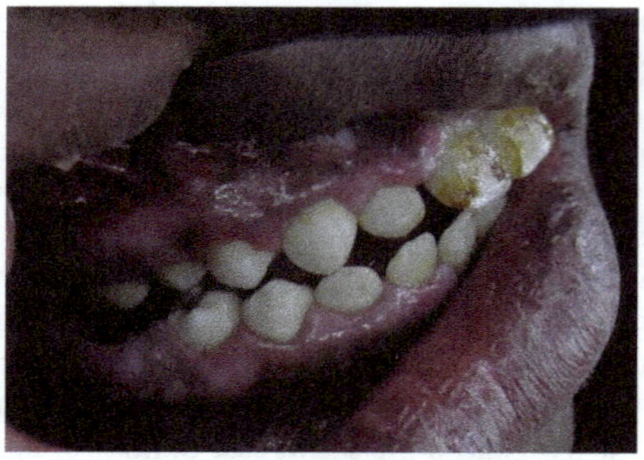

Figure 13: Case 3: small size of teeth which may be due to gingival enlargement or incomplete eruption (right side view).

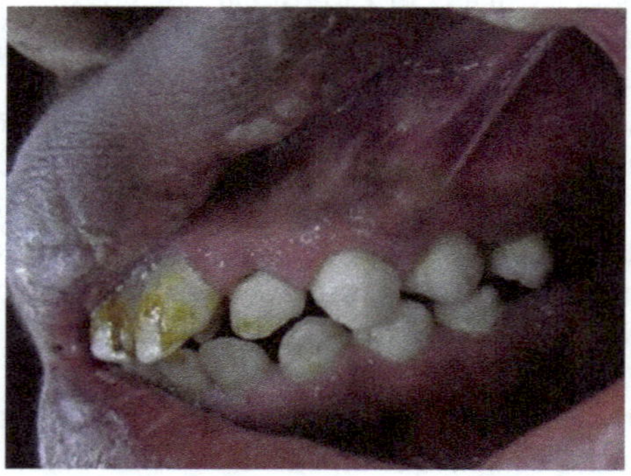

Figure 14: Case 3: small size of teeth which may be due to gingival enlargement or incomplete eruption (left side view).

periapical radiograph or dental panoramic tomography to trace the pulp extension within the cusp. Accordingly, the author has suggested computed tomography before commencing in treatment of some cases of large separated talon cusp. Evaluation of pulp extension within the tubercle will be more accurate this way.

The treatment plan for case 1 was challenging due to the risk of pulp exposure following grinding of the large tubercles in the central incisors. Risk of exposing the pulp is critical for the right central incisor rather than the left as the left central incisor has already been necrotic. Radiographic evaluation

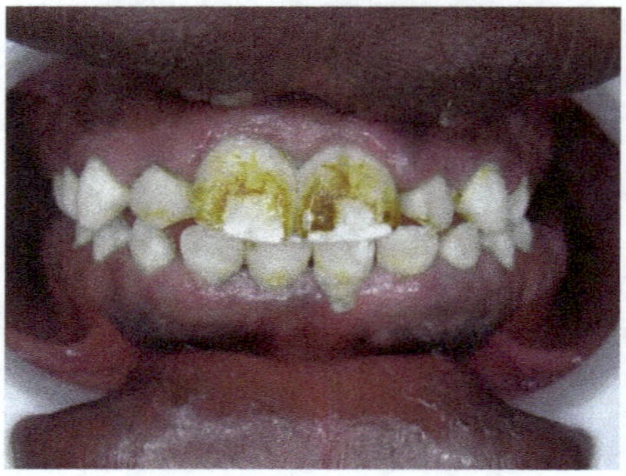

Figure 15: Case 3: small size of teeth which may be due to gingival enlargement or incomplete eruption (labial view).

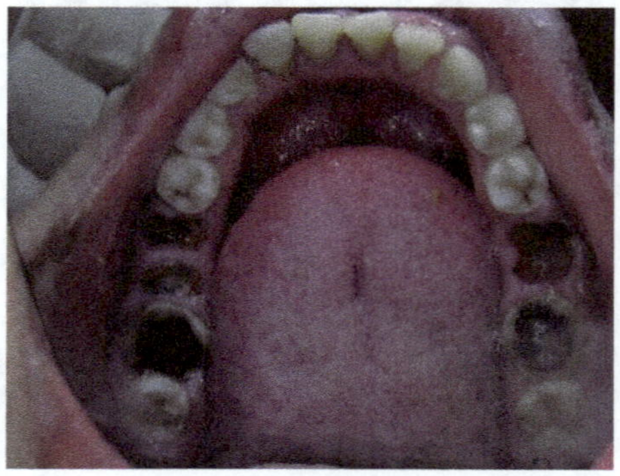

Figure 16: Case 3: shovel-shaped mandibular canines.

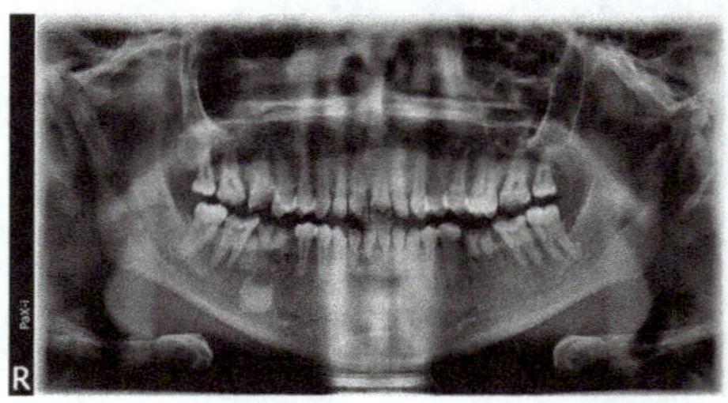

Figure 17: Case 3: dental panoramic tomography (DPT) shows taurodontism in molars.

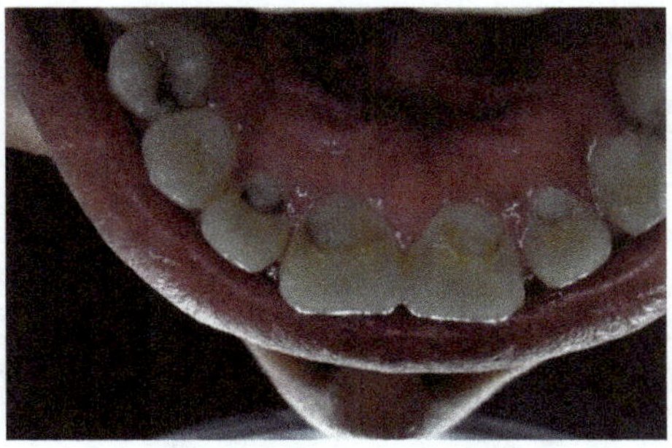

FIGURE 18: Case 4: talon cusps in all upper anterior teeth.

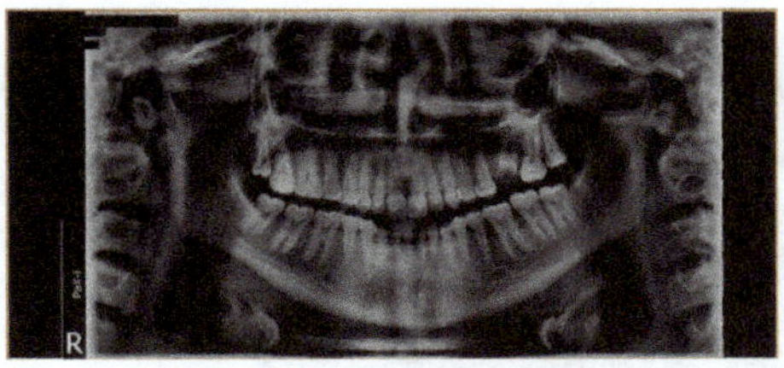

FIGURE 19: Case 4: dental panoramic tomography (DPT) shows taurodontism in molars.

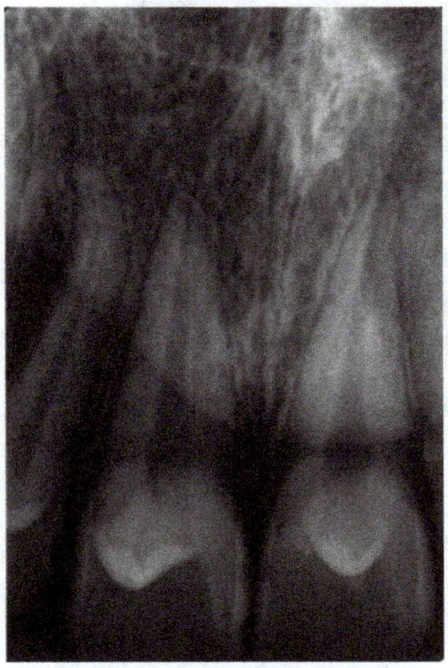

FIGURE 20: Case 4: periapical view for central incisors.

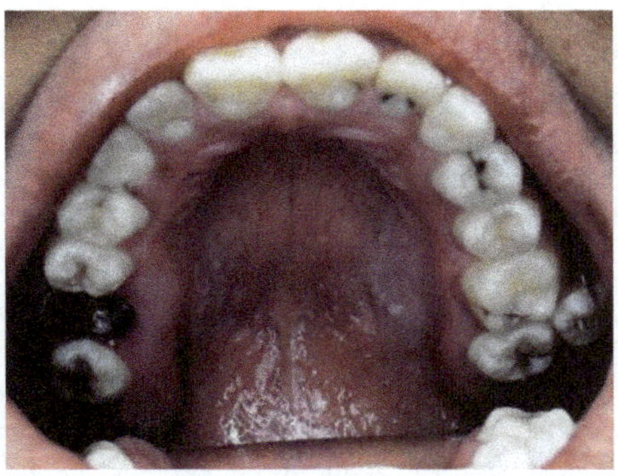

FIGURE 21: Case 4: supernumerary tooth (paramolar) associated with talon cusps (occlusal view).

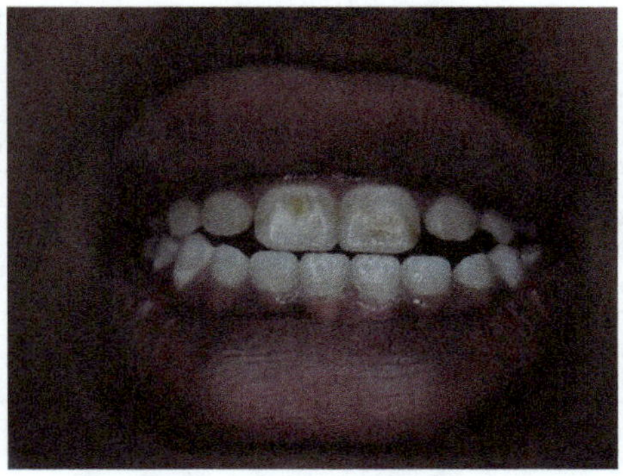

FIGURE 22: Case 4: unusual small teeth due to incomplete eruption (labial view).

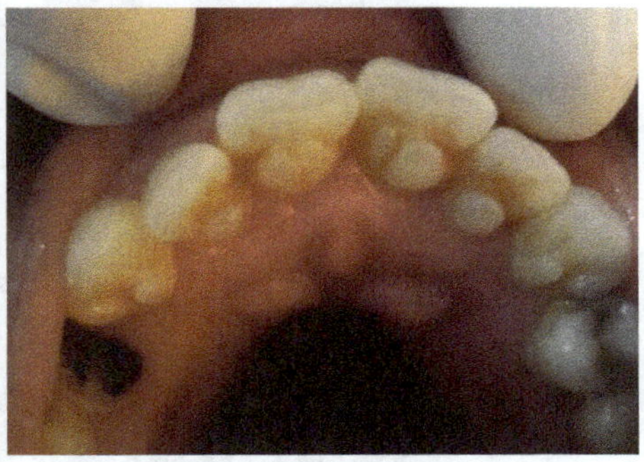

FIGURE 23: Case 5: talon cusps in all upper anterior teeth.

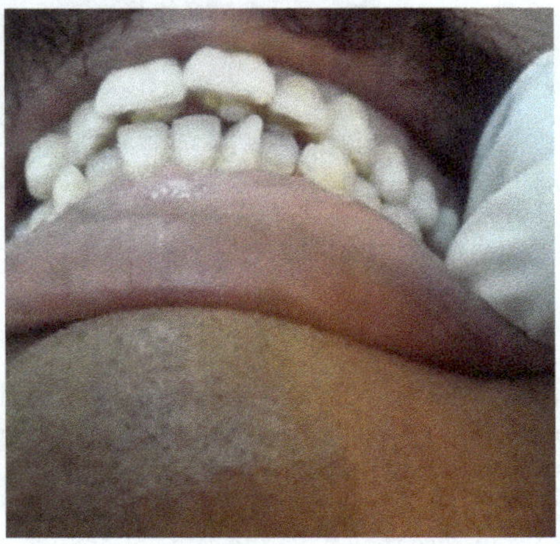

FIGURE 24: Case 5: occlusal interference by talon cusps. Proclination of upper anterior teeth occurs as a result of this interference.

for case 1 has been done using cone beam computed tomography (CBCT) (Figure 25).

The four accessible siblings have been contacted and invited for dental examination. They have poor oral hygiene, gingivitis, and multiple carious teeth. Free dental treatment has been offered in the university clinic. However, they live in remote rural areas making it difficult to follow up with treatment.

4. Conclusion

Talon cusp is a significant anomaly with variant clinical impacts. Early discovery of this anomaly can diminish or

Table 2: Summary of dental anomalies associated with talon cusp in the report.

Case number	Associated dental anomaly		
Case 1	Taurodontism	Dens invaginatus	
Case 2	Taurodontism	Bifid cingula	
Case 3	Taurodontism	Shovel-shaped anterior teeth	Small teeth size (questionable if it is due to incomplete eruption or inflammatory gingival enlargement)
Case 4	Taurodontism	Supernumerary tooth (paramolar)	Small teeth size (questionable if it is due to incomplete eruption or inflammatory gingival enlargement)
Case 5	Clinical examination was not done		

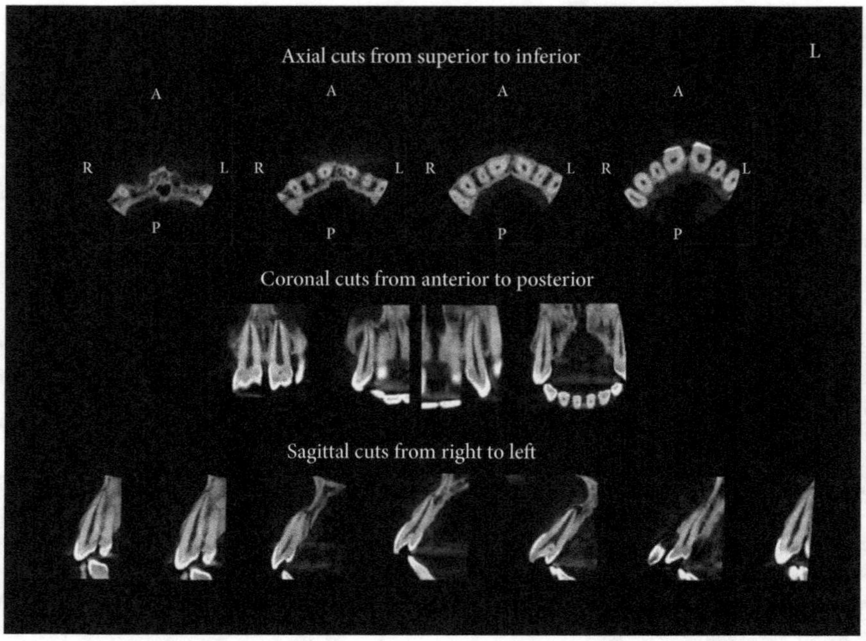

Figure 25: Cone beam computed tomography (CBCT) for the anterior segment of case 1.

prevent the clinical problems which are associated with it. This report is a strong evidence of a genetic background of talon cusp. So, if a patient present with talon cusp, it is advisable to examine his/her siblings to provide an early preventive measure in case they have the same anomaly.

Abbreviations

MD: Mesiodistally
IG: Incisogingivally
DPT: Dental panoramic tomography.

Acknowledgments

I am grateful to my colleague Dr. Musab B. Haga who took all photographs for the first four cases with his camera Nikon D5600. I also have to send my appreciation to Dr. Ezzedin M. Osman in the far distant town (Al Diain) with less dental facilities who used his phone to take photos for case 5.

References

[1] F. N. Hattab, O. M. Yassin, and K. S. al Nimri, "*Talon cusp-clinical significance and management: case reports*," *Quintessence International*, vol. 26, pp. 115–120, 1995.

[2] F. N. Hattab, "Talon cusp in permanent dentition associated with other dental anomalies: review of literature and reports of seven cases," *Journal of Dentistry for Children*, vol. 6, pp. 368–376, I996.

[3] C. L. Mader and S. L. Kellogg, "*Primary talon cusp*," *Journal of Dentistry for Children*, vol. 52, pp. 223–226, 1985.

[4] W. H. Mitchell, "*Case report*," *Dental Cosmos*, vol. 34, p. 1036, 1892.

[5] J. K. Mellor and L. W. Ripa, "*Talon cusp: a clinically significant anomaly*," *Oral Surgery, Oral Medicine, and Oral Pathology*, vol. 29, no. 2, pp. 225–228, 1970.

[6] E. Natkin, D. L. Pitts, and P. Worthington, "A case of talon cusp associated with other odontogenic abnormalities," *Journal of Endodontia*, vol. 9, no. 11, pp. 491–495, 1983.

[7] R. J. Chen and H. S. Chen, "Talon cusp in primary dentition,"

Oral Surgery, Oral Medicine, Oral Pathology, vol. 62, no. 1, pp. 67–72, 1986.

[8] E. Dankner, D. Harari, and I. Rotstein, "Dens evaginatus of anterior teeth," *Oral Surgery, Oral Medicine, Oral Pathology, Oral Radiology, and Endodontics*, vol. 81, no. 4, pp. 472–475, 1996.

[9] D. S. Uyeno and A. Lugo, "*Dens evaginatus: a review*," *ASDC Journal of Dentistry for Children*, vol. 63, no. 5, pp. 328–332, 1996.

[10] M. E. Levitan and V. T. Himel, "Dens evaginatus: literature review, pathophysiology, and comprehensive treatment regimen," *Journal of Endodontia*, vol. 32, no. 1, pp. 1–9, 2006.

[11] S. Vasudev and B. Goel, "*Endodontic management of dens evaginatus of maxillary central incisors: a rare case report*," *Journal of Endodontia*, vol. 31, no. 1, pp. 67–70, 2005.

[12] F. Hattab, "Double talon cusps on supernumerary tooth fused to maxillary central incisor: review of literature and report of case," *Journal of Clinical and Experimental Dentistry*, vol. 6, no. 4, pp. e400–e407, 2014.

[13] J. J. Segura-Egea, A. Jiménez-Rubio, J. V. Ríos-Santos, and E. Velasco-Ortega, "Dens evaginatus of anterior teeth (talon cusp): report of five cases," *Quintessence International*, vol. 34, no. 4, pp. 272–277, 2003.

[14] E. Goldstein and J. L. Medina, "Mohr syndrome or oral-facial-digital II: report of two cases," *Journal of the American Dental Association (1939)*, vol. 89, no. 2, pp. 377–382, 1974.

[15] D. G. Gardner and S. S. Girgis, "*Talon cusps: a dental anomaly in the Rubinstein-Taybi syndrome*," *Oral Surgery, Oral Medicine, and Oral Pathology*, vol. 47, no. 6, pp. 519–521, 1979.

[16] F. N. Hattab, O. M. Yassin, and I. S. Sasa, "*Oral manifestations of Ellis-van Creveld syndrome: report of two siblings with unusual dental anomalies*," *The Journal of Clinical Pediatric Dentistry*, vol. 22, pp. 159–165, 1998.

[17] M. A. O. Al-Omari, F. N. Hat, A. M. G. Darwazeh, and P. M. H. Dummer, "*Clinical problems associated with unusual cases of talon cusp*," *International Endodontic Journal*, vol. 32, no. 3, pp. 183–190, 1999.

[18] D. C. Lee, P. N. King, P. E. Lo, and D. S. Y. Cho, "*Talon cusp in the primary dentition: literature review and report of three rare cases*," *The Journal of Clinical Pediatric Dentistry*, vol. 30, no. 4, pp. 299–305, 2006.

[19] C. M. Stojanowski and K. M. Johnson, "*Labial canine talon cusp from the Early Holocene site of Gobero, Central Sahara Desert, Niger*," *International Journal of Osteoarchaeology*, vol. 21, no. 4, pp. 391–406, 2011.

[20] H. O. Sedano, I. C. Freyre, M. L. G. de la Garza et al., "*Clinical orodental abnormalities in Mexican children*," *Oral Surgery, Oral Medicine, and Oral Pathology*, vol. 68, no. 3, pp. 300–311, 1989.

[21] R. Meon, "Talon cusp in Malaysia," *Australian Dental Journal*, vol. 36, no. 1, pp. 11–14, 1991.

[22] R. Meon, "*Talon cusp in two siblings*," *The New Zealand Dental Journal*, vol. 86, no. 384, pp. 42–44, 1990.

[23] J. F. Liu and L. R. Chen, "*Talon cusp affecting the primary maxillary central incisors in two sets of female twins: report of two cases*," *Pediatric Dentistry*, vol. 17, no. 5, p. 362, 1995.

[24] J. J. Segura and A. Jiménez-Rubio, "*Talon cusp affecting permanent maxillary lateral incisors in 2 family members*," *Oral Surgery, Oral Medicine, Oral Pathology, Oral Radiology, and Endodontics*, vol. 88, no. 1, pp. 90–92, 1999.

[25] A. Sarraf-Shirazi, M. Rezaiefar, and M. Forghani, "*A rare case of multiple talon cusps in three siblings*," *Brazilian Dental Journal*, vol. 21, no. 5, pp. 463–466, 2010.

[26] C. L. Mader, "*Talon cusp*," *Journal of the American Dental Association (1939)*, vol. 103, no. 2, pp. 244–246, 1981.

[27] P. J. Davis and A. H. Brook, "*The presentation of talon cusp: diagnosis, clinical features, associations and possible aetiology*," *British Dental Journal*, vol. 160, no. 3, pp. 84–88, 1986.

[28] J. A. Ferraz, J. R. de Carvalho Júnior, P. C. Saquy, J. D. Pécora, and M. D. Sousa-Neto, "*Dental anomaly: dens evaginatus (talon cusp)*," *Brazilian Dental Journal*, vol. 12, no. 2, pp. 132–134, 2001.

[29] D. L. Pitts and S. H. Hall, "*Talon-cusp management: orthodontic-endodontic considerations*," *Journal of Dentistry for Children*, vol. 50, no. 5, pp. 364–368, 1983.

[30] F. N. Hattab, S. H. Y. Wei, and D. C. N. Chan, "*A scanning electron microscopic study of enamel surface treated with topical fluoride agents in vivo*," *Journal of Dentistry for Children*, vol. 55, pp. 205–209, 1988.

[31] E. Dankner, D. Harari, and I. Rotstein, "*Conservative treatment of dens evaginatus of anterior teeth*," *Endodontics & Dental Traumatology*, vol. 12, no. 4, pp. 206–208, 1996.

[32] F. N. Hattab and A. M. Hazza'a, "*An unusual case of talon cusp on geminated tooth*," *Journal of the Canadian Dental Association*, vol. 67, pp. 263–266, 2001.

25

Long-Term Follow-up of SAPHO Syndrome for 15 Years Led to a Diagnosis of Temporomandibular Joint Pain and Trismus

Koki Takamatsu,[1] Hitoshi Sato,[1,2] Takashi Moriya,[1] Arisa Yasuda,[1] Takaaki Kamatani,[1] and Tatsuo Shirota[1]

[1]*Department of Oral and Maxillofacial Surgery, School of Dentistry, Showa University, Tokyo, Japan*
[2]*Department of Oral Oncology, School of Dentistry, Showa University, Tokyo, Japan*

Correspondence should be addressed to Hitoshi Sato; h.sato@dent.showa-u.ac.jp

Academic Editor: Rui Amaral Mendes

Synovitis, acne, pustulosis, hyperostosis, and osteitis (SAPHO) syndrome is a systemic disease with symptoms of pustular skin disease and sterile osteoarticular lesions. This disease rarely involves the temporomandibular joint (TMJ). Although it is a disease with a good long-term prognosis, its treatment remains challenging. We describe a case with long-term follow-up of SAPHO syndrome for 15 years in which TMJ pain and trismus led to the diagnosis. A 30-year-old woman with TMJ pain and trismus was referred to our department. Her medical history included palmoplantar pustulosis. Sterile inflammation in the left TMJ and diffuse sclerosing osteomyelitis of the mandible were observed. Thus, she was diagnosed with SAPHO syndrome. The symptoms of severe TMJ pain, trismus, and left cheek swelling presented three times in the 15 years. Symptomatic treatment with nonsteroidal anti-inflammatory drugs, antibiotics, corticosteroids, and bisphosphonates was administered several times. There has been no relapse of symptoms over the past nine years. The patient must be continuously kept under observation to look for the relapse of symptoms.

1. Introduction

Synovitis, acne, pustulosis, hyperostosis, and osteitis (SAPHO) syndrome causes inflammatory changes in the bones, joints, and skin. It is a systemic disease manifested by pustular skin disease, aseptic bone, and joint lesions [1]. In particular, bone and joint lesions are classified as osteomyelitis, periostitis, and arthritis. Diffuse sclerosing osteomyelitis of the mandible (DSOM) occurs in approximately 10% of cases of SAPHO syndrome but rarely involves the temporomandibular joint (TMJ) [2].

Usually, symptomatic treatment is provided for bone and joint lesions. Nonsteroidal anti-inflammatory drugs (NSAIDs) such as indomethacin and diclofenac sodium are effective [3, 4]. Although SAPHO syndrome causes aseptic inflammation, secondary infections may occur from nearby tissues, and antibiotics such as azithromycin and doxycycline are mainly used. Steroid therapy has also been reported to be effective, but the details are unknown. Indications of antibacterial agents and bisphosphonates for cases that are difficult to control with NSAIDs may be considered [5]. Here, we report the case of a patient with SAPHO syndrome who was treated with NSAIDs, antibacterial drugs, corticosteroid hormones, and bisphosphonates and was followed up for a long period.

2. Case Presentation

The patient was a 30-year-old woman. Her medical history included palmoplantar pustulosis. The first consultation was in September 2004, and the chief complaint was left TMJ pain. Extraoral findings showed tenderness in the left TMJ and pain at the time of opening. The maximum painless opening is 13 mm. The facial appearance was asymmetrical, and a slight bulge was observed from the left cheek to

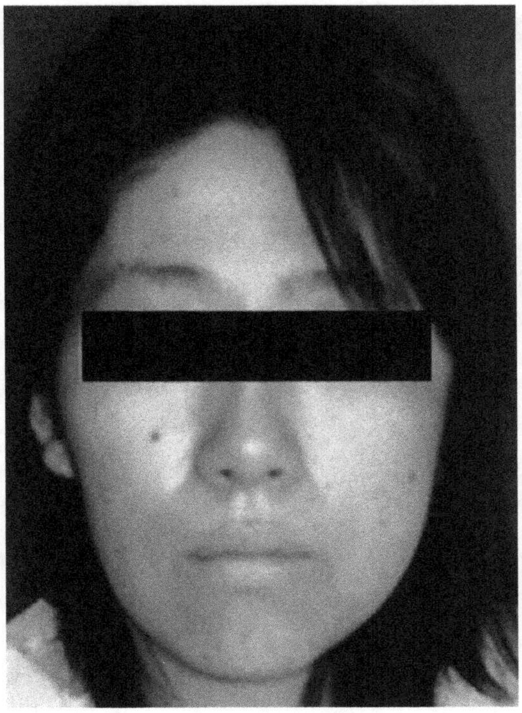

FIGURE 1: A slight bulge is observed from the left cheek to the lower jaw.

the lower jaw, but no major abnormalities were observed in the oral cavity (Figure 1).

The panoramic radiography findings showed absorptive changes of the left mandibular condyle (Figure 2). Computed tomography (CT) findings showed swelling in the buccal side of the mandibular bone and sclerosing changes in the bone marrow from the body to the ramus of the left mandible (Figure 3). Based on these results, we diagnosed left mandibular osteomyelitis and associated trismus.

2.1. Treatment Time and Course

2.1.1. 2004. Although the dental infection was suspected as the primary disease of left mandibular osteomyelitis, the cause of infection could not be identified from a panoramic radiograph and oral findings. Administration of NSAIDs (loxoprofen sodium) showed a tendency to improve TMJ pain and trismus, but swelling of the left TMJ persisted. Therefore, fine needle aspiration of the upper joint cavity was performed. Since the synovial fluid was colorless, transparent, and odorless, the patient was diagnosed with noninfectious jaw arthritis. When 3.3 mg of dexamethasone was injected into the upper joint cavity of the left TMJ, pain disappeared completely, and the maximum mouth opening amount increased to 29 mm. Since the patient had a history of palmoplantar pustulosis and CT images showed diffuse sclerotic changes in the left mandible, it was considered to correspond to bone and joint lesions associated with palmoplantar pustulosis according to Benhamou's diagnostic criteria. In addition, since there were no diseases that met the exclusion criteria, the patient was diagnosed with SAPHO syndrome.

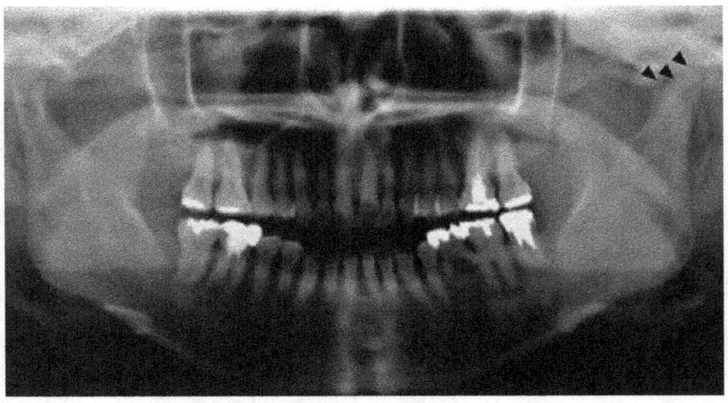

FIGURE 2: The panoramic radiograph showing absorption changes in the left mandibular condyle (arrowhead).

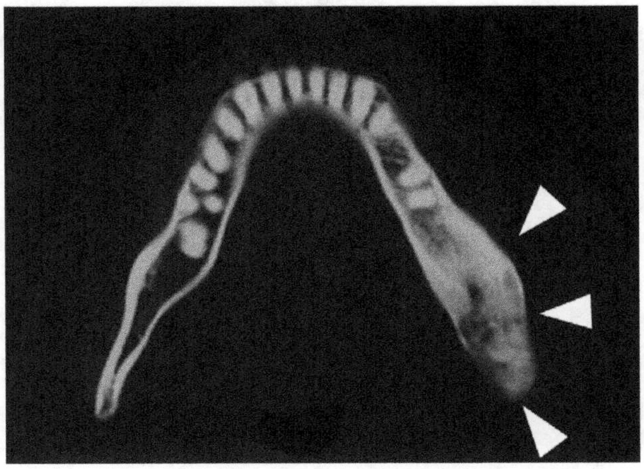

FIGURE 3: Computed tomography showing a bulge with an osteosclerosis was observed from the left mandibular branch to the mandibular condyle (arrowhead).

2.1.2. 2005. Pain in the left TMJ during jaw movement recurred, and painful swelling of the left TMJ to the cheek was observed. The maximum painless mouth opening is 8 mm. Laboratory test showed a white blood cell count of 5,800/μL and CRP level of 2.1 mg/dL. The condition was diagnosed as relapse of chronic mandibular osteomyelitis associated with SAPHO syndrome, and clindamycin 600 mg/day and cefazolin sodium 1 g/day were administered. In addition, a single intravenous dose of 30 mg disodium pamidronate, a bisphosphonate (BP) preparation, was administered. The swelling of the left cheek and pain of the left TMJ improved, and the maximum painless mouth opening increased to 30 mm.

2.1.3. 2010. Left TMJ pain and trismus recurred during jaw movement. Laboratory tests showed no abnormal white blood cell count or CRP. Bone scintigraphy showed accumulation of technetium-99m hydroxymethylene diphosphonate (99mTc-HMDP) in the left mandible, including the TMJ (Figure 4(a)), and accumulation in both thoracic rib joints and sternum (Figure 4(b)). In August of the same year, a biopsy of the left mandible was performed under hospitalization and general anesthesia.

Pathological findings showed sclerotic changes in the trabecular bone, inflammatory granulation tissue, and

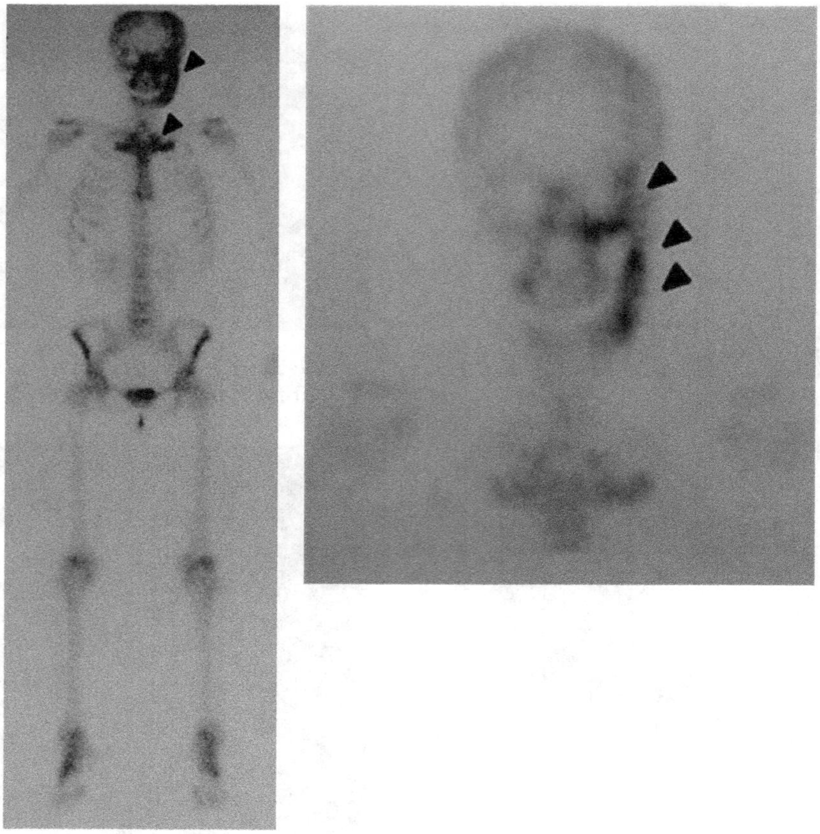

(a) (b)

FIGURE 4: (a) Bone scintigraphy showing abnormal accumulation in the bilateral thoracic rib joints and sternum (arrowhead). It presents with the so-called bull's head sign. (b) Abnormal accumulation is observed in the temporal bone, cheekbone, sphenoid bone, and mandible (arrowhead).

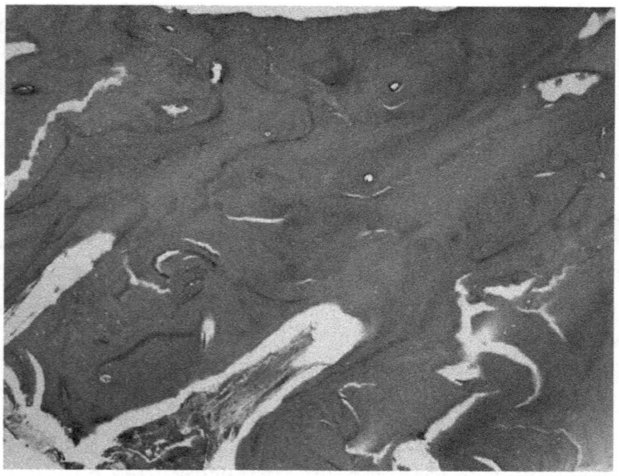

FIGURE 5: H-E staining showing sclerosing changes and bone cell defects in the trabecular bone.

fibrous connective tissue with lymphocyte infiltration (Figure 5). Therefore, we made a histopathological diagnosis of sclerosing mandibular osteomyelitis.

2.2. Additional Treatment and Course. Hyperbaric oxygen therapy was performed 10 times in total, and clarithromycin 400 mg/day was administered; however, no improvement

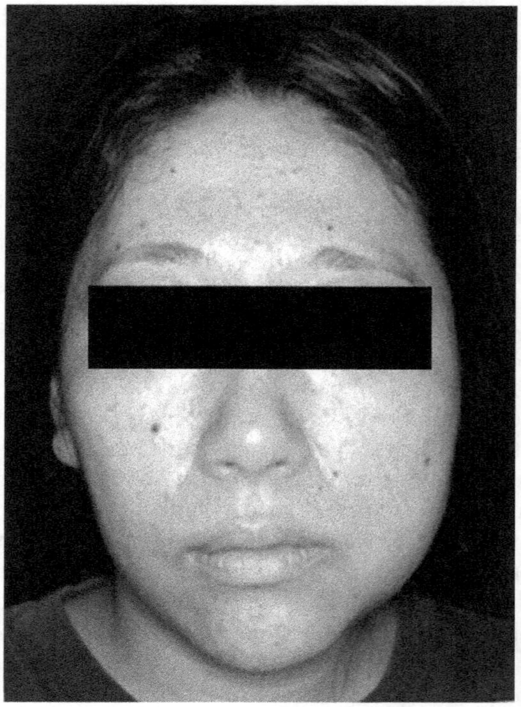

FIGURE 6: Image showing facial asymmetry with bulging of the left mandible of the patient in 2010.

Table 1: Reported cases of SAPHO syndrome including the temporomandibular joint.

No.	Reporter	Sex	Age	Lesions			Trismus	Swelling	Treatment		Follow-up (month)
				Temporomandibular joint	Chest	Skin			No effect	Effect	
1	Kodama et al. [5] 2013	M	50	O	O	—	O	O	—	NSAIDs, BP, steroids	60
2	Kotaki et al. [8] 2020	M	37	O	O	O	O	—	Antibiotic, coronoid process removal	BP	12
3	Takamatsu et al. 2021	F	30	O	O	O	O	O	Antibiotic	NSAIDs, BP, steroids	180

NSAIDs: nonsteroidal anti-inflammatory drugs; BP: bisphosphonate.

was observed. Administration of prednisolone 40 mg/day eliminated left TMJ pain and improved trismus. Since then, the patient continued to visit our department regularly, and although his facial asymmetry remained (Figure 6), her symptoms did not recur.

3. Discussion

The diagnostic criteria for SAPHO syndrome include (1) bone-related lesions associated with severe acne, (2) bone/joint lesions associated with palmoplantar pustulosis, (3) bone hyperplasia, and (4) chronic recurrent multimyelitis [1]. The mandible is the most common site for bone and joint lesions associated with SAPHO syndrome in the oral and maxillofacial regions. DSOM occurs in approximately 10% of cases of SAPHO syndrome, and most of them are intractable [2, 6, 7]. In this case, it is possible that the inflammation of the DSOM associated with SAPHO syndrome spread to the left mandibular condyle and caused absorptive changes. The affected area rarely included the TMJ since 2010 (Table 1).

Mandibular osteomyelitis associated with SAPHO syndrome needs to be differentiated from purulent mandibular osteomyelitis associated with dental infections [9–11]. This patient had a history of palmoplantar pustulosis, and there was no lesion that could be the source of infection, and resorption of the mandibular condyle and sclerotic changes in the mandible were observed. Therefore, the above diagnostic criteria (2) were met. The applicable exclusion criteria were purulent osteomyelitis, chest wall arthritis due to infection, infectious palmoplantar pustulosis, palmar keratosis, diffuse idiopathic osteoproliferative disorder (DISH), and osteoarthritis associated with retinoid therapy. Therefore, the patient was diagnosed with SAPHO syndrome.

In the treatment, the symptoms improved noninvasively by using drugs such as NSAIDs and BP preparation. In previous reports on nonbacterial osteomyelitis, aggressive surgical treatment resulted in a relapse of symptoms and reports recommending noninvasive treatment [3, 4]. To date, no definitive treatment method has been established, but noninvasive treatment methods such as those using drugs may be effective.

In this case, 15 years have passed since the diagnosis of SAPHO syndrome, and the follow-up period is the longest in the previously reported cases, including the TMJ in the affected area (Table 1). The symptoms did not recur from 2010 to the present. It is necessary to carefully continue the follow-up and consider resection of the mandibular condyle and total replacement of the TMJ when the symptoms recur.

4. Conclusion

In this study, we report a case of SAPHO syndrome, which was diagnosed by pain in the left temporomandibular joint and difficulty in opening the mouth and treated with NSAIDs, antimicrobial agents, corticosteroid hormones, and BP preparations, with long-term follow-up. In the results of long-term follow-up, we consider that conservative treatment of osteomyelitis in SAPHO syndrome is preferable to surgical invasion.

Abbreviations

SAPHO: Synovitis, acne, pustulosis, hyperostosis, and osteitis
TMJ: Temporomandibular joint
NSAIDs: Nonsteroidal anti-inflammatory drugs.

Acknowledgments

We would like to thank Editage (http://www.editage.com) for English language editing.

References

[1] S. Biuden, K. Maatallah, H. Riahi, H. Ferjani, M. D. Kaffel, and W. Hamdi, "SAPHO syndrome mimicking infectious spondylodiscitis and bone metastasis," *Case Reports in Rheumatology*, vol. 2021, Article ID 5577257, 7 pages, 2021.

[2] I. Rukavina, "SAPHO syndrome: a review," *Journal of Children's Orthopaedics*, vol. 9, no. 1, pp. 19–27, 2015.

[3] L. F. Reichardt, P. Pitak-Arnnop, A. Hemprich, K. Dhanuthai, and N. C. Pausch, "Chronic refractory osteomyelitis as a part of synovitis, acne, pustulosis, hyperostosis and osteitis (SAPHO) syndrome: a diagnostic challenge," *ANZ Journal of Surgery*, vol. 81, no. 9, pp. 642-643, 2011.

[4] M. Timme, L. Bohner, S. Huss, J. Kleinheinz, and M. Hanisch, "Response of different treatment protocols to treat chronic non-bacterial osteomyelitis (CNO) of the mandible in adult patients: a systematic review," *International Journal of Environmental Research and Public Health*, vol. 17, no. 5, p. 1737, 2020.

[5] Y. Kodama, R. Tanaka, A. Kurokawa et al., "Severe destruction of the temporomandibular joint with complete resorption of the condyle associated with synovitis, acne, pustulosis, hyperostosis, and osteitis syndrome," *Oral Surgery, Oral Medicine, Oral Pathology, Oral Radiology*, vol. 116, no. 2, pp. e128–e133, 2013.

[6] W. Zemann, M. Pau, M. Feichtinger, B. Ferra-Matschy, and H. Kaercher, "SAPHO syndrome with affection of the mandible: diagnosis, treatment, and review of literature," *Oral Surgery, Oral Medicine, Oral Pathology, Oral Radiology, and Endodontics*, vol. 111, no. 2, pp. 190–195, 2011.

[7] Z. Fu, M. Liu, Z. Li et al., "Is the bullhead sign on bone scintigraphy really common in the patient with SAPHO syndrome? A single-center study of a 16-year experience," *Nuclear Medicine Communications*, vol. 37, no. 4, pp. 387–392, 2016.

[8] S. Kotaki, S. Gamoh, H. Yoshida et al., "SAPHO syndrome of the temporomandibular joint associated with trismus: a case report and review of the literature," *Oral Radiology*, vol. 36, no. 2, pp. 197–202, 2020.

[9] P. Pottecher, R. Loffroy, L. Estivalet et al., "SAPHO syndrome revealed by sclerosing mandibular osteomyelitis," *Diagnostic and Interventional Imaging*, vol. 95, no. 9, pp. 885–887, 2014.

[10] A. Q. Rasmussen, U. B. Andersen, N. R. Jørgensen, and P. Schwarz, "Non-infectious osteomyelitis of the mandible in a young woman: a case report," *Journal of Medical Case Reports*, vol. 8, no. 1, p. 44, 2014.

[11] A. Marí, A. Morla, M. Melero, R. Schiavone, and J. Rodríguez, "Diffuse sclerosing osteomyelitis (DSO) of the mandible in SAPHO syndrome: a novel approach with anti-TNF therapy. Systematic review," *Journal of Cranio-Maxillofacial Surgery*, vol. 42, no. 8, pp. 1990–1996, 2014.

Early Creeping Attachment Noted after Mandibular Labial Frenuloplasty

P. Stylianou,[1] N. Soldatos,[1] E. K. Edmondson,[2] N. Angelov,[1] and R. Weltman[1]

[1]*Department of Periodontics and Dental Hygiene, School of Dentistry, University of Texas, Health Science Center at Houston, Houston, TX, USA*
[2]*Private Practice, San Antonio, TX, USA*

Correspondence should be addressed to N. Soldatos; nikolaos.k.soldatos@uth.tmc.edu

Academic Editor: John H. Campbell

Recession of the mandibular central incisors is frequently associated with high frenum insertion. Often times, this recession is accompanied by a lack of sufficient amount of keratinized tissue and absence of attached gingiva. In this case report, an ASA I patient presented with Cairo Recession Type 2 (RT2) and a minimal amount of keratinized tissue on the mandibular central incisors and underwent frenuloplasty in the anterior mandible with the use of a conventional scalpel technique due to high frenum attachment. The results demonstrated creeping attachment of 1.0 mm as early as 10 days postoperatively resulting in complete root coverage and closure of the interproximal space between teeth #24 and 25. A second soft tissue surgery was avoided due to complete root coverage which remained stable at the 6-month follow-up appointment.

1. Introduction

Labial, buccal, and tongue frenal attachments are considered normal anatomical structures of the oral cavity providing stability of the lips, cheeks, and tongue, respectively [1]. The frenum attachment is composed of an orthokeratinized or parakeratinized stratified epithelium, nerve fibers, and elastic and collagen fibers that are derived from the orbicularis oris muscle [2]. Abnormal frenum attachments have been implicated in diastema formation between teeth, especially the maxillary and mandibular central incisors, recession of the gingival margins around teeth with subsequent root exposure, shallow vestibule, difficulty in brushing, loss of teeth alignment, and restricted tongue movement [3]. Moreover, abnormal oral frena have been associated with different syndromes such as Ehlers-Danlos syndrome, infantile hypertrophic pyloric stenosis (IHPS), Ellis-van Creveld syndrome, oral-facial-digital syndrome, and holoprosencephaly (HPE), as well as nonsyndromic disorders [1].

Sewerin in 1971 evaluated in a Danish population the different morphological types of maxillary labial frenum. Eight categories were described: (i) simple frenum, (ii) persistent tectolabial frenum, (iii) simple frenum with appendix, (iv) simple frenum with nodule, (v) double frenum, (vi) frenum with nichum, (vii) bifid frenum, and (viii) frenum with two or more variations at a time [4]. In 1974, Placek et al. introduced a classification system for the labial frenum attachment [5]. Typically, the labial frenum inserts in the mucogingival junction. However, gingival, papillary, or papilla penetrating attachments were described by Placek et al. [5] In addition, as a separate parameter, the "pull syndrome" was described as the frequency of the movement of the interdental papilla resulting from the pull of the frenum. The mucosal attachment was found to be more prominent in upper and lower frena followed by the gingival attachment [5]. The "pull syndrome" was found to be associated with gingival, papillary, and papilla penetrating attachments. The presence of the various types of attachments was not associated with age or sex. One very common finding, associated with abnormal frenum attachment, is the shallow vestibule in the anterior mandible, often accompanied by plaque accumulation, inflammation, gingival recession, and root

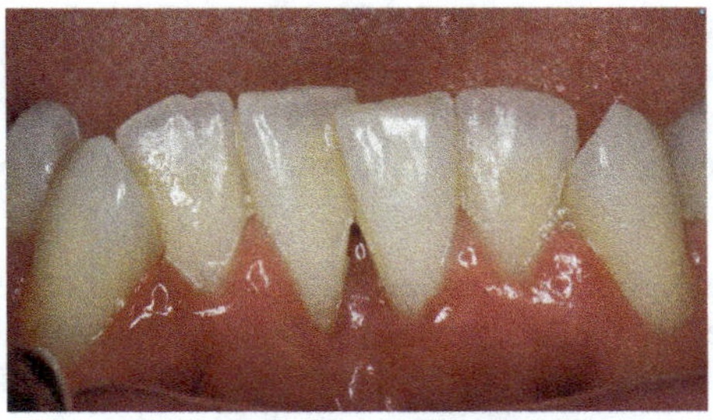

Figure 1: Preoperative picture of tooth #25 presented with 1 mm of recession and 1 mm of keratinized tissue with no attached gingiva. Interproximal loss of papilla and high frenum attachment were noted between #24 and #25.

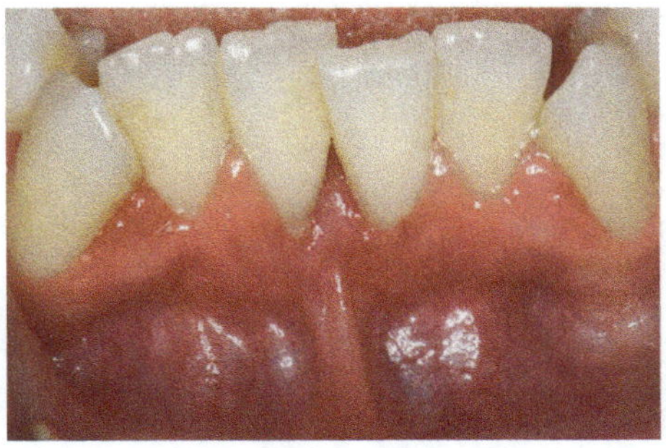

Figure 2: Simple high frenum with gingival attachment was noted between #24 and 25.

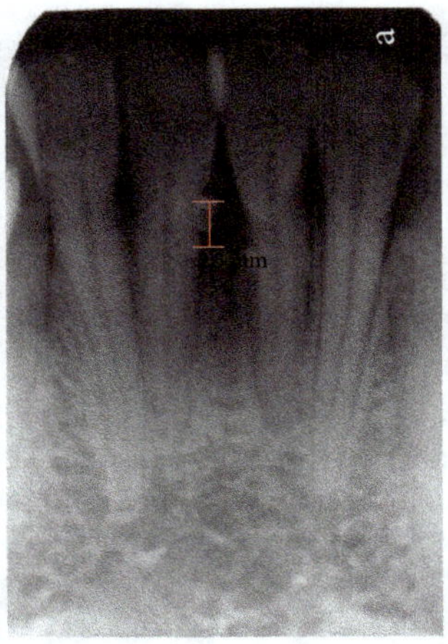

Figure 3: Radiographically 2.3 mm bone loss was noted between #24 and 25.

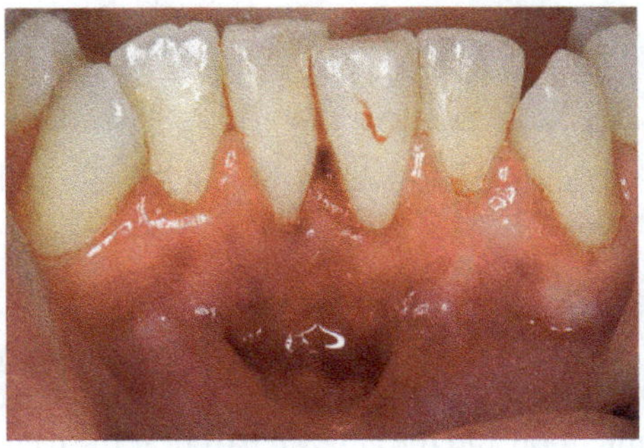

Figure 4: A diamond-shape flap was created using a 15C blade between #24 and 25. The depth of the incision was such to allow for a partial-thickness flap.

exposure of the mandibular central incisors, especially where the "pull syndrome" is noted. In addition, these teeth also present with a minimal amount or lack of keratinized tissue and attached gingiva [5].

"Creeping attachment" was first reported in 1964 by Goldman et al. and refers to the coronal migration of the gingival margin after a mucogingival surgery in a coronal direction over portions of a previously denuded root [6]. The coronal migration of the gingival margin does not occur at a constant rate but seemed to be the result of successive episodes of recession and creeping. Biologically, the mechanism could be explained through the functional arrangement and maturation of connective tissue [6].

The purpose of this case report is to demonstrate early creeping attachment after frenuloplasty only, with the use of the conventional scalpel technique.

2. Case Description

A 25-year-old ASA I Caucasian female patient presented with a chief concern of sensitivity on the mandibular central incisors. Upon clinical evaluation, teeth #22-27 showed crowding. Tooth #24 presented with no recession and 1.0 mm of keratinized tissue but no attached gingiva, and tooth #25 presented with 1.0 mm of recession and 1.0 mm of keratinized tissue with no attached gingiva. The probing depths and clinical attachment levels on teeth #24 and 25 ranged between 1 and 3 mm. The case was diagnosed with plaque-induced gingivitis on a reduced periodontium and acquired mucogingival deformities around teeth. After the treatment, the patient was placed under regular periodontal maintenance every 6 months. Moreover, on tooth #25, interproximal loss of papilla and a simple high frenum with gingival attachment were noted (Figures 1 and 2). The area between teeth #24 and 25 was diagnosed with "pull syndrome." Radiographically 2.3 mm of bone loss was noted (Figure 3), and the defect was characterized as Cairo Recession Type 2 (RT2) or Miller class III due to interproximal periodontal attachment loss. Clinically, the probing depths ranged from 1 to 2 mm without BOP. The treatment plan included frenuloplasty, and further assessment for future soft tissue grafting, based on the healing process [7, 8].

At the day of the surgery, informed consent was obtained for frenuloplasty via a conventional scalpel approach. The area of #24-25 was anesthetized on the labial aspect by means of local infiltrations with one carpule of lidocaine 2% with epinephrine 1 : 100,000. Supragingival scaling was completed on teeth #23-26 for the preparation and smoothing of the root surfaces removing any plaque deposits. A diamond-shape flap was created using a 15C blade. Initially, a "reverse V-shape" incision was made starting from the most coronal aspect of the frenum near its gingival insertion, following the fiber insertion towards the apex, near the vestibule. The depth of the incision was such to allow for a partial-thickness flap (Figure 4). After the initial "reverse V-shape" incision was made, a diamond-shape bed was created, and

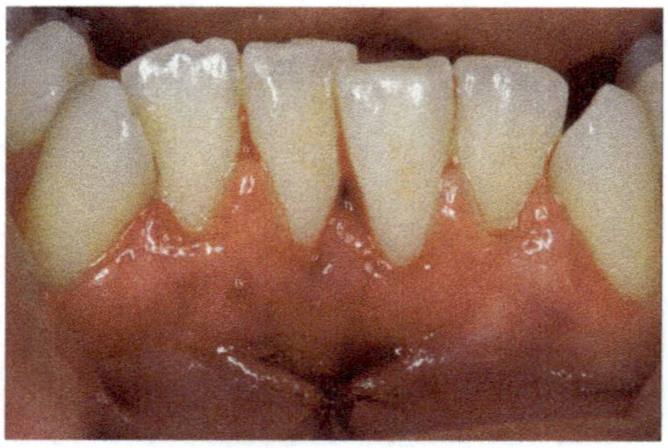

Figure 5: Postoperative picture showed a diamond-shape flap which was secured using 5-0 chromic gut single interrupted suture.

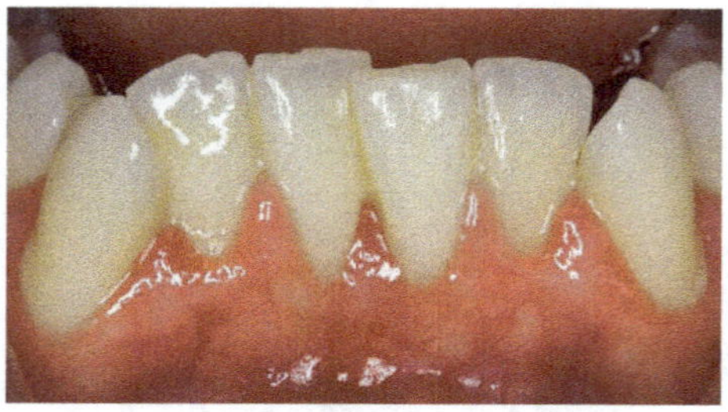

Figure 6: Ten-day postoperative picture showed creeping attachment of 1 mm at #25 and complete closure of the interproximal space, which resulted in complete root coverage.

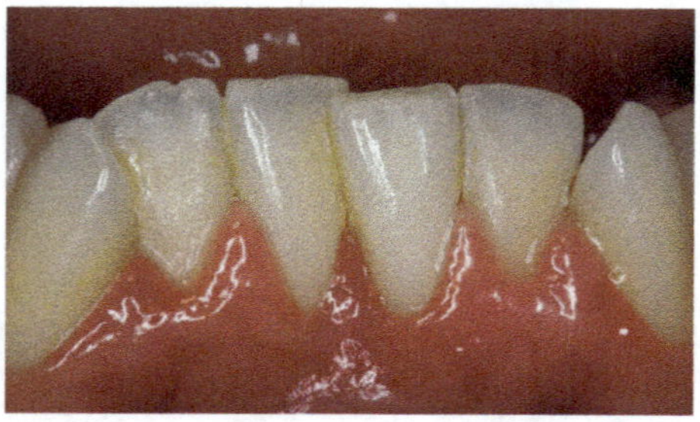

Figure 7: Six-month postoperative picture showed stable clinical results between #24 and 25.

the vestibular part of the diamond was secured using 5-0 chromic gut single interrupted sutures. With this technique, the vestibular aspect of the diamond flap was left to heal via primary intention and the gingival part near the teeth was left to heal via secondary intention (Figure 5).

The patient returned at 10 days for a postoperative appointment, and complete root coverage and closure of the interproximal space between #24 and 25 were noted. Additionally, creeping attachment of 1.0 mm was noted on #25, which resulted in elimination of sensitivity issues. The site was healing uneventfully without any signs of infection or inflammation (Figure 6). The patient returned for a follow-up at 1- and 6-month postoperative appointments with stable clinical results (Figure 7). Therefore, a second soft tissue surgery was avoided due to complete root coverage.

3. Discussion

It is very important to evaluate the frenal attachments of the patients during routine assessment. Proper diagnosis using the Placek and Sewerin classification systems will result in successful treatment and will prevent severe mucogingival problems like recession and interproximal loss of papilla, teeth malalignment, diastema, and accumulation of plaque due to difficulty in brushing [4, 5].

Labial frenectomy can be performed with a conventional scalpel technique, electrosurgery, or soft tissue lasers [9, 10]. The problem associated with the conventional scalpel technique is the postsurgical pain and discomfort. The increased use of soft tissue lasers in dentistry has also increased patient acceptance [10–12]. Various lasers including CO_2, diode, Nd:YAG, Er:YSGG, and Er:YAG have been successfully used for the aforementioned procedure [11].

Creeping attachment is frequently observed after mucogingival surgeries, but it does not occur in a constant rate, and the amount is not predictable [6, 13]. Matter in 1980 reported an average of 0.89 mm of creeping attachment 1 year after a free gingival graft surgery [14]. Nelson in 1987 first described creeping attachment of 1-2 mm, during the first postoperative year, in certain cases of subpedicle connective tissue grafting [15]. Similar findings have been reported by Harris, when a connective tissue graft was coupled with partial-thickness double-pedicle flaps, resulting in a mean creeping attachment of 0.8 mm [16]. Most recently, creeping attachment has been reported after a coronally advanced flap and the use of a xenogeneic graft [17]. The creeping attachment reported ranged between 0.5 and 2 mm at 1 year postoperatively [17].

In a similar case report, Fowler and Breault reported a creeping attachment of 1.0 mm after frenectomy with the scalpel technique in the anterior mandible after 4 weeks [3]. In the present case report, the same protocol with Fowler and Breault was followed but the creeping attachment was noted as early as 10 days postoperatively. Furthermore, full coverage of the root surface was noted along with the interproximal soft tissue fill. The results remained stable for 6 months, and a second soft tissue surgery was avoided. Our incidental findings are in accordance with the existing literature and indicate a potential of coronal creeping attachment after removal of high frenal insertions in the anterior mandible which can result in complete root coverage preventing further need for mucogingival surgeries.

4. Conclusions

Early creeping attachment of 1.0 mm was noted after removal of high frenum insertion in the anterior mandible which resulted in complete root coverage, preventing further need for mucogingival surgery.

Authors' Contributions

P. Stylianou and N. Soldatos are sharing the first authorship.

References

[1] S. M. Mintz, M. A. Siegel, and P. J. Seider, "An overview of oral frena and their association with multiple syndromic and non-syndromic conditions," *Oral Surgery, Oral Medicine, Oral Pathology, Oral Radiology, and Endodontology*, vol. 99, no. 3, pp. 321–324, 2005.

[2] K. S. Saladin, *Anatomy & Physiology: The Unity of Form and Function*, McGraw Hill, 5th edition, 2004.

[3] E. B. Fowler and L. G. Breault, "Early creeping attachment after frenectomy: a case report," *General Dentistry*, vol. 48, no. 5, pp. 591–593, 2000.

[4] I. Sewerin, "Prevalence of variations and anomalies of the upper labial frenum," *Acta Odontologica Scandinavica*, vol. 29, no. 4, pp. 487–496, 1971.

[5] P. Mirko, S. Miroslav, and M. Lubor, "Significance of the labial frenum attachment in periodontal disease in man. Part 1. Classification and epidemiology of the labial frenum attachment," *Journal of Periodontology*, vol. 45, no. 12, pp. 891–894, 1974.

[6] H. M. Goldman, S. Schluger, L. Fox, and D. W. Cohen, *Periodontal Therapy*, C. V. Mosby Co, St. Louis, MO, USA, 3rd edition, 1964.

[7] F. Cairo, M. Nieri, S. Cincinelli, J. Mervelt, and U. Pagliaro, "The interproximal clinical attachment level to classify gingival recessions and predict root coverage outcomes: an explorative and reliability study," *Journal of Clinical Periodontology*, vol. 38, no. 7, pp. 661–666, 2011.

[8] P. Miller, "A classification of marginal tissue recession," *International Journal of Periodontics & Restorative Dentistry*, vol. 5, no. 2, pp. 8–13, 1985.

[9] D. DE Santis, R. Gerosa, P. F. Graziani et al., "Lingual frenectomy: a comparison between the conventional surgical and laser procedure," *Minerva Stomatologica*, vol. 62, no. 8, Supplement 1, pp. 45–53, 2013.

[10] M. Haytac and O. Ozcelik, "Evaluation of patient perceptions after frenectomy operations: a comparison of carbon dioxide laser and scalpel techniques," *Journal of Periodontology*, vol. 77, no. 11, pp. 1815–1819, 2006.

[11] H. A. Wigdor, J. T. Walsh, J. D. B. Featherstone, S. R. Visuri, D. Fried, and J. L. Waldvogel, "Lasers in dentistry," *Lasers in Surgery and Medicine*, vol. 16, no. 2, pp. 103–133, 1995.

[12] F. Schwarz, A. Aoki, A. Sculean, and J. Becker, "The impact of laser application on periodontal and peri-implant wound healing," *Periodontology 2000*, vol. 51, no. 1, pp. 79–108, 2009.

[13] R. J. Harris, "A comparison of two techniques of obtaining a connective tissue graft from the palate," *International Journal of Periodontics & Restorative Dentistry*, vol. 17, no. 3, pp. 261–272, 1997.

[14] J. Matter, "Creeping attachment of free gingival grafts: a five-year follow-up study," *Journal of Periodontology*, vol. 51, no. 12, pp. 681–685, 1980.

[15] S. Nelson, "The subpedicle connective tissue graft. A bilaminar reconstructive procedure for the coverage of denuded root surfaces," *Journal of Periodontology*, vol. 58, no. 2, pp. 95–102, 1987.

[16] R. J. Harris, "Creeping attachment associated with the connective tissue with partial-thickness double pedicle graft," *Journal of Periodontology*, vol. 68, no. 9, pp. 890–899, 1997.

[17] N. K. Soldatos, K. Font, and C. A. Powell, "Creeping attachment after xenogeneic collagen matrix placement for multiple recessions treatment: a discussion of two case reports," *Journal of Implant and Advanced Clinical Dentistry*, vol. 8, no. 6, pp. 6–14, 2016.

27

Oral Lichenoid Reaction: An Uncommon Side Effect of Rituximab

Amerigo Giudice, Francesco Liborio, Fiorella Averta, Selene Barone, and Leonzio Fortunato

School of Dentistry, Department of Health Sciences, Magna Graecia University of Catanzaro, Catanzaro, Italy

Correspondence should be addressed to Amerigo Giudice; a.giudice@unicz.it

Academic Editor: Ronald S. Brown

Oral lichenoid reactions (OLR) can be caused by systemic drug exposure. To the best of our knowledge, this is the second report describing a case of OLR induced by rituximab administration in a patient with a diagnosis of non-Hodgkin B-cell lymphoma. After 5 doses of rituximab, a typical pattern of OLP was identified with bilateral and symmetrical lesions on the buccal mucosa and on the right lingual margin. This temporal relationship suggested a probable association between oral lesions and drug therapy. The clinical diagnosis of a rituximab-induced OLR was confirmed by an incisional biopsy reporting a histopathological result of lichenoid mucositis consistent with oral lichen planus. Because of the increasing use of rituximab, it is necessary to know and recognize this uncommon side effect.

1. Introduction

Lichen planus-like lesion can be an uncommon cutaneous and mucosal adverse effect of several drugs. Despite the different etiology, it can be very challenging to distinguish oral lichenoid drug reactions (OLDRs) from oral lichen planus (OLP) with immune-mediated pathogenesis [1]. Histology can also be similar although some evidences suggest that neutrophils, eosinophils, and plasma cells can be found more in depth in drug-induced lesions [2–4].

In literature, few cases of cutaneous lichenoid reactions have been reported after administration of different anti-CD20 monoclonal antibodies [5]. Among these, rituximab is a monoclonal antibody usually used in the treatment of non-Hodgkin's lymphoma in the last 20 years [6, 7]. It is generally well-tolerated by most patients even after a long-term administration [6, 8, 9].

In this study, we present a case of rituximab-induced OLDR.

2. Case

A 40-year-old woman was early diagnosed with non-Hodgkin extranodal marginal-zone B-cell lymphoma of the parotid glands. She was immediately treated with 375 mg infusion of rituximab (Truxima, Mundipharma Pharmaceuticals S.r.l.) including 8 administrations: the first four doses every 15 days and the remaining ones given every month. After the 5th dose the patient presented a diffuse stomatitis, together with joint pain and pink papules on her trunk and legs. A decrement of ferritin was also observed. Her past medical history was unremarkable, and before therapy, she did not report lesions or symptoms to the mouth, skin, neither genitals. Furthermore, she also did not use oral hygiene products or assume any other drug compatible with such clinical findings.

During the intraoral examination, carried out one month after the therapy conclusion, ulcers with white keratotic halos and peripheral erythema were found. A typical pattern of OLP was identified with bilateral and symmetrical lesions on the buccal mucosa (Figure 1) and on the right lingual margin (Figure 2).

Symptomatology was exacerbated by the assumption of certain acid foods. Based on the chronological order of the appearance of lesions, the clinical diagnosis of a rituximab-induced OLDR was confirmed by an incisional biopsy. Indeed, histopathological result reported a CD8 T-lymphocyte bandlike infiltrate close to the basal membrane, an alteration of the dermoepidermal junction and several

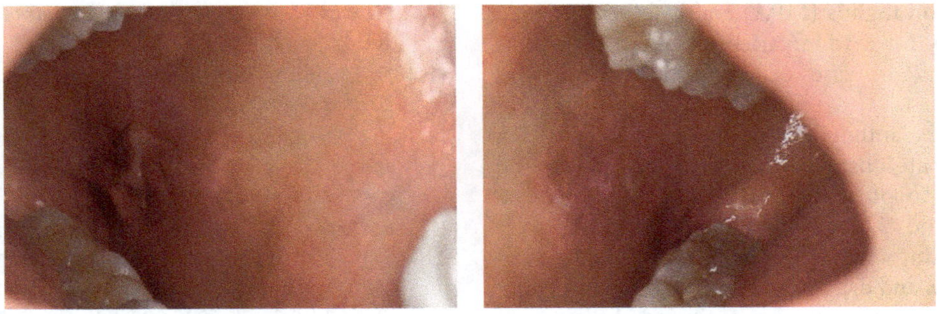

(a) (b)

FIGURE 1: After rituximab therapy, ulcers surrounded by white reticulation and erythema on the left buccal mucosa (a), right buccal mucosa (b), can be observed.

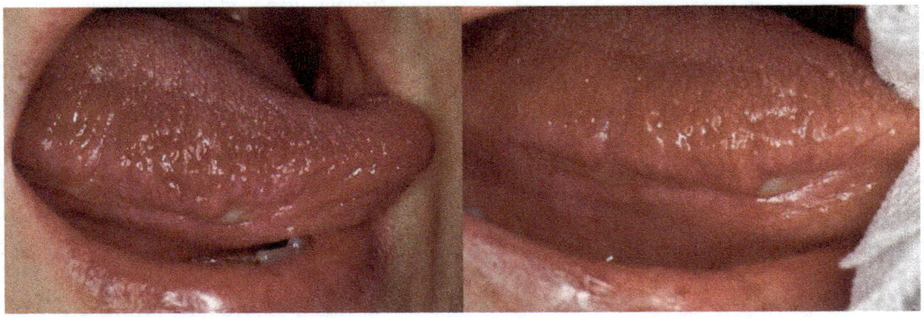

FIGURE 2: Extensive ulcer localized on the right margin of the tongue.

areas of keratinocyte necrosis; few CD4 T-lymphocytes and rare CD20 B-cells were also found.

Despite the appearance of OLDR as side effects, the therapy with rituximab was effective; indeed, PET exam showed a tumor regression one month after the last administration of the drug.

The patient was treated with intralesional injections of 0.5 mL triamcinolone acetonide (Kenacort 40 mg/mL; HanAll Biopharma). The injection was carried out on both buccal mucosae once a week for 8 weeks, until the complete remission of symptomatology and almost 50% decrease in ulcer size overall. It was decided not to administer systemic corticosteroid. At 6-month follow-up, 9 months after rituximab withdrawal, oral symptomatology did not relapse; skin lesions and joint pain have autonomously healed while oral ulcers did not completely disappear.

3. Discussion

Oral lichenoid reactions may result from systemic drug exposure involving the skin, oral mucosa, or both. A temporal relationship between initiation of medication and onset of OLDRs may not be readily apparent: for this reason, a thorough history of systemic medication use over the preceding 12-14 months should be obtained [10–12]. OLDRs have been reported in association with many systemic medications, the most common of which include nonsteroidal anti-inflammatory drugs, antihypertensives, oral hypoglycemic agents, beta-blockers, and HIV antiretrovirals [3, 13, 14]. These lesions can be symptomatic or not, and drug withdrawal does not ensure healing.

OLDR is less common than cutaneous lichenoid drug reaction and may occur without skin involvement [3, 11]. OLDRs are common in adults but have been rarely reported in pediatric patients [15, 16].

In 2012, a case study conducted by Bakkour and Coulson reported a widespread cutaneous lichenoid eruption related to the administration of obinutuzumab, a new anti-CD20 monoclonal antibody, in a patient with relapsed follicular lymphoma previously treated with rituximab [5]. Two years later, Kuten-Shorrer et al. reported the first case of OLDR in a patient treated with rituximab for a stage IIIA follicular lymphoma [17].

Rituximab, a chimeric monoclonal antibody whose target is the B-cell CD20 antigen, is a type I monoclonal anti-CD20 antibody that has been approved for the treatment of non-Hodgkin lymphoma [18]. It showed few adverse effects, and the onset of the reaction in the reported cases ranged from 1 to 13 weeks [11, 18]. The most common side effects with rituximab intravenous administration are infusion-related alterations (such as fever, nausea, headache, chills, and rigors) while other less common reactions include infections, hypotension, hypoxia, bronchospasm, rash, and pruritus [6, 9, 11, 18].

Initially used as an antitumoral agent, rituximab became an encouraging treatment choice in B-cell-driven systemic inflammatory and autoimmune diseases (SIADs) and it is now approved for treatment of rheumatoid arthritis (RA), granulomatosis with polyangiitis (GPA), and microscopic polyangiitis (MPA) and is frequently used as off-label therapy for a wide variety of other SIADs like pemphigus vulgaris, in case of conventional treatment failure [9, 19, 20].

In this paper, the authors describe a rare case of OLDR where the rituximab dose administered was lower and shorter compared to other reports. Side effects appeared after 3 months and 5 doses totally administered. This temporal relationship suggested a probable association between oral lesions and drug administration. In that period, the patient did not receive any other antitumoral therapy. It is noteworthy that rituximab activity leads to the suppression of antigen presentation, the inhibition of T-cell recruitment, and the IFN-alpha pathway preventing, eventually, B-cell expansion [6, 12]. For this beneficial effect, recently, it has been used to treat severe and persistent lichenoid drug reaction [12, 21, 22].

Rituximab has been widely used in patients diagnosed with lymphoma, and its use is increasing in cases of a wide spread of autoimmune diseases. The authors presenting this unusual side effect believe its recognition is crucial and should not be underestimated in order to achieve a better clinical management of the patient.

References

[1] C. Scully and M. Carrozzo, "Oral mucosal disease: lichen planus," *British Journal of Oral and Maxillofacial Surgery*, vol. 46, no. 1, article S0266435607003725, pp. 15–21, 2008.

[2] M. Mravak-Stipetić, B. Lončar-Brzak, I. Bakale-Hodak et al., "Clinicopathologic correlation of oral lichen planus and oral lichenoid lesions: a preliminary study," *The Scientific World Journal*, vol. 2014, Article ID 746874, 6 pages, 2014.

[3] B. E. McCartan and C. E. McCreary, "Oral lichenoid drug eruptions," *Oral Diseases*, vol. 3, no. 2, pp. 58–63, 1997.

[4] L. Fortunato, S. Barone, F. Bennardo, and A. Giudice, "Management of facial pyoderma gangrenosum using platelet-rich fibrin: a technical report," *Journal of Oral and Maxillofacial Surgery*, vol. 76, no. 7, pp. 1460–1463, 2018.

[5] W. Bakkour and I. H. Coulson, "GA101 (a novel anti-CD20 monoclonal antibody) induced lichenoid eruption," *Dermatology and Therapy*, vol. 2, no. 1, p. 3, 2012.

[6] G. Salles, M. Barrett, R. Foà et al., "Rituximab in B-cell hematologic malignancies: a review of 20 years of clinical experience," *Advances in Therapy*, vol. 34, no. 10, pp. 2232–2273, 2017.

[7] S. Guastafierro, U. Falcone, M. Celentano, S. Cappabianca, A. Giudice, and G. Colella, "Primary mantle-cell non-Hodgkin's lymphoma of the tongue," *International Journal of Hematology*, vol. 88, no. 2, pp. 206–208, 2008.

[8] Q. Chen, T. Ayer, L. J. Nastoupil et al., "Initial management strategies for follicular lymphoma," *International Journal of Hematologic Oncology*, vol. 1, no. 1, pp. 35–45, 2012.

[9] J. Vikse, K. Jonsdottir, J. T. Kvaløy, K. Wildhagen, and R. Omdal, "Tolerability and safety of long-term rituximab treatment in systemic inflammatory and autoimmune diseases," *Rheumatology International*, vol. 39, no. 6, pp. 1083–1090, 2019.

[10] P. B. Sugerman and N. W. Sabage, "Oral lichen planus: causes, diagnosis and management," *Australian Dental Journal*, vol. 47, no. 4, pp. 290–297, 2002.

[11] N. Scheinfeld, "A review of rituximab in cutaneous medicine," *Dermatology Online Journal*, vol. 12, no. 1, 2006.

[12] K. El-Reshaid and S. Al-Bader, "Rituximab therapy for severe and persistent lichenoid drug reaction," *Journal of Drug Delivery and Therapeutics*, vol. 9, no. 3-s, pp. 751–753, 2019.

[13] R. Clayton, S. Chaudhry, I. Ali, S. Cooper, T. Hodgson, and F. Wojnarowska, "Mucosal (oral and vulval) lichen planus in women: are angiotensin-converting enzyme inhibitors protective, and beta-blockers and non-steroidal anti-inflammatory drugs associated with the condition?," *Clinical and Experimental Dermatology*, vol. 35, no. 4, pp. 384–387, 2010.

[14] A. T. Güneš, E. Fetil, T. İlknur, B. Birgin, and Ş. Özkan, "Naproxen-induced lichen planus: report of 55 cases," *International Journal of Dermatology*, vol. 45, no. 6, pp. 709–712, 2006.

[15] V. Woo, J. Bonks, L. Borukhova, and D. Zegarelli, "Oral lichenoid drug eruption: a report of a pediatric case and review of the literature," *Pediatric Dermatology*, vol. 26, no. 4, pp. 458–464, 2009.

[16] V. Ridola, E. Mahe, O. Fawaz, L. Galmiche, C. Patte, and J. Grill, "Dactinomycin-Induced, Severe Lichenoid Eruption in a Child," *Pediatric Dermatology*, vol. 23, no. 5, pp. 503–506, 2006.

[17] M. Kuten-Shorrer, E. P. Hochberg, and S. B. Woo, "Lichenoid mucosal reaction to rituximab," *The Oncologist*, vol. 19, no. 10, pp. e12–e13, 2014.

[18] E. Kimby, "Tolerability and safety of rituximab (MabThera®)," *Cancer Treatment Reviews*, vol. 31, no. 6, pp. 456–473, 2005.

[19] K. Muhammad, P. Roll, H. Einsele, T. Dörner, and H. P. Tony, "Delayed acquisition of somatic hypermutations in repopulated IGD+CD27+ memory B cell receptors after rituximab treatment," *Arthritis & Rheumatism*, vol. 60, no. 8, pp. 2284–2293, 2009.

[20] H. H. Wang, C. W. Liu, Y. C. Li, and Y. C. Huang, "Efficacy of rituximab for pemphigus: a systematic review and meta-analysis of different regimens," *Acta Dermato-Venereologica*, vol. 95, no. 8, pp. 928–932, 2015.

[21] K. Heelan, M. A. McAleer, L. Roche, C. McCreary, and M. Murphy, "Intractable erosive lichen planus treated successfully with rituximab," *British Journal of Dermatology*, vol. 172, no. 2, pp. 538–540, 2015.

[22] L. Parmentier, B. A. Bron, C. Prins, J. Samson, I. Masouyé, and L. Borradori, "Mucocutaneous lichen planus with esophageal involvement," *Archives of Dermatology*, vol. 144, no. 11, pp. 1427–1430, 2008.

An Uncommon Case of Plasma Cell Mucositis of the Tongue in a Young Man

Alessandro Antonelli,[1] Fiorella Averta,[1] Federica Diodati,[1] Danila Muraca,[1] Ylenia Brancaccio,[1] Chiara Mignogna,[2] and Amerigo Giudice[1]

[1]*School of Dentistry, Department of Health Sciences, "Magna Graecia" University of Catanzaro, Italy*
[2]*Interdepartmental Service Center, "Magna Graecia" University of Catanzaro, Italy*

Correspondence should be addressed to Alessandro Antonelli; antonellicz@gmail.com

Academic Editor: Evanthia Chrysomali

Plasma cell mucositis (PCM) is an unusual plasma cell proliferative disorder of the upper aerodigestive tract. It is a rare disease, and its etiology is not yet known with variable clinical features. Symptoms include dysphagia, oral pain, and swelling. We described a case of PCM involving the tongue of a 14-year-old man. In the first place, several diagnostic hypotheses were proposed, most of them discarded for incompatibility with blood and laboratory tests. This disease rarely manifests itself on the tongue, especially in young patients with no comorbidities. The management of PCM is mainly aimed at reducing the symptoms, and in our report, the treatment involved the use of systemic prednisone with an improvement of the quality of life. At 1-year follow-up, there was no recurrence of the disease. Many therapeutic treatments are able to stabilize but not able to induce a complete remission. PCM is considered an uncommon benign disorder with a favorable prognosis and should be considered in the differential diagnosis with other inflammatory or neoplastic conditions.

1. Introduction

Plasma cell mucositis (PCM) is an unusual plasma cell proliferative disorder of the upper aerodigestive tract [1]. In the past, this pathology has been reported under various names. The name indicated the anatomical structure involved together with the component of plasma cells, such as idiopathic plasmacytosis of the gingiva, plasma cell vulvitis, oral papillary plasmacytosis, or mucous membrane plasmacytosis of the upper aerodigestive tract [2]. It is a rare disease, and its etiology is not yet known; it is considered a benign condition of adults, and there are no correlations in literature with the development of plasma cell neoplasm. Clinical features are an intensely erythematous mucosa with papillomatous, cobblestone, nodular, or velvety surface changes. Symptoms include dysphagia, oral pain, sore throat, and pharyngitis [2]. PCM can be treated with corticosteroids, administrated topically, systemically, or intralesionally. Usually, the treatment is not resolutive; however, the main outcome is the improvement of the symptoms. Generally, PCM patients have a previous history of an autoimmune or immunologically mediated disease like Sjögren syndrome or possible autoimmune hepatitis; however, these are not present in all cases and no single disease is consistently associated.

2. Case Report

We described a case of PCM involving the tongue of a 14-year-old man. The patient was referred to the Oral Pathology Unit at the Faculty of Dentistry, Magna Graecia University of Catanzaro, in August 2019. The referring practitioner suspected squamous cell carcinoma. His past medical history was not relevant, and the patient was a nonsmoker and nonalcohol user. The patient had previously used a nocturnal bite to control bruxism. He reported a burning sensation in his mouth, local dysgeusia, and pain on the tip and on the right lingual border for 1 year. The patient also referred that he was unable to eat or drink any hot or spicy foods

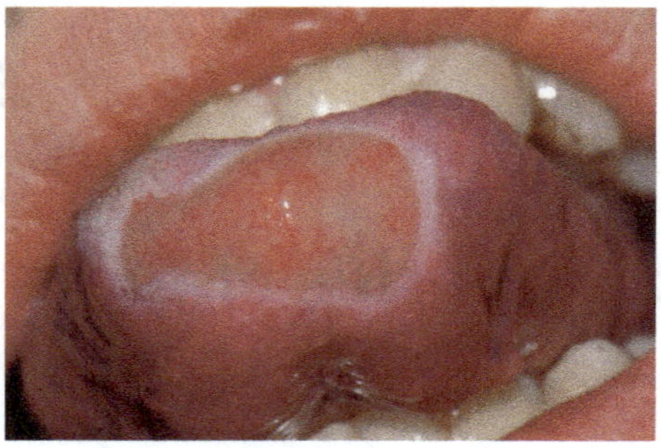

Figure 1: Ulceration on the tip of the tongue.

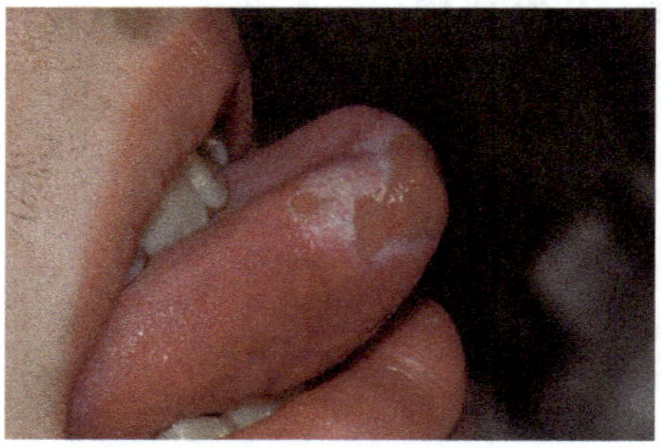

Figure 2: Lateral view of the tongue.

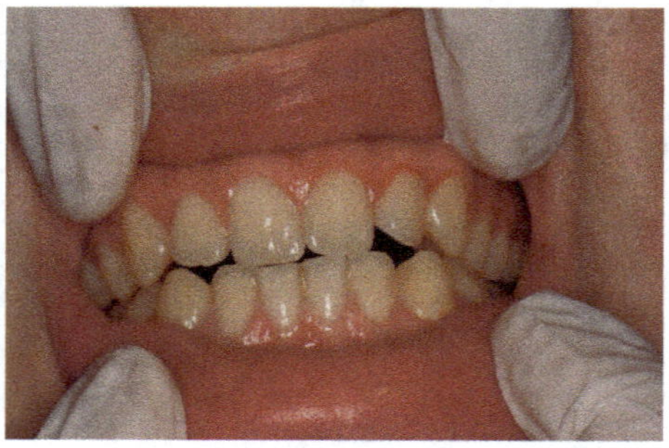

Figure 3: Gingival edema and erythema.

due to burning and pain on his tongue. He stated persistent hoarseness, sore throat, and difficulty sleeping due to continuous oral pain.

Extraoral examination was unremarkable, while intraoral examination revealed the presence of an ulcer and intense erythema of the tongue (Figures 1 and 2) and gingival edema and erythema (Figure 3); however, the other parts of the oral mucosa was clinically normal. In the first place, several diagnostic hypotheses were proposed, most of them discarded for incompatibility with full blood count, serum B12 and folate, urea and electrolytes, liver function tests, glucose, antinuclear antibody, and syphilis IgG that were normal or negative. The patient underwent an incisional biopsy under local anesthesia. The specimen was stored in a tube containing formalin 10% and sent to a laboratory for histopathological analysis. Microscopically, a large area of ulceration of the coating epithelium subtended by dense plasma cell infiltrate was observed (Figures 4 and 5). CD20 and CD3 showed focal positivity for B and T cells, respectively. The plasma cell

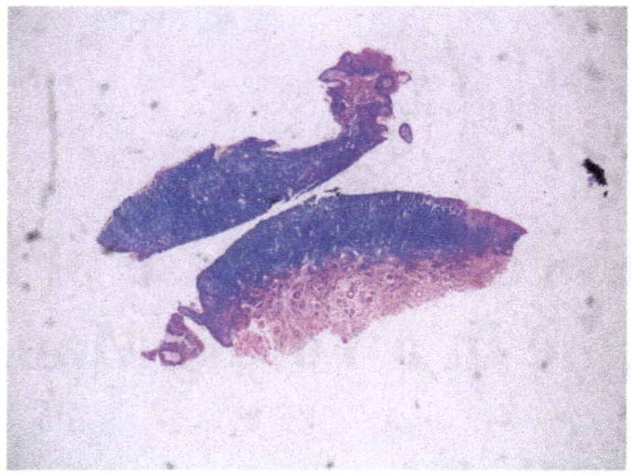

Figure 4: Medium-power hematoxylin and eosine-stained biopsy sample from the tongue mucosa showing a dense polyclonal plasmacytic inflammatory infiltrate throughout the connective tissue.

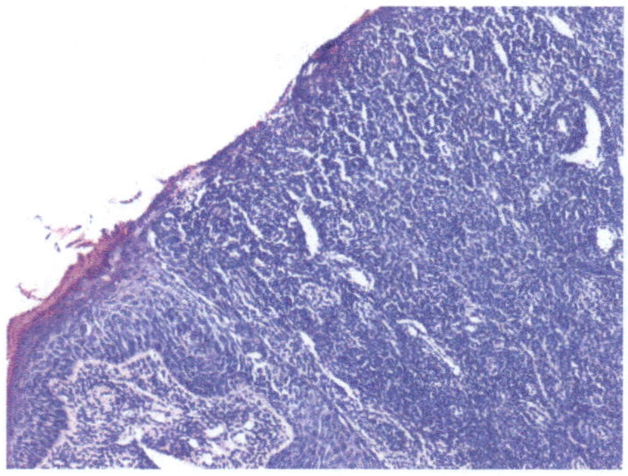

Figure 5: Histological examination of a biopsy taken from the tongue showed a denuded surface epithelium with the superficial and mid dermis demonstrating a dense infiltration of plasma cells.

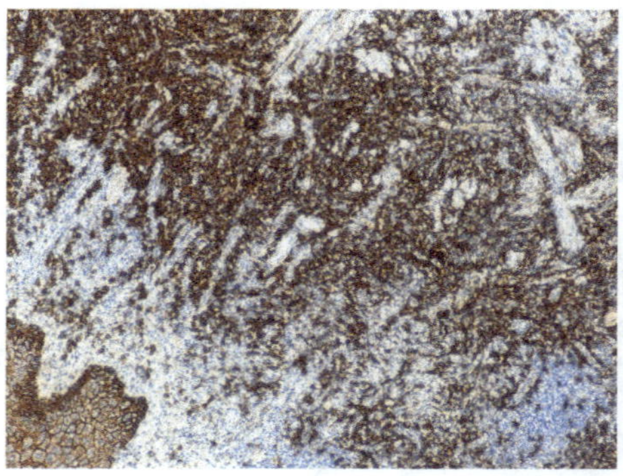

Figure 6: CD138. A high-power view shows a monomorphic population of mature plasma cells (×10).

infiltrate was positive for CD138 (Figures 6 and 7) and showed kappa light chain restriction (Figures 8 and 9) with a kappa/-lambda ratio of 20 : 1 (Figures 10 and 11). The final histopathological diagnosis was "plasmacytosis of the mucous membranes with restriction for the kappa chains." Initial pharmacotherapy with prednisone began with 50 mg/day for two weeks, and the patient referred an improvement of his conditions (reduction of pain and swelling). He repeated this treatment one month later, and he experienced a partial

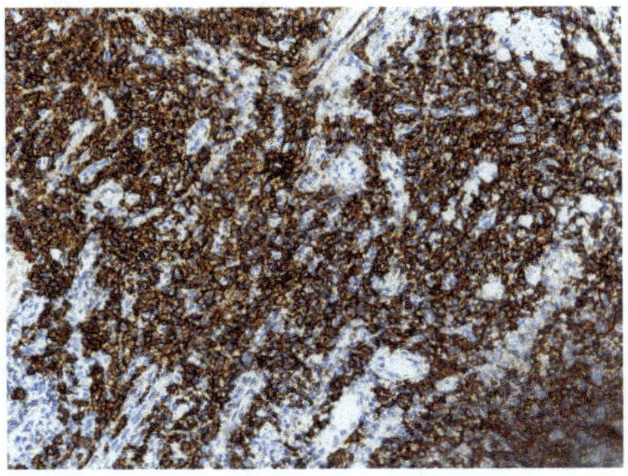

FIGURE 7: CD138. A high-power view shows a monomorphic population of mature plasma cells (×20).

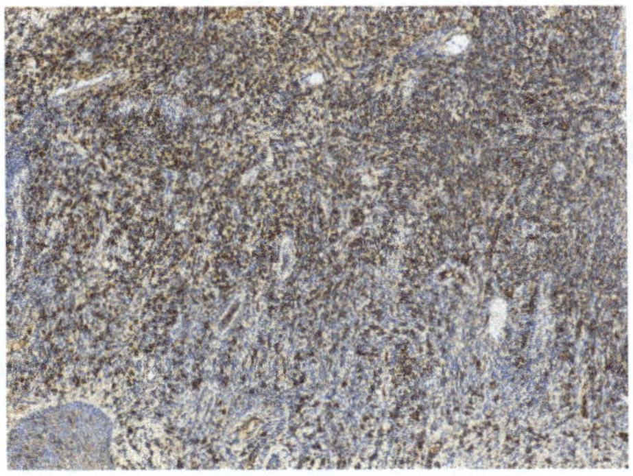

FIGURE 8: Plasma cells showing kappa light chain restriction (×10).

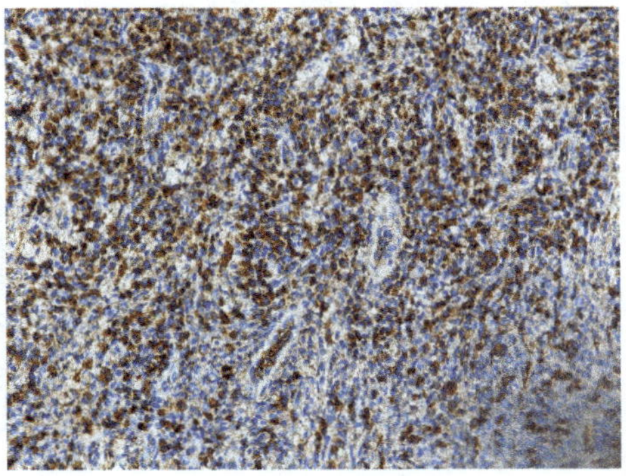

FIGURE 9: Plasma cells showing kappa light chain restriction (×20).

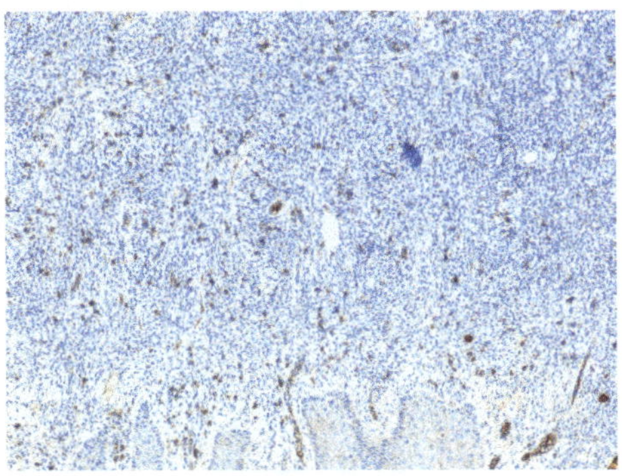

FIGURE 10: Plasma cells showing lambda light chain restriction (×10).

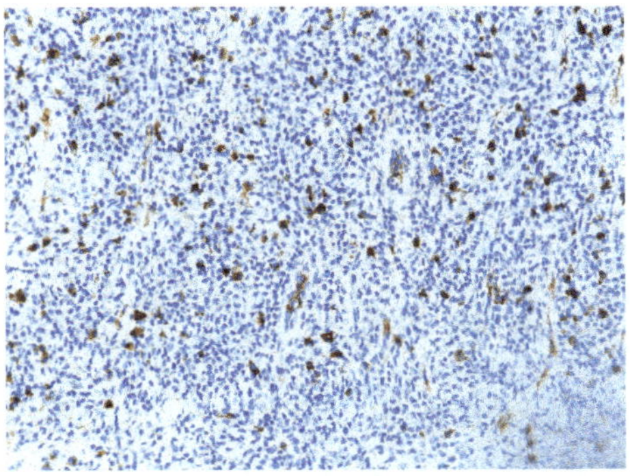

FIGURE 11: Plasma cells showing lambda light chain restriction (×20).

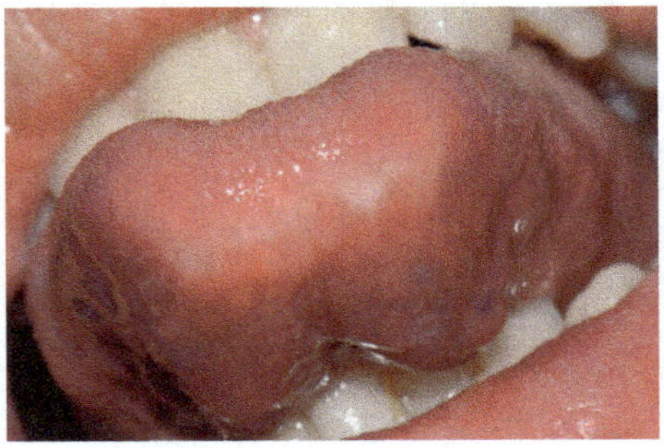

FIGURE 12: Follow-up at 1 year.

regression of the lesions. At 1-year follow-up, there was no regression of the disease and no recurrence of the lesions (Figure 12).

3. Discussion

Plasma cell mucositis (PCM) is an idiopathic disorder histologically characterized by dense infiltrates of lymphocytes and plasma cells in submucosa. Usually, the lesions are mainly observed on the mucosal surfaces, vulva and penis, gingiva, lips, tongue, buccal mucosa, epiglottis, and larynx.

A review of the English-language literature was performed. The keywords "plasma cell mucositis" and "oral" were entered in the search fields of PubMed. 103 results were identified. Another research was performed including the keywords "plasmacytosis" and "oral." 40 results were identified. The research was conducted by considering the articles published until November 2019. Excluded were cases that were not about the oral cavity, not in English, not human study, and not compatible with the PCM diagnosis or report lacking immunohistochemical analysis. According to the exclusion criteria, we selected 26 studies [1–26] that included 45 cases of PCM. We analysed patients' age, gender, symptoms, lesion location, treatment, and follow-up. The principal features and data pertaining the selected cases are compiled in Table 1. Age data were available in all selected studies, and the average age was 56.06 ± 16.33 years. The youngest patient was 13 years old [17] and the oldest 83 years old [20]. All studies included in our review reported the gender of the subjects. The analysis of the data collected

Table 1: Review of PCM.

Study/year of publication	Age*	Gender	Symptoms	Location of the lesions	Treatment	Follow-up
Poswillo et al. [7]/1967	37	F	Redness, swelling	Gingiva	Resection, oral hygiene programme	AWD, 2 years
	39	F	Redness, hypertrophy	Gingiva	Resection	Not available
	21	F	Hyperplastic red lesion, hypertrophy, erythema	Maxillary labial vestibule, gingiva	Resection, oral hygiene programme	Not available
White et al. [3]/1986	47	F	Dysphonia, sore throat	Lips, mouth, tongue, supraglottic larynx	Resection, prednisone	AWD, 9 years (f/u reported by Ferreiro et al. [1])
Timms et al. [8]/1988	70	F	Hoarseness, cough, stridor	Gingiva, supraglottic, hard palate	CO_2 laser, prednisolone, topical steroid spray	AWD, 1 year
Timms and Sloan [9]/1991	32	F	Hoarseness, sore throat	Gingiva, false cord, mucobuccal	Systemic and topical steroids	Marginal improvement, no f/u epiglottis
Ferreiro et al. [1]/1994	60	F	Dysphonia, dysphagia	Supraglottic larynx	CO_2 laser, prednisone, antibiotics, beclomethasone (Vanceril) spray	AWD, 1 year
	41	M	Dysphonia, stridor	Supraglottic, glottic larynx, nose, pharynx	Antibiotics	AWD, 7 years; tracheostomy
	62	F	Dysphonia, stridor, dry eyes, dysphagia	Supraglottic, glottic larynx, trachea	Not available	AWD, 16 years; tracheostomy
	54	M	Dysphonia	Supraglottic, glottic larynx	Resection	AWD, 1 year
	40	M	Dysphonia, sore mouth	Lips, tongue, palate, pharynx, supraglottic & glottic larynx	Prednisone, isotretinoin (Accutane), CO_2 laser	AWD, 15 years; sleep apnea
	67	M	Sore mouth	Lips, mouth, tongue, palate	Prednisone	AWD, 3 years
	61	M	Unknown	Lips through larynx	Not available	Not available
	56	M	Unknown	Nose, palate, pharynx	Resection	Not available
Van de Kerkhof and Van Baar [26]/1995	80	F	Pain, soreness, erythema, swelling	Lips	Betamethasone dipropionate	Partial symptomatic relief, f/u not available
	57	F	Sore throat	Gingiva, supraglottic larynx	Topical steroids	Gingival improvement, no f/u
Khan et al. [5]/1997	69	M	Hoarseness, dysphagia, hemoptysis	Left faucial pillar, hypopharynx, epiglottis, larynx	Beclomethasone spray, Corsodyl mouthwash	No recurrence, 20 months f/u
Noorily [25]/1997	67	M	Induration, erythema, crusting	Lower lip	Resection, primary closure	Not available
Smith et al. [4]/1999	59	M	Swelling, hoarseness, sore throat, erythema	Soft palate, gingiva, oropharynx, nasopharynx	None	Asymptomatic, 6 months f/u

Table 1: Continued.

Study/year of publication	Age*	Gender	Symptoms	Location of the lesions	Treatment	Follow-up
Kaur et al. [24]/2001	47	M	Swelling, erythema, inflammation	Upper lip	Triamcinolone acetonide injections	No recurrence, 3 months f/u
Bharti and Smith [10]/2003	42	F	Pain, dysphagia	Buccal mucosa, palate	Topical and systemic antifungals, corticosteroids	Partial symptomatic relief, no regression of the disease, no f/u
Heinemann et al. [23]/2006	61	F	Pain, ulcerations, erythema, erosions	Tongue, lips, buccal mucosa, vulvae	Prednisolone, cyclosporin	Complete remission, 6 months f/u
Solomon et al. [2]/2008	60	F	Pain, sore throat, erosions, swelling, erythema	Gingiva, lips, ventral tongue, hard palate	Prednisone	Disease remission, f/u not available
Senol et al. [11]/2008	46	M	Inflammation, maceration, pruritic, eczema	Oral commissures, gingivobuccal mucosa, toe-webs, groins, preputium, perineum, umbilicus	Prednisolone	No recurrence, 1 year f/u
Najarian et al. [12]/2008	56	M	Pain, impetigo, bleeding	Lower lip	Topical and systemic glucocorticosteroid, cryotherapy	No recurrence, 6 months f/u
Pepper et al. [13]/2009	77	M	Atrophy, hyperkeratosis, erosion, pain	Commissure, lips, cheek	Tacrolimus, methotrexate, betamethasone mouthwash, CO_2 laser, radiotherapy	Onset of squamous cell carcinoma, partial resolution of mucosal plasmacytosis
Puvanendran et al. [22]/2012	74	M	Ulceration, erythema	Uvula, hypopharyngeal wall	Resection	Lesion resolved, 6 months f/u
Gupta et al. [21]/2014	72	M	Difficulty in swallowing, soreness, burning sensation, sore throat, ulcerations, swelling, bleeding gums, erosions	Buccal mucosa, palate, tongue, pharynx, gingiva	Topical corticosteroids (betamethasone 1 mg, triamcinolone acetonide gel 0.1%), prednisolone, topical antifungals	Partial symptomatic relief, no regression of the disease, no f/u
Madhavarajan and Tighe [15]/2015	63	M	Pain, ulceration	Commissure, buccal mucosa, gingiva	No treatment	Spontaneous resolving, 6 months f/u
Cottom et al. [20]/2015	54	F	Erythema	Soft palate	Not available	Not available
	51	M	Erythema, ulceration, erosions	Border of tongue	Not available	Not available
	50	M	Inflammation	Gingiva	Not available	Not available
	67	M	Pain, bleeding, erosions	Gingiva	Not available	Not available
	83	F	Erosions	Gingiva	Not available	Not available
	65	M	Inflammation	Gingiva, hard palate	Not available	Not available
	72	M	Inflammation	Gingiva	Not available	Not available

Table 1: Continued.

Study/year of publication	Age*	Gender	Symptoms	Location of the lesions	Treatment	Follow-up
Galvin et al. [14]/2016	68	F	Erythema, ulceration	Alveolar ridges, palate, buccal mucosa, gingiva	Oral fluconazole, chlorhexidine mouthwash, betamethasone cream and tablets	AWD, 7 years
	61	F	Sore mouth, ulceration, erythema, edema	Gingiva, buccal mucosa	Prednisolone, adalimumab	No recurrence, 18 months
	69	M	Oropharynx congestion	Gingiva, dorsum and borders of the tongue, soft palate, uvula	Mycophenolate mofetil, prednisolone	Partial symptomatic relief, no regression of the disease, no f/u
Trehan et al. [19]/2016	39	M	Ulceration, dysphagia, erosions	Lips, buccal mucosa, gingiva	Prednisolone	Good response, f/u not available
Arun et al. [17]/2017	13	M	Swelling, bleeding, erythema,	Upper lip, gingiva	Triamcinolone acetonide injections,	No recurrence, 1 year f/u
Liu et al. [18]/2017	18	F	Swelling, bleeding, erosions, pain	Lips	Methylprednisolone, dapsone, hydroxychloroquine, antibiotics	Symptoms decreasing, 6 months f/u
Gasparro et al. [6]/2019	78	F	Pain, erythema, ulcerations, erosions	Buccal mucosa	Injectable platelet-rich fibrin (i-PRF)	No complete healing, inflammation reduction, 6 months f/u
Shanahan et al. [16]/2019	62	F	Dry mouth, ulceration, swelling, dysphagia, hoarseness	Soft palate, buccal mucosa	Prednisolone, dapsone, mycophenolate mofetil	No recurrence of symptoms, 1 year f/u

AWD: alive with disease; F: female; f/u: follow-up; M: male. *Age at presentation (years).

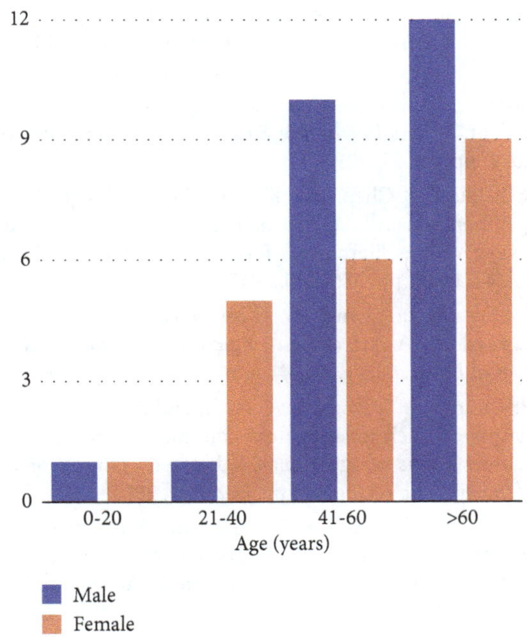

FIGURE 13: Distribution of age and sex in the 45 cases of PCM of the oral cavity reviewed.

suggested a male predilection with a male-to-female ratio of 1.25 : 1 (45 cases: 25 M, 20 F). A graph of the age and gender distribution is reported in Figure 13. Rarely the lesions are isolated, and in 45 cases reviewed, the oral cavity zones most affected by the lesions were the gingiva (20 cases), the lips (14 cases), the upper aerodigestive tract (13 cases), the palate (12 cases), the buccal mucosa (11 cases), and the tongue (8 cases). In our review, the symptoms most present are typical of inflammation with a particular interest of the oropharynx; the main symptoms are erythema (13 cases), pain (10 cases), swelling (9 cases), sore throat (7 cases), dysphonia, and dysphagia (6 cases). The analysis of the treatment evidenced 24 cases (53.3%) treated with corticosteroids in different forms (systemic, topical, and injections), and in 10 cases of these, there was no recurrence of the disease.

Plasma cell mucositis (PCM) is classified as idiopathic and rarely manifests itself on the tongue, especially in young patients with no comorbidities. Despite the fact that plasma cell mucositis often involves the oral and genital mucosa [3], there was no genital involvement in this circumstance. Since it is a very rare pathology, in the diagnosis of PCM, it is important to exclude other pathologies with similar pathological features, such as erosive lichen planus, mucous membrane pemphigoid, sarcoidosis, allergic gingivostomatitis, extramedullary plasmacytoma, rhinoscleroma, pemphigus, erythroplasia, squamous cell carcinoma, and fungal infections [4, 5]. Lichen planus is a chronic-relapsing inflammatory disease, with cutaneous and mucous involvement. It can be distinguished in oral lichen planus (OLP) and oral lichenoid drug reactions (OLDRs). The lesions may cause pain and, generally, appear as white patches with erosive aspects. A typical OLP model is identified with bilateral and symmetrical lesions; moreover, a hyperkeratosis is observed in the lower epidermis and in the upper dermis [27]. Pemphigoid of the mucous membranes affects mainly older individuals, as well as the plasma cell mucositis. Unlike the PCM, it presents itself with erosions to the mucous membranes of variable gravity that are mainly located in the oral cavity [5]. Sarcoidosis is a rare acquired systemic granulomatous disease. The respiratory system is more interested, but in a smaller number of cases, there is the involvement of the oral and perioral mucosa. Oral lesions can be solitary or multiple; they appear as a well-delimited and occasionally ulcerated red swelling [28]. Allergic gingivostomatitis is the result of an immunologic injury reaction; it is a complex disease which can have more than one etiologic factor [29]. Extramedullary plasmacytoma is a tumor that rarely affects the head and neck, especially the upper airways, and the lesions are generally polypoidal in appearance [5]. Primary Non-Hodgkin's Lymphoma (NHL) can rarely arise from lymphoid tissue of the tongue and give manifestations that mimic PCM [30].

Several times, PCM lesions can enter into differential diagnosis with squamous cell carcinoma (SCC) [4–22]; in literature, there are cases in which a differential diagnosis was made with oral carcinoma and there is a case report where a SCC arose from a mucosal plasmacytosis [13]. Therefore, a correct diagnosis and adequate management of the disease are essential.

The management of PCM is mainly aimed at reducing the symptoms; in fact, the patient treatment involved the use of systemic prednisone 50 mg/day to improve his quality of life.

However, in literature, there are some reported cases where the use of PRF injections is associated with cortisone therapy [6]. The benefit of PRF is to allow a continuous release of growth factors, inducing neoangiogenesis and fibroblast activations. Therefore, PRF creates an optimal scaffold for the tissue healing process, with the advantage of low cost and easy to prepare [31].

Although many therapeutic treatments are able to stabilize the disease, they are not able to induce a complete remission. The condition is generally of long-standing duration and the disease has a significant impact on the patient's quality of life. The disease treatment is mainly targeted to the management of symptoms. PCM is considered an uncommon benign disorder with a favorable prognosis. The distinctions between the conditions that are present in the oral cavity with the histologic finding of a dense submucosal plasma cell infiltrate are not well documented in oral pathology literature.

4. Conclusion

It is important that PCM is recognized in the dental community, because diagnosis is dependent on clinical pathologic correlation. Only close communication between specialists in several disciplines prevented inappropriate treatment of a patient with an extremely rare condition. Nevertheless, it is very important to differentiate the PCM disease from other neoplastic conditions in order to achieve a better clinical management of the patients, so it is necessary to investigate this disease in depth.

References

[1] J. A. Ferreiro, E. V. Egorshin, K. D. Olsen, P. M. Banks, and L. H. Weiland, "Mucous membrane plasmacytosis of the upper aerodigestive tract. A clinicopathologic study," *The American Journal of Surgical Pathology*, vol. 18, no. 10, pp. 1048–1053, 1994.

[2] L. W. Solomon, R. O. Wein, I. Rosenwald, and N. Laver, "Plasma cell mucositis of the oral cavity: report of a case and review of the literature," *Oral Surgery, Oral Medicine, Oral Pathology, Oral Radiology, and Endodontics*, vol. 106, no. 6, pp. 853–860, 2008.

[3] J. W. White Jr., K. D. Olsen, and P. M. Banks, "Plasma cell orificial mucositis: report of a case and review of the literature," *Archives of Dermatology*, vol. 122, no. 11, pp. 1321–1324, 1986.

[4] M. E. Smith, A. J. Crighton, D. M. Chisholm, and R. E. Mountain, "Plasma cell mucositis: a review and case report," *Journal of Oral Pathology & Medicine*, vol. 28, no. 4, pp. 183–186, 1999.

[5] N. A. Khan, W. S. McKerrow, and T. J. Palmer, "Mucous membrane plasmacytosis of the upper aerodigestive tract. A case report with effective treatment," *The Journal of Laryngology & Otology*, vol. 111, no. 3, pp. 293–295, 1997.

[6] R. Gasparro, D. Adamo, M. Masucci, G. Sammartino, and M. D. Mignogna, "Use of injectable platelet-rich fibrin in the treatment of plasma cell mucositis of the oral cavity refractory to corticosteroid therapy: a case report," *Dermatologic Therapy*, vol. 32, no. 5, article 13062, 2019.

[7] D. Poswillo, "Plasmacytosis of the gingiva," *British Journal of Oral Surgery*, vol. 5, no. 3, article S0007117X67800611, pp. 194–202, 1967.

[8] M. S. Timms, P. Sloan, and A. Pace Balzan, "Idiopathic plasmacytosis of the oral and supraglottic mucosa," *The Journal of Laryngology & Otology*, vol. 102, no. 7, pp. 646–648, 1988.

[9] M. S. Timms and P. Sloan, "Association of supraglottic and gingival idiopathic plasmacytosis," *Oral Surgery, Oral Medicine, Oral Pathology*, vol. 71, no. 4, pp. 451–453, 1991.

[10] R. Bharti and D. R. Smith, "Mucous membrane plasmacytosis: a case report and review of the literature," *Dermatology Online Journal.*, vol. 9, no. 5, p. 15, 2003.

[11] M. Senol, A. Ozcan, N. E. Aydin, E. Hazneci, and N. Turan, "Intertriginous plasmacytosis with plasmoacanthoma: report of a typical case and review of the literature," *International Journal of Dermatology*, vol. 47, no. 3, pp. 265–268, 2008.

[12] D. J. Najarian, B. K. Rao, and A. S. Pappert, "A case of mucous membrane plasmacytosis successfully treated with cryotherapy," *Dermatology Online Journal*, vol. 14, no. 2, p. 6, 2008.

[13] T. Pepper, K. Shekar, M. Singh, and P. A. Brennan, "Squamous cell carcinoma arising in mucosal plasmacytosis," *British Journal of Oral and Maxillofacial Surgery*, vol. 48, no. 3, pp. 208–210, 2010.

[14] S. Galvin, C. Bowe, E. M. O. Regan, N. Conlon, S. R. Flint, and C. M. Healy, "Circumorificial plasmacytosis/plasma cell orificial mucositis: a case series and a review of the literature," *Oral Surgery, Oral Medicine, Oral Pathology and Oral Radiology*, vol. 122, no. 3, pp. e77–e81, 2016.

[15] S. Madhavarajan and J. Tighe, "Orofacial plasmacytosis: a management conundrum," *British Journal of Oral and Maxillofacial Surgery*, vol. 53, no. 4, pp. 399–402, 2015.

[16] D. Shanahan, D. Shipley, and K. Staines, "Plasma cell mucositis," *Ear, Nose, & Throat Journal*, article 145561319849001, 2019.

[17] K. Arun, M. Ambooken, S. S. Varghese, T. Varghese, and J. J. Mathew, "A rare case of plasma cell mucositis in a young patient," *Journal of Indian Society of Periodontology*, vol. 21, no. 1, pp. 63–65, 2017.

[18] R.-F. Liu, C. B. Chen, T. T. Kuo, and W. H. Chung, "Idiopathic lymphoplasmacellular mucositis of the lips: a case report and review of the literature," *Journal of Cutaneous Pathology*, vol. 44, no. 9, pp. 776–780, 2017.

[19] P. Trehan, E. Pang, N. Khirwadkar, A. Alsharqi, and R. Parslew, "A rare cause of mucositis," *Clinical and Experimental Dermatology*, vol. 41, no. 8, pp. 951-952, 2016.

[20] H. Cottom, A. J. Mighell, A. High, and A. C. Bateman, "Are plasma cell-rich inflammatory conditions of the oral mucosa manifestations of IgG4-related disease?," *Journal of Clinical Pathology*, vol. 68, no. 10, pp. 802–807, 2015.

[21] S. R. Gupta, R. Gupta, R. K. Saran, and S. Krishnan, "Plasma cell mucositis with gingival enlargement and severe periodontitis," *Journal of Indian Society of Periodontology*, vol. 18, no. 3, p. 379, 2014.

[22] M. Puvanendran, A. Lieder, and W. Issing, "Plasma Cell Mucositis of Oro- and Hypopharynx: A Case Report," *Case Reports in Otolaryngology*, vol. 2012, Article ID 304136, 3 pages, 2012.

[23] C. Heinemann, T. Fischer, U. Barta, A. Michaelides, and P. Elsner, "Plasma cell mucositis with oral and genital involvement–successful treatment with topical cyclosporin," *Journal of the European Academy of Dermatology and Venereology*, vol. 20, no. 6, pp. 739-740, 2006.

[24] C. Kaur, G. P. Thami, R. Sarkar, and A. J. Kanwar, "Plasma cell mucositis," *Journal of the European Academy of Dermatology and Venereology*, vol. 15, no. 6, pp. 566-567, 2001.

[25] A. D. Noorily, "Plasma cell orificial mucositis," *Otolaryngology - Head and Neck Surgery*, vol. 116, no. 3, pp. 416-417, 1997.

[26] P. C. M. Van de Kerkhof and H. M. J. Van Baar, "Co-occurrence of plasma cell orificial mucositis and plasmoacanthoma," *Dermatology*, vol. 191, no. 1, pp. 52–55, 1995.

[27] A. Giudice, F. Liborio, F. Averta, S. Barone, and L. Fortunato, "Oral lichenoid reaction: an uncommon side effect of rituximab," *Case Reports in Dentistry*, vol. 2019, Article ID 3154856, 3 pages, 2019.

[28] A. E. Kolokotronis, M. A. Belazi, G. Haidemenos, T. K. Zaraboukas, and D. Z. Antoniades, "Sarcoidosis: oral and perioral manifestations," *Hippokratia*, vol. 13, no. 2, pp. 119–121, 2009.

[29] R. E. Paul, D. Hoover, C. Dunlap, R. Gier, and T. Alms, "An immunologic investigation of atypical gingivostomatitis," *Journal of Periodontology*, vol. 49, no. 6, pp. 301–306, 1978.

[30] S. Guastafierro, U. Falcone, M. Celentano, S. Cappabianca, A. Giudice, and G. Colella, "Primary mantle-cell non-Hodgkin's lymphoma of the tongue," *International Journal of Hematology*, vol. 88, no. 2, pp. 206–208, 2008.

[31] L. Fortunato, S. Barone, F. Bennardo, and A. Giudice, "Management of facial pyoderma gangrenosum using platelet-rich fibrin: a technical report," *Journal of Oral and Maxillofacial Surgery*, vol. 76, no. 7, pp. 1460–1463, 2018.

29

Closure of Orocutaneous Fistula using Submandibular Gland as a Pedicled Flap

Erol Cansiz[1] **Emine Deniz Gozen,**[2] **and Murat Yener**[2]

[1]*Istanbul University, Faculty of Dentistry, Department of Oral and Maxillofacial Surgery, Turkey*
[2]*Istanbul Cerrahpasa University, Medical Faculty, Department of Otorhinolaryngology, Turkey*

Correspondence should be addressed to Erol Cansiz; erol.cansiz@istanbul.edu.tr

Academic Editor: Sukumaran Anil

Orocutaneous fistulas in the maxillofacial region may be due to tumor resection, osteoradionecrosis, or trauma, and these defects limit the function of the patients and effect aesthetic and also psychological condition. Articulation and nutrition are also affected by these fistulas. Local flaps can be used for the reconstruction of small- and medium-sized defects with ease. Submandibular gland with its rich blood supply from the facial artery is a practical and useful choice for the reconstruction of mandibular region defects.

1. Introduction

Orocutaneous (or orofacial) fistula is a pathological pathway between the oral cavity and the cutaneous surface of the face. The most common causes of the orocutaneous fistulas are malignancy, inflammation, and trauma, and they may lead to functional, aesthetic, and psychological problems due to the irrepressible leakage of saliva from the oral cavity to the face [1].

Literature search on this topic, by using "orocutaneous, fistula, closure" keywords, does not reveal convincing results about treatment options or incidence. There are few reports about the management of orocutaneous fistula. Balakrishnan et al. successfully used pedicled expanded deltopectoral flap to repair fistula in a patient with previous neck dissection and radiotherapy [2]. Another method is tissue plug technique in which the dermal component of a pedicle flap is advanced through the fistula, and with external traction, the tissue obliterates the tract [3]. Tian et al. used a vacuum-assisted closure system for the management of orocutaneous fistula and were able to treat most of their patients [4]. There are other techniques for the closure of orocutaneous fistulas. Local rotational flaps and advancement flaps, transpositional flaps, autogenous, alloplastic, or allogenic grafting techniques may be used for the reconstruction [5]. Each technique has pros and cons, and it is important to choose the right technique in the right situation.

As most of the orocutaneous fistula closes by conservative methods like antibiotic therapy, decrease of salivary secretions, packing, and nasogastric tube feeding, the orocutaneous fistulas are not regarded as a major complication. However, in the situation of a persistent fistula, great discomfort may occur both for the patient and the operator [6]. In this technical note, the closure of a resistant orocutaneous fistula by using submandibular gland as a pedicled flap is presented.

2. Case Report

A 56-year-old male patient, whose plasmacytoma was enucleated 3 years ago from the medial side of the left mandible, was referred to our clinic due to his complaints of persistent orocutaneous fistula (Figures 1–3). Past medical history revealed that the patient was operated three times to close the orocutaneous fistula by local flaps; however, none of these operations were successful. CT images of the patient demonstrated that the medial side of the left mandible was missing and there was a 3×2 cm diameter defect located between the left side of the mouth floor and the basis of the left mandible neighboring the left submandibular gland. The main

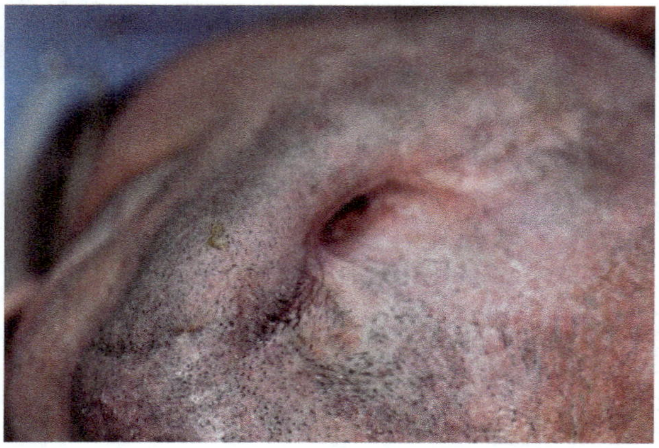

Figure 1: Pre-op view of the orocutaneous mandibular fistula from the bottom.

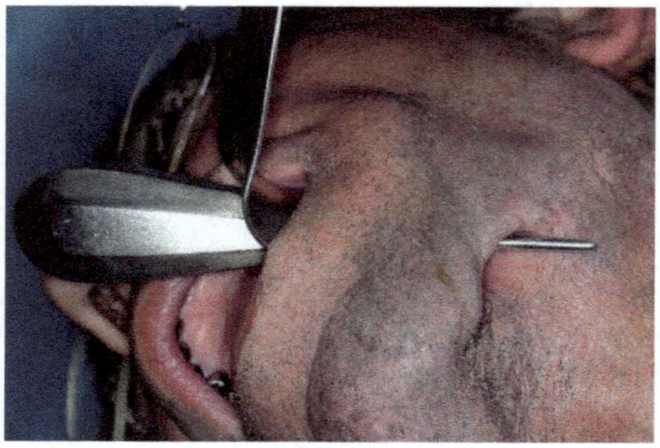

Figure 2: Figure shows the relation of defect with oral cavity.

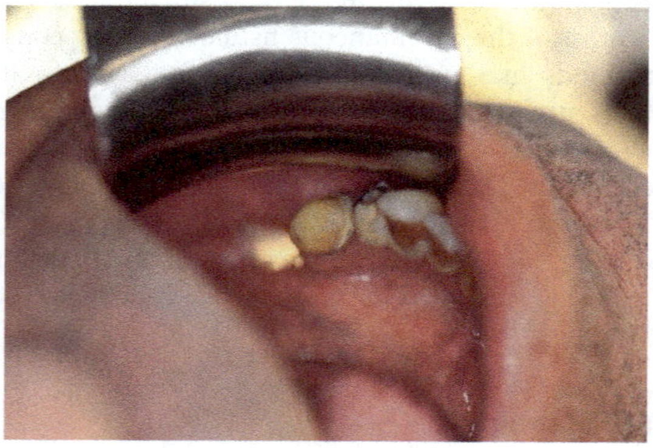

Figure 3: Intraoral view of the fistula; the light from outside can be seen through the defect hollow.

reason of the failed attempts to close the fistula was considered to be the ineffective management of dead space surrounding the fistula. Consequently, it was decided to use the submandibular gland as a pedicled flap to fill the defect and support the oral and the cutaneous flaps.

Under general anesthesia, the fistula was excised initially and the oral and the cutaneous healthy soft tissues were prepared. At the extraoral site, the incision was extended to the posterior and anterior directions, following the previous incision lines. In the subplatysmal plane, the superficial layer of

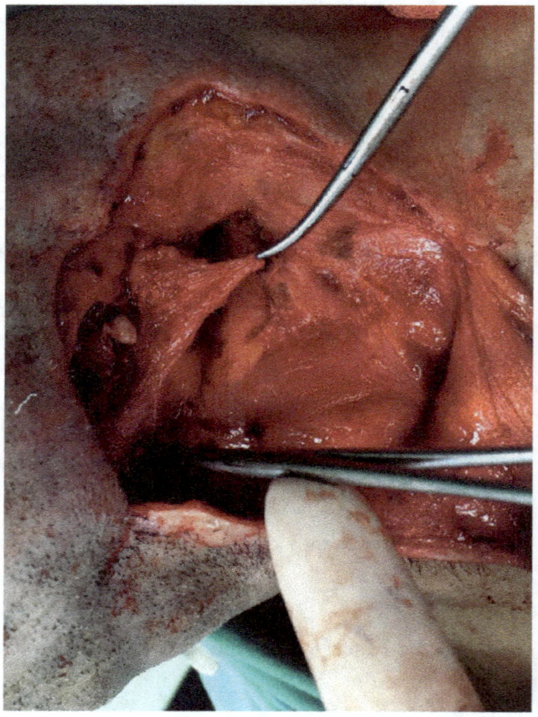

Figure 4: The rotation of the submandibular pedicled flap to the defected site.

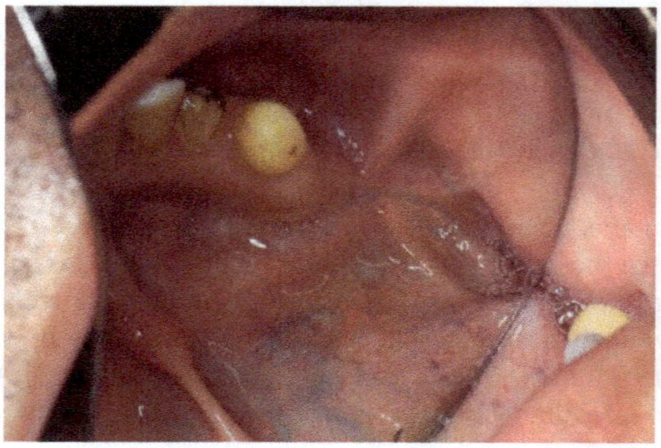

Figure 5: Post-op 6 months; closure of the fistula could be seen from the intraoral view.

the neck fascia was dissected to reach the base of the mandible. After the dissection of the fascia, the submandibular gland and the base of the mandible were exposed, the soft tissues surrounding the submandibular gland were dissected, and the gland was mobilized by protecting the arteriovenous supply and the duct. At the oral site, the margins of the wound were released by blunt dissection and were closed by mattress sutures via 5/0 polypropylene. Following the mobilization of the gland, a soft tissue tunnel was prepared between the submandibular space and the defect area and the submandibular gland was rotated by passing the gland through the soft tissue tunnel by preserving the pedicle (Figure 4). The rotated gland was sutured to the recipient site with 3/0 reabsorbable polyglaction sutures for the stabilization. At the cutaneous site, the flap was closed layer by layer by using 3/0 resorbable polyglaction for the facia and

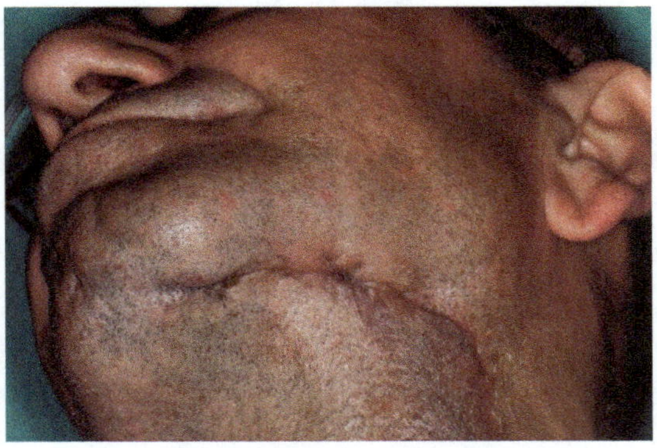

FIGURE 6: Extraoral operation site in 6 months.

the subcutaneous layers and 3/0 polypropylene sutures for the skin. After the surgery, pressure bandage was applied for the edema control externally and the patient was ordered soft diet for a week. The postoperative healing was uneventful, and at the sixth month follow-up visit, ideal closure of the fistula was observed (Figures 5 and 6).

3. Discussion

An orofacial or orocutaneous fistula is a pathological communication between the cutaneous surface of the face and the oral cavity. These defects can cause aesthetic and functional problems due to the continuous leakage of saliva. The common causes are malignancy, osteoradionecrosis (ORN), residual lesions of the cyst and tumors of the jaws, inflammation, and trauma [5].

The reconstruction of the defects in the maxillofacial region should be based on the principles of function and aesthetic. For this aim, free flaps, pedicled flaps, local regional flaps, and rotation flaps can be used. Local flaps have some advantages like providing the same skin texture and color, and also morbidity is less because there is no other donor site [7].

Submandibular gland flap which has its own blood supply from facial artery was first introduced by Mozolewski et al. [8] in the reconstruction following partial laryngectomy. Yang et al. [9] used the submandibular gland flap successfully for the reconstruction of the defects in the infratemporal region after tumor resection. In addition, Zhang et al. reported the usage of submandibular gland flap for the reconstruction of oral cavity [10].

In general, if the donor site is far from the recipient site, the success of the local flap can be hazardous. The pedicle of the flap should be handled and placed gently without any tension. The pedicled submandibular gland flap has some advantages like being near the orofacial zones so it can be rotated to a desirable place without tension. With this type of flap, spaces (like defects or fistulas) can be filled with minimal morbidity and no loss of function of the gland.

In comparison to allografts, the submandibular flap has no risk of tissue rejection, no potential transmission of disease from the donor of the allograft, or no prolonged healing response.

It also has some pros when comparing with free flaps. The main disadvantage of a free flap depends on the technical difficulties related to the microsurgery [11]. In free flaps, if the revascularization is unsuccessful flap, failure is inevitable. The presence of two operation sites and increased operation time is the other cons of the free flaps. Rotation of the pedicled submandibular gland flap is accomplished from the same incision, and there is no need to wait for the revascularization or microsurgery.

On the contrary, as the pedicle of the submandibular gland flap is relatively short, the flap is suitable in the submandibular region. Careful and rigorous surgery must be performed in order to avoid gland obstruction which results in functional loss. Ranula formation and atrophy of a gland are other possible complications of this flap. The pedicled submandibular gland flap is a good choice in defects near the mandibular region, and it is also a good alternative when other rotational flaps failed.

References

[1] I. B. Bender and S. Seltzer, "The oral fistula: Its diagnosis and treatment," *Oral Surgery, Oral Medicine, Oral Pathology*, vol. 14, no. 11, pp. 1367–1376, 1961.

[2] C. Balakrishnan, K. Narasimhan, T. Gursel, O. Jackson, and A. Schaffner, "Closure of orocutanous fistula using a pedicled expanded deltopectoral flap," *Canadian Journal of Plastic Surgery*, vol. 16, no. 3, pp. 178–180, 2008.

[3] C. J. Salgado, S. Mardini, H. C. Chen, and S. Chen, "Critical oropharyngocutaneous fistulas after microsurgical head and neck reconstruction: indications for management using the "tissue-plug" technique," *Plastic and Reconstructive Surgery*, vol. 112, no. 4, pp. 957–963, 2003.

[4] B. Tian, D. Khoo, A. C. Tay et al., "Management of orocutaneous fistulas using a vacuum-assisted closure system," *Head & Neck*, vol. 36, no. 6, pp. 873–881, 2014.

[5] E. Cansiz, A. Gultekin, M. Koltuk, and S. Cakarer, "Treatment of Oral fistulas," in *A textbook of advanced Oral and maxillofacial surgery volume 3. s.L.: Chapter 17*, M. H. K. Motamedi, Ed., Intech Open, 2016.

[6] D. A. Föll, A. Jokuszies, C. Radtke, and P. M. Vogt, "Successful closure of persistent oro-cutaneous fistulas by injection of autologous adipose-derived stem cells: a case report," *GMS German Plastic, Reconstructive and Aesthetic Surgery*, vol. 3, 2013.

[7] M. A. Mashrah, S.-h. Zhou, A. Abdelrehem et al., "Oropharyngeal reconstruction with a pedicled submandibular gland flap," *British Journal of Oral and Maxillofacial Surgery*, vol. 54, no. 4, pp. 388–393, 2016.

[8] E. Mozolewski, P. Maj, J. Kordowski, S. Szostak, and C. Tarnowska, "Vascular pedicle flap of the thyroid or submandibular gland in the reconstruction following partial laryngectomy," *Otolaryngologia Polska*, vol. 53, no. 4, pp. 387–396, 1999.

[9] B. Yang, M. Su, H. Li, J. Li, J. Ouyang, and Z. Han, "Use of submandibular gland flap for repairing defects after tumor

resection in the infratemporal region," *Journal of Cranio-Maxillofacial Surgery*, vol. 43, no. 1, pp. 87–91, 2015.

[10] X. Zhang, F. Liu, X. Lan, and S. Li, "Combined submandibular gland flap and sternocleidomastoid musculocutaneous flap for postoperative reconstruction in older aged patients with oral cavity and oropharyngeal cancers," *World Journal of Surgical Oncology*, vol. 12, no. 1, p. 259, 2014.

[11] A. Torroni, "Engineered bone grafts and bone flaps for maxillofacial defects: state of the art," *Journal of Oral and Maxillofacial Surgery*, vol. 67, no. 5, pp. 1121–1127, 2009.

Parosmia, Dysgeusia and Tongue Features Changes in a Patient with Post-Acute COVID-19 Syndrome

Aliaa Abdelmoniem Bedeir Eita

Faculty of Dentistry, Oral Medicine, Periodontology, Diagnosis and Radiology Department, Alexandria University, Alexandria, Egypt

Correspondence should be addressed to Aliaa Abdelmoniem Bedeir Eita; aliaa_bedeir@hotmail.com

Academic Editor: Sreekanth Kumar Mallineni

Coronavirus disease 2019 (COVID-19) is the pandemic of major global concern that has been causing several tragic events ever since December 2019. Infection with COVID-19 varies from being asymptomatic or mild with general unwellness to severe with difficulty in breathing and even mortality. Recently, several reports signified the persistence of symptoms or the development of new ones for weeks or months after the virus has gone, the so-called "post-acute COVID-19 syndrome." This article presents a 31-year-old female with post-acute COVID-19 syndrome showing parosmia, dysgeusia, and tongue feature changes as simultaneous newly developed manifestations after the viral clearance. Follow-up revealed complete remission of manifestations after one month. Post-acute COVID-19 syndrome can show oral manifestations. Despite the lack of evidence regarding the etiology, risk factors, and consequences of post-COVID-19 syndrome, it is important to monitor COVID-19 survivors to avoid complications during their recovery period.

1. Introduction

Coronavirus disease 2019 is caused by severe acute respiratory syndrome coronavirus 2 (SARS-CoV-2), an enveloped RNA virus and a member of the *Coronaviridae* family [1]. Infection with SARS-CoV-2 elicits an array of clinical manifestations that mostly include fatigue, fever, dry cough, and others ranging from mild to severe [2]. Several oral manifestations have also been reported in patients with acute COVID-19 infection. Dysgeusia (altered taste sensation) is considered an early recognized symptom which is believed to help in the early diagnosis of the disease. Other oral findings include ulcers, vesiculo-bullous eruptions, petechiae, erythema, tongue coat changes (white, yellow, and/or greasy tongue), and more [3–5].

Post-acute COVID-19 syndrome, also called "long COVID," "COVID long haul syndrome," and "post-COVID syndrome" (PCS), is known as the persistence of symptoms or the development of complications for more than three to four weeks after the onset of acute viral symptoms and where SARS-CoV-2 is not isolated [6, 7]. Fatigue, insomnia, compromised memory and concentration, palpitations, gastrointestinal manifestations, parosmia, and dysgeusia are all common symptoms of long COVID-19 [7]. Serious manifestations as acute renal injury, diabetic ketoacidosis, and multisystem involvement were also reported [6].

The aim of this report is to contribute to the current literature by presenting a case of the newly described entity post-acute COVID-19 syndrome showing parosmia (altered smell sensation), dysgeusia, and greasy white coated tongue with prominent papillae as simultaneous newly developed manifestations for four weeks after polymerase chain reaction (PCR) negativity. To the best of our knowledge, this is the first case report to document tongue manifestations in PCS.

2. Case Report

A 31-year-old female patient presented to the oral medicine clinic complaining of dysgeusia; she lost the ability to distinguish food with the retention of sweet and salty sensations only. Moreover, she was concerned about an unpleasant

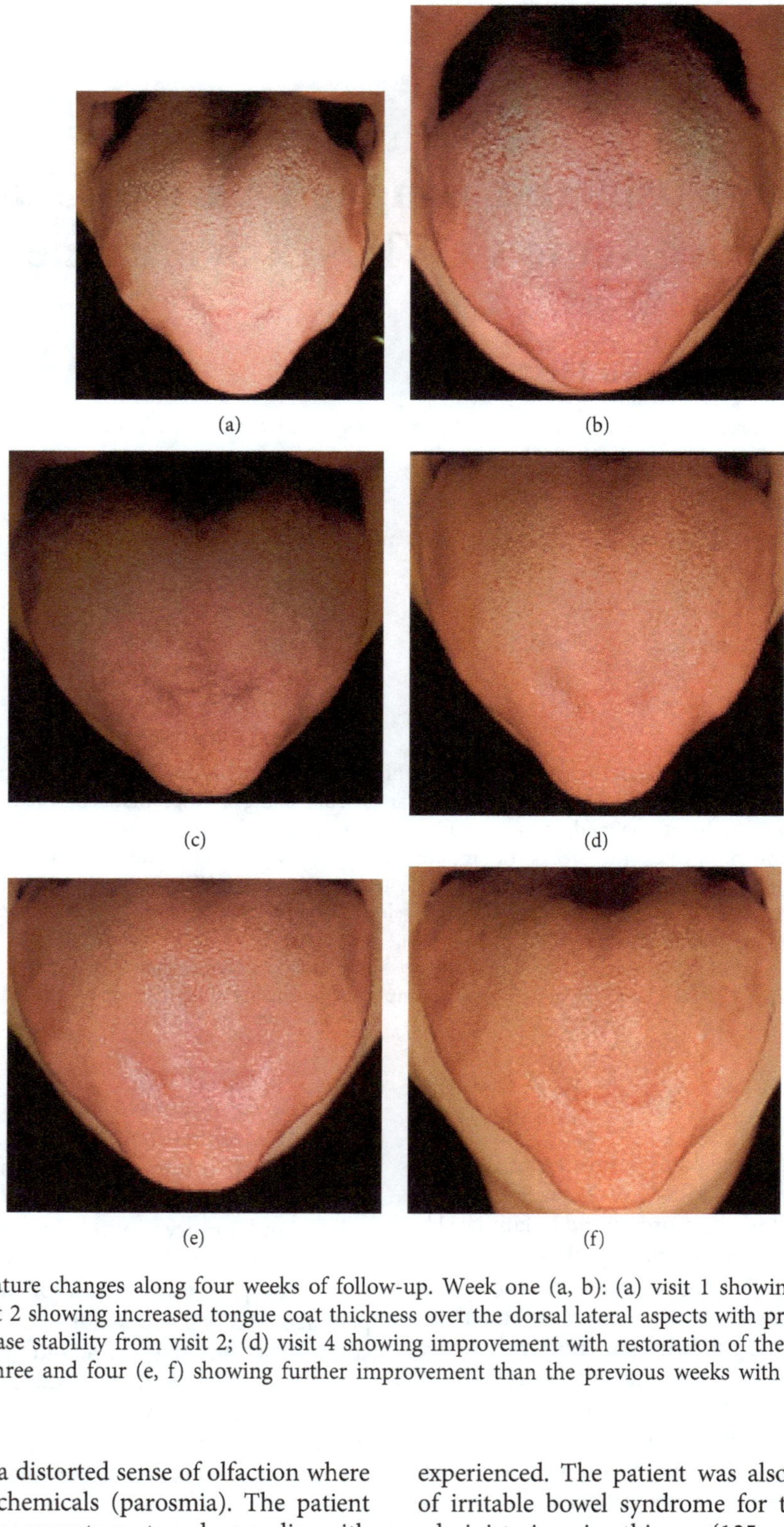

FIGURE 1: (a–f) Tongue feature changes along four weeks of follow-up. Week one (a, b): (a) visit 1 showing white coated tongue with prominent papillae; (b) visit 2 showing increased tongue coat thickness over the dorsal lateral aspects with prominent papillae. Week two (c, d): (c) visit 3 showing case stability from visit 2; (d) visit 4 showing improvement with restoration of the normal tongue coating and papillary features. Weeks three and four (e, f) showing further improvement than the previous weeks with normal tongue coating and papillae.

greasy white tongue and a distorted sense of olfaction where everything smelled like chemicals (parosmia). The patient reported the onset of these symptoms two days earlier with significant worsening. The condition was persistent and affected her quality of life, the thing that made her seek professional assistance.

2.1. History, Clinical Examination, and Diagnosis. Past medical history revealed that the patient is atopic; she reported occasional administration of antihistamines (loratadine 10 mg once daily) whenever hypersensitivity reactions are experienced. The patient was also suffering from episodes of irritable bowel syndrome for ten years. She is used to administering simethicone (125 mg 2-3 times daily) during exacerbations to relief bloating. Dental and family histories were negative.

Fourteen days earlier, the patient was COVID-19 positive. She suffered from sore throat, persistent low-grade fever (38°C), nasal congestion and itching, conjunctivitis, nausea, abdominal pain, diarrhea, fatigue, and severe joint pain. Chest computed tomography and all the relevant laboratory investigations were normal. The patient was scheduled on a

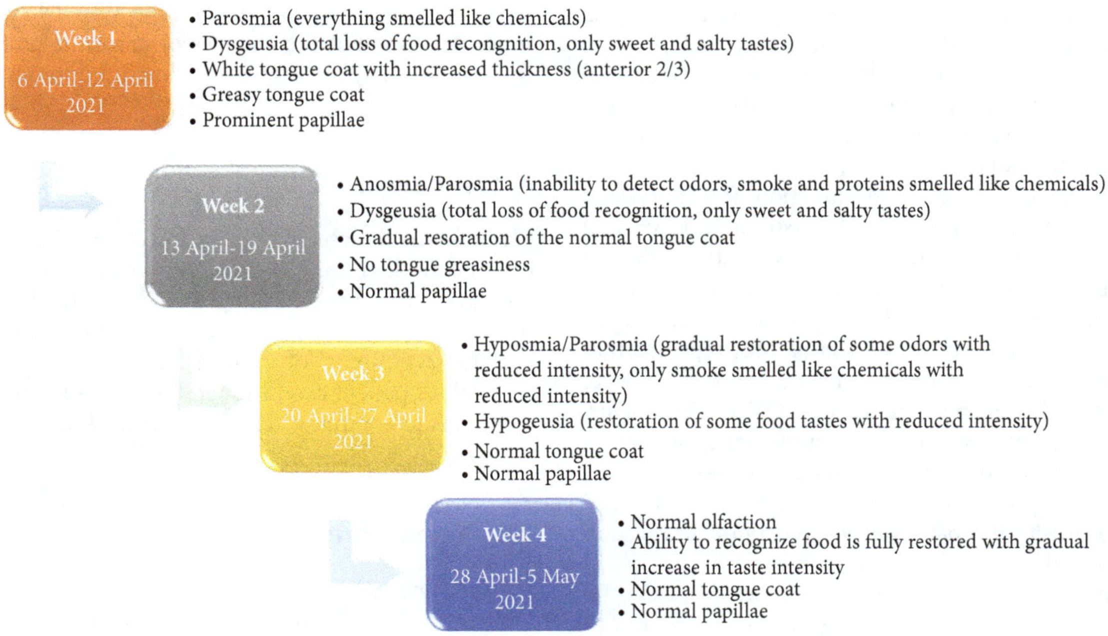

FIGURE 2: Timeline of the patient's symptoms throughout four weeks of post-acute COVID-19 syndrome.

treatment protocol for COVID-19 in accordance to her current medical condition following the guidelines set by the Egyptian Ministry of Health and Population [8] and under the supervision of a physician. Therapy included azithromycin 500 mg/day, paracetamol 500 mg 2 tablets ×3 times daily, zinc (50 mg), and vitamin C (1000 mg) supplements once daily. Throughout the treatment phase, symptom improvement was noted. After 12 days of infection, a nasopharyngeal swab was collected, and real-time PCR for COVID-19 detection was negative. At that time, all the reported COVID-19 symptoms disappeared, and treatment was discontinued.

Extraoral examination was normal. Intraoral examination revealed an unscrapable white coat over the dorsum of the tongue with prominent papillae. Bilateral indentation marks from reported continuous tongue sucking were also noted (Figure 1(a)). Tongue sucking was an established oral habit ever since childhood; underlying medical conditions and psychological impairment were ruled out.

Based on history and clinical examination, the patient was diagnosed with post-acute COVID-19 syndrome.

2.2. Treatment and Follow-Up. The patient was reassured, and a comprehensive explanation about her condition was performed. She was instructed about the appropriate oral hygiene measures, and prophylactic medications were prescribed to prevent superimposed infections (0.12% chlorhexidine mouth rinse and nystatin oral drops 100.000 I.U/ml 2-3 times daily). Daily vitamin C (1000 mg) and zinc (50 mg) supplements were also prescribed to enhance recovery.

Follow-up appointments were scheduled at short intervals (one to two visits per week throughout four weeks) to monitor manifestation improvement (Figures 1(a)–1(f)). Phone calls were arranged every other day from the start of treatment to ensure patient's compliance with the scheduled protocol. A second PCR test for COVID-19 detection was performed by the end of week one follow-up and confirmed the previous negative result.

After one month of treatment (4 weeks from viral clearance), the tongue features were restored to normal, and the patient reported complete resolution of parosmia and dysgeusia. No adverse side effects were noted. A detailed documentation of the changes in all manifestations of PCS is shown as a timeline in Figure 2. The patient was followed up after another month from PCS recovery (8 weeks from viral clearance) and showed no complication or symptom recurrence.

3. Discussion

Coronavirus disease 2019 outbreak has been gaining the world's attention to date. Several studies have discussed the nature and manifestations of COVID-19. However, scientists cannot predict its course and sequelae in patients during and after the viral infection [1].

There is a growing body of evidence about the symptoms and risk factors of PCS. In the present case, the patient's sex and some of the clinical features at the viral stage as persistent fever and infection duration are coincident with the emerging literature. Mahmud et al. [9] in their cohort study reported fatigue as the most prevalent symptom. Moreover, they reported female sex, lethargy, respiratory distress, and long infection durations (14 days from PCR diagnosis) as risk factors for PCS. In the same study, patients with fever were found to be more susceptible to develop PCS.

Olfactory dysfunction and dysgeusia have been notably discussed in the context of SARS-CoV-2 infection. The pathogenesis of anosmia (loss of smell sensation) in COVID-19 can be explained by several mechanisms like nasal airway obstruction, olfactory center and sensory neural damage, olfactory epithelium, and supporting cell dysfunction. On the other hand, it was found that salivary glands and the oral mucosa are vulnerable to being attacked by SARS-CoV-2 through angiotensin converting enzyme 2 receptors (ACE2) leading to dysgeusia. Other mechanisms for dysgeusia have been proposed as zinc deficiency, cranial nerve dysfunction, and others [10].

In general, chemosensory dysfunction (olfactory and gustatory) was found to be linked to stress, anxiety, and depression. Depression was found to be associated with high levels of glucocorticoids and inflammatory cytokines which can result in compromised olfactory neural proliferation [11]. Moreover, a study by Al'Absi et al. [12] reported that stress-related changes in the adrenocortical activity were linked to altered taste perception. In COVID-19 patients, Speth et al. [13] revealed a positive and specific association between the severity of taste and smell loss and depressed mood and anxiety from viral infection. The authors raised attention to direct viral pathogenesis as a possible cause of such an association.

Different tongue coat changes were reported in COVID-19 patients. Pang et al. [4] found that light red tongue with white coating is commonly seen in mild to moderate SARS-CoV-2 infection. Furthermore, they reported greasy coating as a significant characteristic in all patients. White coated tongue is usually a normal physiologic change. Regardless, white and red oral mucosal patches or plaques seen in COVID-19 patients could be attributed to superimposed fungal infection from long-term treatments or difficulties in complying with the meticulous oral hygiene measures from health deterioration [3]. Oxidative stress and dysbiosis have been linked to both COVID-19 infection and greasy tongue coating [14, 15]. It was suggested that the resultant cellular damage from oxidant-antioxidant imbalance as well as dysbiosis could be possible causes for greasy tongue coating in COVID-19 patients [3].

To date, the exact pathophysiology of PCS is not well established. Nonetheless, the implication of physiologic viral changes, host immune, and inflammatory response to the invading pathogen and critical illness have all been proposed as possible mechanisms of PCS [6]. The present patient suffered from persistent nasal itching and fever throughout the acute viral phase. Besides, she was tired and unable to follow the appropriate measures of care. The reported manifestations of PCS in this article could be the sequelae of such compromisations, the result of the patient's body response to face COVID-19, or a composite of all proposed mechanisms.

Due to the increasing sequelae of COVID-19 in the post-viral stages on a multiorgan scale, studies highlighted the importance of monitoring COVID-19 patients for longer durations after the viral clearance. This would help understand more about this pandemic through rigorous investigation, management, and documentation of the newly evolving symptoms. The provided care should involve multidisciplinary cooperation in both inpatient and outpatient settings in accordance to the prevailing symptoms and their severity [6].

One possible limitation of the present case is the lack of reagents and materials used for olfactory and taste function tests. Chemosensory function testing would have provided more details about the changes of parosmia and dysgeusia throughout the treatment and follow-up durations.

4. Conclusion

Coronavirus disease 2019 is an infectious disease with heterogeneous literature and international health challenges. New symptoms can develop post-COVID-19 clearance. Parosmia, dysgeusia, and white tongue coating with greasiness can be symptoms of post-acute COVID-19 syndrome. Meticulous patient care through long-term follow-up is crucial to avoid complications during convalescence.

Additional Points

Patient Perspective. The patient reported overall satisfaction at the end of follow-up. The odor of chemicals and the greasy tongue feeling have completely disappeared. Also, she was able to distinguish between all food types.

Consent

The patient signed an informed consent regarding publishing the present data and photographs in an online publication.

Authors' Contributions

Aliaa A.B. Eita contributed to the diagnosis, investigation, follow-up, data curation, resources, writing original draft, and writing review and editing.

Acknowledgments

The author would like to acknowledge Dr. Doaa Gaber Hegazy for her scientific support.

References

[1] H. Harapan, N. Itoh, A. Yufika et al., "Coronavirus disease 2019 (COVID-19): a literature review," *Journal of Infection and Public Health*, vol. 13, no. 5, pp. 667–673, 2020.

[2] D. Wang, B. Hu, C. Hu, F. Zhu, X. Liu, and J. Zhang, "Clinical characteristics of 138 hospitalized patients with 2019 novel coronavirus-infected pneumonia in Wuhan, China," *JAMA*, vol. 323, no. 11, pp. 1061–1069, 2020.

[3] B. Iranmanesh, M. Khalili, R. Amiri, H. Zartab, and M. Aflatoonian, "Oral manifestations of COVID-19 disease: a review article," *Dermatologic Therapy*, vol. 34, p. e14578, 2021.

[4] W. Pang, D. Zhang, J. Zhang et al., "Tongue features of patients with coronavirus disease 2019: a retrospective cross-sectional study," *Integ Med Res.*, vol. 9, no. 3, p. 100493, 2020.

[5] J. A. dos Santos, A. G. C. Normando, R. L. C. da Silva et al., "Oral mucosal lesions in a COVID-19 patient: new signs or secondary manifestations?," *International Journal of Infectious Diseases*, vol. 97, pp. 326–328, 2020.

[6] A. Nalbandian, K. Sehgal, A. Gupta et al., "Post-acute COVID-19 syndrome," *Nature Medicine*, vol. 27, no. 4, pp. 601–615, 2021.

[7] NHS, *Long-term effects of coronavirus (long COVID)*, 2021, https://www.nhs.uk/conditions/coronavirus-covid-19/.

[8] The Egyptian Ministry of Health and Population, *Egyptian National Guidelines forCOVID-19*, 2020, https://hiph.alexu.edu.eg/images/egyptian_national_guidelines_covid-19.pdf.pdf.pdf.

[9] R. Mahmud, M. M. Rahman, M. A. Rassel et al., "Post-COVID-19 syndrome among symptomatic COVID-19 patients: a prospective cohort study in a tertiary care center of Bangladesh," *PLoS One*, vol. 16, no. 4, p. e0249644, 2021.

[10] E. Mutiawati, M. Fahriani, S. S. Mamada et al., "Anosmia and dysgeusia in SARS-CoV-2 infection: incidence and effects on COVID-19 severity and mortality, and the possible pathobiology mechanisms - a systematic review and meta-analysis," *F1000Research*, vol. 10, 2021.

[11] T. F. Yuan, G. Hou, and O. Arias-Carrion, "Chronic stress impacts on olfactory system," *CNS & Neurological Disorders Drug Targets*, vol. 14, no. 4, pp. 486–491, 2015.

[12] M. Al'Absi, M. Nakajima, S. Hooker, L. Wittmers, and T. Cragin, "Exposure to acute stress is associated with attenuated sweet taste," *Psychophysiology*, vol. 49, no. 1, pp. 96–103, 2012.

[13] M. M. Speth, T. Singer-Cornelius, M. Oberle, I. Gengler, S. J. Brockmeier, and A. R. Sedaghat, "Mood, anxiety and olfactory dysfunction in COVID-19: evidence of central nervous system involvement?," *The Laryngoscope*, vol. 130, no. 11, pp. 2520–2525, 2020.

[14] B. V. Chernyak, E. N. Popova, A. S. Prikhodko, O. A. Grebenchikov, L. A. Zinovkina, and R. A. Zinovkin, "COVID-19 and oxidative stress," *Biochemistry (Moscow)*, vol. 85, pp. 1543–1553, 2020.

[15] L. He, L. Ren, J. Li, Y. Wu, X. Li, and L. Zhang, "Intestinal flora as a potential strategy to fight SARS-CoV-2 infection," *Frontiers in Microbiology*, vol. 11, p. 1388, 2020.

31

Maxillomandibular Transverse Osteodistraction: A Multidisciplinary Case Report with 30-Month Follow-up

G. Turatti,[1] A. Bruni,[2,3] M. Savoini,[4] M. Giordano,[1] and G. Gerbino[4]

[1]*Odontostomatology OU, Martini Hospital, Via Tofane 71, Turin 10141, Italy*
[2]*CIR Dental School, Department of Surgical Sciences, Università degli Studi di Torino, Via Nizza 230, Turin 10126, Italy*
[3]*Department of Mechanical and Aerospatial Engineering (DIMEAS), Politecnico di Torino, C.so Duca degli Abruzzi 24, Turin 10129, Italy*
[4]*Division of Maxillofacial Surgery, Department of Surgical Sciences, Università degli studi di Torino, Città della Salute e delle Scienza Hospital, Corso A.M. Dogliotti 14, Turin 10126, Italy*

Correspondence should be addressed to A. Bruni; alessandro.bruni@polito.it

G. Turatti and A. Bruni contributed equally to this work.

Academic Editor: Hüsamettin Oktay

Aim. To describe a multidisciplinary treatment to correct a severe II class malocclusion with reduced both maxillary and mandibular transverse dimensions and dental crowding. *Case Report.* A 17-year-old young woman presented with an increased overjet complaining chiefly of forwardly placed upper front teeth and unpleasant smile aesthetics. The patient facially exhibited a gently convex profile, severe mentalis strain on lip closure, and dark buccal corridors. The intraoral assessment indicates Class II molar relationship bilaterally, mandibular and maxillary anterior crowding, and narrow shape of upper and lower arches. The cephalometric evaluation of the lateral radiograph of the skull evidences a skeletal Class II with a reduction of lower face height. Based upon the diagnostic records and consultation with the patient, surgically assisted expansion of both arches using bone-borne distractors, comprehensive orthodontic treatment, and combined jaw surgery was planned. *Results.* This approach permitted achieving most of the desired objectives in approximately 30 months. The follow-up records 30 months after treatment conclusion showed a stable occlusion. No complications were clinically and radiographically noticeable during the follow-up.

1. Introduction

Transverse deficiencies are a common finding among populations [1]: in selected patients, concurrent osteodistraction of both arches represents a viable option [2–4] to treat severe maxillomandibular transverse deficiency and dental crowding.

Historically, the mandibular arch dimension has always been considered immutable.

The synostosis of the mandibular symphysis occurs during the first year after delivery, and the use of orthodontic devices (e.g., lingual arches [5], functional appliances [6], Schwarz plates, and archwires [7]) has proved inadequate to gain more than 6-8 mm in the lower arch [8, 9]. Several methods exist to overcome this limit (e.g., through interproximal enamel reduction, extracting teeth, or even using bone anchorages to lower the lateral sectors [8]). However, the stability of these treatments is often unpredictable and can result in adverse side effects [10].

Distraction osteogenesis is the biological process of new bone formation between bone segments that are gradually separated by incremental traction after an intentional surgical bone fracture [10].

The first *Mandibular Symphyseal Distraction Osteogenesis* (MSDO) was performed by Guerrero in 1997 [11] and subsequently described under various nomenclature, e.g., Mandibular Midline (Osteo-) Distraction (MMD) and Transmandibular Symphyseal (Osteo-) Distraction (TMSD).

This treatment modality, compared to the abovementioned ones, improves aesthetics and function, shortens treatment time, and appears stable over time [11].

The fusion of midpalatal suture has a variable timing: it occurs generally after the age of 15 [12].

Surgically Assisted Rapid Palatal Expansion (SARPE), also mentioned as *Surgically Assisted Rapid Maxillary Expansion* (SARME), is a widely accepted procedure for skeletally mature patients with maxillary transverse deficiency.

The first *SARPE* was performed by Brown in 1938 [13, 14] to prevent unwanted effects of orthopedic or orthodontic expansion in skeletally mature patients (e.g., buccal tipping of posterior teeth, extrusion, periodontal membrane compression, buccal root resorption, alveolar bone bending, fenestration of the buccal cortex, palatal tissue necrosis, pain, and instability of the expansion [15]) by surgically releasing the closed sutures resisting the expansion forces.

The most frequent indications for a simultaneous bimaxillary osteodistraction, mentioned as *Maxillomandibular Transverse Osteodistraction* (MMTOD), are severe (maxillary-) mandibular transverse deficiency, severe (maxillary-) mandibular anterior crowding [11], uni- [16] and bilateral buccal crossbite, impacted anterior teeth with insufficient space and hugely tipped teeth [17], and obstructive sleep apnea syndrome [18].

In this case report, the focus is on the orthodontic and surgical procedure, the distractor devices, the distraction sequence, the skeletal and aesthetic outcome, the stability after a 30-month follow-up, treatment-related difficulties, and complications.

2. Case Report

In September 2013, a 17-year-old female came to the Department of Orthodontics at the Martini Hospital in Torino with the chief complaint of prominent upper teeth and crooked mandibular and maxillary incisors with difficulty in maintenance of oral hygiene.

2.1. History. She reported CCE (common childhood exanthemas) when she was a child. She was in good general health, without any allergies. The patient's oral health was good. Before treatment, complete orthodontic and radiographic documentation was requested. No previous orthodontic treatment was performed; no TMJ problems were reported. The first step was to conduct thorough extraoral and intraoral examinations.

2.2. Assessment

2.2.1. Extraoral Assessment. During the extraoral clinical examination, a mandibular retrusion and severe mentalis strain on lip closure were verified; the profile was reasonably convex; and the nasolabial angle was moderately closed. The face shape was oval with moderate mandibular asymmetry to the right side; smile arch appeared to be flattened with an excessive amount of gingival display during forced smiling; and dark buccal corridors were found (Figure 1).

2.2.2. Intraoral Assessment. Intraorally, a narrow shape of the upper arch and the lower arch, a bilateral Class II molar and canine relationship, increased overjet (OVJ: 12.7 mm) and overbite (OVB: 7.2 mm), a dental crowding in both dental arches (slight in the upper, severe in the lower), and deviation of the superior midline to the right of 4 mm and inferior midline to the right of 6 mm were detected. In the mandibular arch, lack of space was noted (Figure 1).

2.2.3. Dental Cast Assessment. The dental cast analysis also showed an increased OVJ and OVB and enhanced Spee's curve (Figure 2).

2.2.4. Radiographic Assessment. Radiographically, a complete permanent dentition with unerupted third molars was observed (Figure 1).

The cephalometric evaluation of the lateral radiograph of the skull (Figure 3(a); Table 1, T0) showed that the patient had a skeletal Class II pattern (Wits: 5.7 mm) with a slightly retruded position of the maxilla (SNA: 77.1°) and mandible (SNB: 75.8°). The occlusal plane was significantly anteriorly upward pitched (Mand plane-Occ plane: 23.6°).

The maxillary incisors were protruded (A1 to APo plane: 2.3 mm) and proclinate (U1-Occ plane: 50.0°; U1-palatal plane: 131.0°), and the mandibular incisors were slightly retruded (L1 to Apo plane: 12.4 mm) and reclined (IMPA: 83.5°).

The cephalometric evaluation of the skull radiograph in the posteroanterior (PA) view showed good symmetry overall (Figure 3(b)).

2.2.5. Diagnosis. No symptoms of TMJ dysfunction were referred (there were neither noises from the joint nor pain identified during mandibular movement; there was a good range of mandibular movement).

The patient was diagnosed as having a skeletal Class II pattern with dental deep bite and severe dental Class II combined with dental crowding, in particular in the anterior part of the lower arch. The accentuated Spee's curve, resulting from an overeruption of lower incisors in association with the anterior labial flaring of the upper incisors, led to the tilting of the occlusal plane anteriorly upward.

2.3. Treatment

2.3.1. Treatment aim. The following treatment objectives were established:

(1) To obtain space in the arches to accommodate the teeth

(2) To expand the maxillary arch to obtain harmony with the mandibular arch

(3) To expand the mandibular arch

(4) To reduce OVJ and OVB

(5) To correct molar and canine Class II dental malocclusion

(6) To restore lip competence at rest and to reduce the mentalis habit

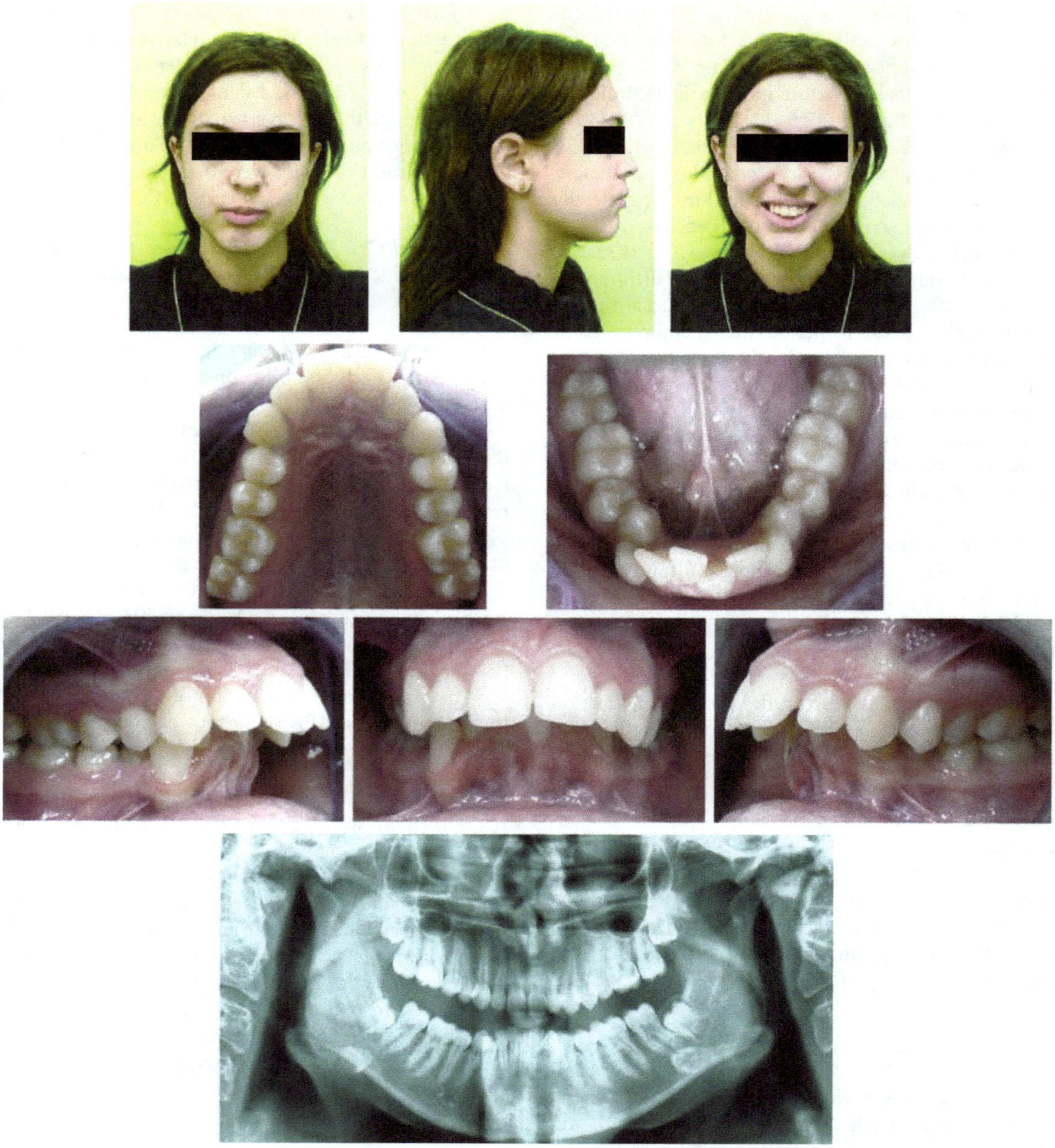

Figure 1: Extraoral photographs (T0), intraoral photographs (T0), and orthopantomogram (T0); T0=pretreatment.

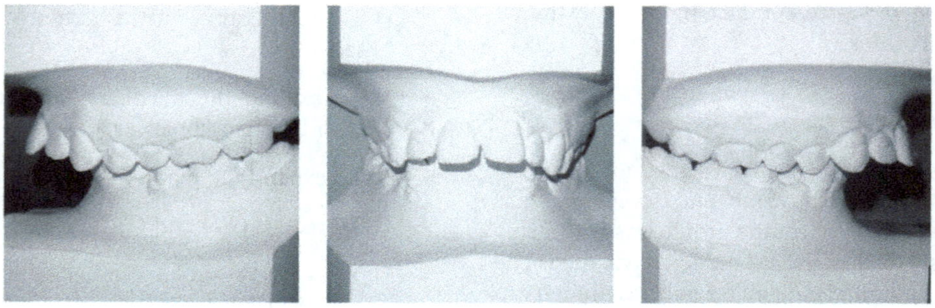

Figure 2: Dental cast models (T0); T0=pretreatment.

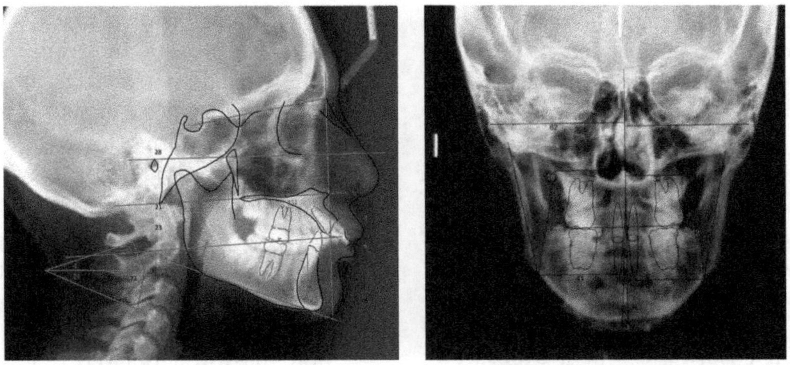

(a) (b)

Figure 3: Cephalometric tracing (T0): (a) cephalometric evaluation of the lateral radiograph of the skull and (b) cephalometric evaluation of the posteroanterior radiograph of the skull; T0=pretreatment.

Table 1: Cephalometric analysis (T0-T2): T0=pretreatment, T2=treatment progress (18 months), and T4=follow-up (30 months after the end of the treatment).

	Measured value T0	Measured value T2	Measured value T4	Norm
SNA	**77.1°**	**83.6°**	***83.1°***	82° ± 3.5°
SNB	**75.8°**	**86.1°**	***80.9°***	80° ± 3°
ANB	**1.4°**	**-2.6°**	***2.2°***	2° ± 2.4°
Maxillary skeletal (A-Na Perp)	**-3.0°**	**5.1°**	***1.6°***	0° ± 3.1°
Mand. skeletal (Pg-Na Perp)	**-5.0°**	**16.5°**	***1.1°***	0° ± 5.3°
Wits appraisal	**5.7** mm	**-4.2** mm	***-0.1°***	0 *mm* ± 1 *mm*
FMA (MP-FH)	**21.1°**	**10.9°**	***20.7°***	26° ± 5°
MP-SN	**30.6°**	**23.3°**	***29.2°***	33° ± 6°
Palatal-Mand angle	**22.7°**	**22.8°**	***23.0°***	28° ± 6°
Palatal-Occ plane	**-1.0°**	**6.3°**	***7.0°***	10° ± 4°
Mand plane-Occ plane	**23.6°**	**16.5°**	***16.0°***	17.4° ± 5°
U1 protrusion (U1-APo)	**2.3** mm	**8.9** mm	***8.6*** mm	0.4 ± 2.0 *mm*
L1 protrusion (L1-Apo)	**12.4** mm	**7.4** mm	***4.5*** mm	3.5 ± 2.3 *mm*
U1-palatal plane	**131.0°**	**120.2°**	***118.4°***	110° ± 5°
U1-Occ plane	**50.0°**	**53.4°**	***54.6°***	57.5° ± 7°
L1-Occ plane	**72.9°**	**58.6°**	***60.6°***	72° ± 5°
IMPA	**83.5°**	**105.0°**	***103.4°***	95° ± 7°

(7) To improve facial and smile aesthetics reducing buccal corridors

The expected compliance was good.

2.3.2. Treatment Plan. Based on the diagnostic records and consultation with the patient, the following plan was developed:

(1) Extraction of 1.8, 2.8, 3.8, and 4.8

(2) Surgically Assisted Rapid Palatal Expansion (SARPE) using bone-borne transpalatal distractor (TPD) and MMD using bone-borne transmandibular distractor (TMD).

(3) Comprehensive orthodontic treatment with particular attention paid to anterior teeth position and relationship

(4) Surgical planning reevaluation of the orthodontic results

(5) Corrective combined jaw surgery: usual bimaxillary advancement procedure with deliberate counterclockwise rotation of the occlusal plane including LeFort I osteotomy of the maxilla for anterior maxillary impaction and advancing; Bilateral Sagittal Split Osteotomy (BSSO) for increasing lower jaw length to provide better balance to the facial features

(6) Postsurgical orthodontics and periodontal follow-up

2.3.3. Treatment Progress. After the removal of the wisdom teeth, a Surgically Assisted Rapid Palatal Expansion using bone-anchored TPD and a Surgically Assisted Mandibular Midline Distraction procedure using bone-anchored TMD were performed.

Both surgical procedures were carried out under general anesthesia with nasotracheal intubation.

The surgical technique and distraction protocol used for SARPE was performed according to Ramieri et al. [19].

A flattened horseshoe-shaped incision was executed high in the vestibule from approximately the second premolar to the second premolar ensuring excellent exposure of the osteotomy site. The surgical cutting of the bone was performed from the piriform aperture to the pterygomaxillary suture, approximately 8 mm above the apices of the teeth. A vertical corticotomy from the anterior nasal spine to the alveolar crest was made using a surgical bur. The maxilla was downfractured sagittaly using a thin, straight osteotome. Pterygomaxillary suture disjunction was obtained using curved osteotomes.

A bone-borne distraction device (TPD™, Surgi-Tec NV, Brugge, Belgium) was subsequently placed to the palatal vault, through small mucosal incisions nearby second premolars, and fixed with 7 mm screws.

The surgical technique used for Surgically Assisted Rapid Mandibular Expansion was performed according to Mommaerts et al. [4]. A labial vestibular incision was carried out in order to gain access for the step osteotomy, consisting of two vertical osteotomies (interdental between canine and later incisor; in the basal bony midline) connected by a horizontal subapical osteotomy. A bone-borne distraction device (TMD™, Surgi-Tec NV, Bruges, Belgium) was subsequently placed on the mandibular symphysis.

The whole surgical procedure had taken approximately 80 minutes.

The patient was hospitalized for one night and was discharged the next morning with antibiotic, analgesic, and corticosteroid therapy. No complication after surgical procedures was reported.

After seven days, the maxillary distractor was activated (0.33 mm/day for the first ten days; 0.66/day thenceforth for an additional seven days); concomitant activation of the mandibular distraction device was performed (2 × 0.5 mm/day for ten days).

After starting the expansion procedure, the amount of the widening was clinically evaluated weekly: the spacing between the maxillary central incisors, the mandibular lateral incisor, and canines was the first sign of disjunction of the bone halves.

Total expansion of 8 mm, assessed by measuring the maxillary intermolar width as the distance between the mesial fossae of the maxillary first molars, was achieved in the upper arch. Total expansion of 5 mm, assessed by measuring the mandibular intercanine width as the distance from cusp tip to cusp tip of the mandibular canines, was achieved in the lower arch.

After the postoperative activation phase, both expansion devices were locked with a securing screw to prevent their deactivation (Figure 4) and to ensure the consolidation phase.

The patient's clinical status was assessed 15 days after expansion in progress: no teeth mobility, no gingival recession, no periodontal pockets, unaltered teeth vitality, and good hygiene with a suitable plaque without bleeding on probing control were detected.

After the surgically assisted widening of both the maxilla and the mandible, a fixed appliance (SW Roth prescription, $0.022'' \times 0.028''$ slots) was used to align the dentition during the consolidation phase. Before starting the active orthodontic treatment, a segmented arch-wire was used to control undesired movements of the lower incisors.

Both the distractors were removed under local anesthesia: the mandibular one was removed after about 120 days, and the maxillary one was removed after about 180 days. The orthodontic treatment continued following these stages:

(1) *Aligning stage*: a lingual arch was mounted mandibulary after removing the upper and lower distractors to control the intermolar width and rotations. In both arches, .012 NiTi archwires were used. During this stage, an active coil was positioned between 35 and 33 and between 45 and 43 to create space for 34 and 44

(2) *Levelling stage*: a TPB was mounted maxillary. NiTi archwires of successive cross-sections were used for about ten months in order to complete the alignment

(3) *Working stage*: the maxillary and mandibular arches were coordinated, the maxillary and mandibular midlines were aligned, spaces were closed, and the maxillary and mandibular occlusal planes were paralleled. The OVJ and OVB were improved

A panoramic radiograph to evaluate the position of the roots and a lateral radiograph of the skull that showed a clockwise rotation of the maxillomandibular complex were taken. Also, the clinical examination showed excessive incisal exposure during the smile (Figure 5).

Presurgical orthodontic results were reevaluated together with the orthognathic surgery team of the University of Turin to decide the proper treatment plan.

In order to improve aesthetics (correction of excessive tooth exposure at rest and increase of soft tissue support with skeletal facial expansion) and improve dental and occlusal relationship, maxillomandibular osteotomies were planned with the agreement of the patient. A total of 4 mm of maxillary impaction and 7 mm of mandibular advancement were programmed. The following corrective combined jaw surgery was performed: LeFort I osteotomy of the maxilla with differential maxillary impaction and advancing simultaneously with a *Bilateral Sagittal Split Osteotomy* (BSSO), achieving a slight counterclockwise rotation of the occlusal plane.

A lateral radiograph of the skull was requested to do tracing for cephalometric evaluation: comparison of the cephalometric analysis before and after surgery demonstrated an improvement in the sagittal skeletal and dental values (Figure 6; Table 1, T2).

(4) *Detailing and finishing stage*: after surgery, the patient was monitored closely for one month and

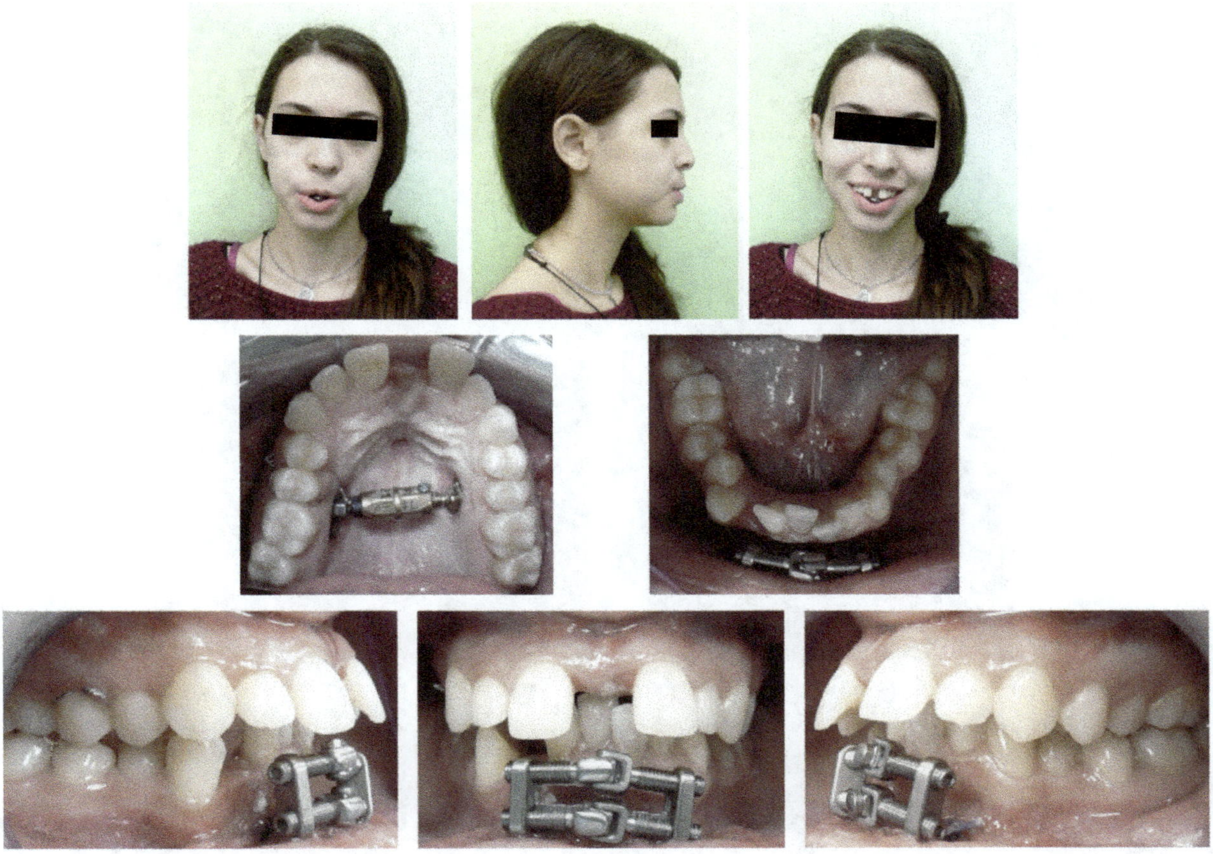

FIGURE 4: Extraoral photographs (T1) and intraoral photographs (T1); T1=treatment progress (1 month).

was then referred for postsurgical orthodontics. At that point, with the same archwires placed, she wore light posterior vertical elastics and bilateral II class elastics full time for three months. The postoperative stage was aimed at additional finalization; therefore, coordination of the maxillary and mandibular arches were followed by finishing and detailing of the occlusion

It was decided that the treatment goals were achieved, and active treatment could be completed. Approximately 30 months spread out over 62 appointments was the comprehensive active treatment time.

2.4. Summary

2.4.1. Treatment Results. On the day of debonding, extra- and intraoral photographs were taken along with impressions and occlusion wax to build the final plaster models. For the retention, it was decided to use a Hawley appliance for the upper teeth and a bonded retainer for the lower teeth.

Review of the treatment outcome with clinical examination, extra- and intraoral photographs (Figure 7), and the final plaster models showed the following outcomes:

(i) Mandibular symmetrization, improvement of smile arch aesthetic, reduction of buccal corridors, and an improved lower third projection

(ii) Correction of the dental Class II was achieved

(iii) Correction of arch shapes was observed

(iv) Significant reduction of the lip incompetence was obtained

(v) Mentalis habit was reduced

2.4.2. Follow-Up. Approximately 30 months after debonding, the shapes of the arches and occlusion appeared to be stable, even though a moderate amount of relapse occurred (Figure 8). Both cephalometric evaluations of the lateral radiograph of the skull (Figure 9(a); Table 1, T4) and the posteroanterior radiograph of the skull (Figure 9(b)) showed a nonsignificant difference compared to postsurgery assessment except for sagittal jaw relationship that exhibited a considerable relapse (Table 1, T2 and T4).

3. Discussion

In selected adult patients, the simultaneous osteodistraction of both the maxilla and mandible represent a viable option to obtain satisfactory and stable outcomes.

The basic requirements for an optimal result of osteodistraction are minimally traumatic osteotomies, stable mechanical fixation across osteotomies, an adequate latency period before lengthening (to establish repair processes), suitable rhythm and amplitude of lengthening, a realistic goal

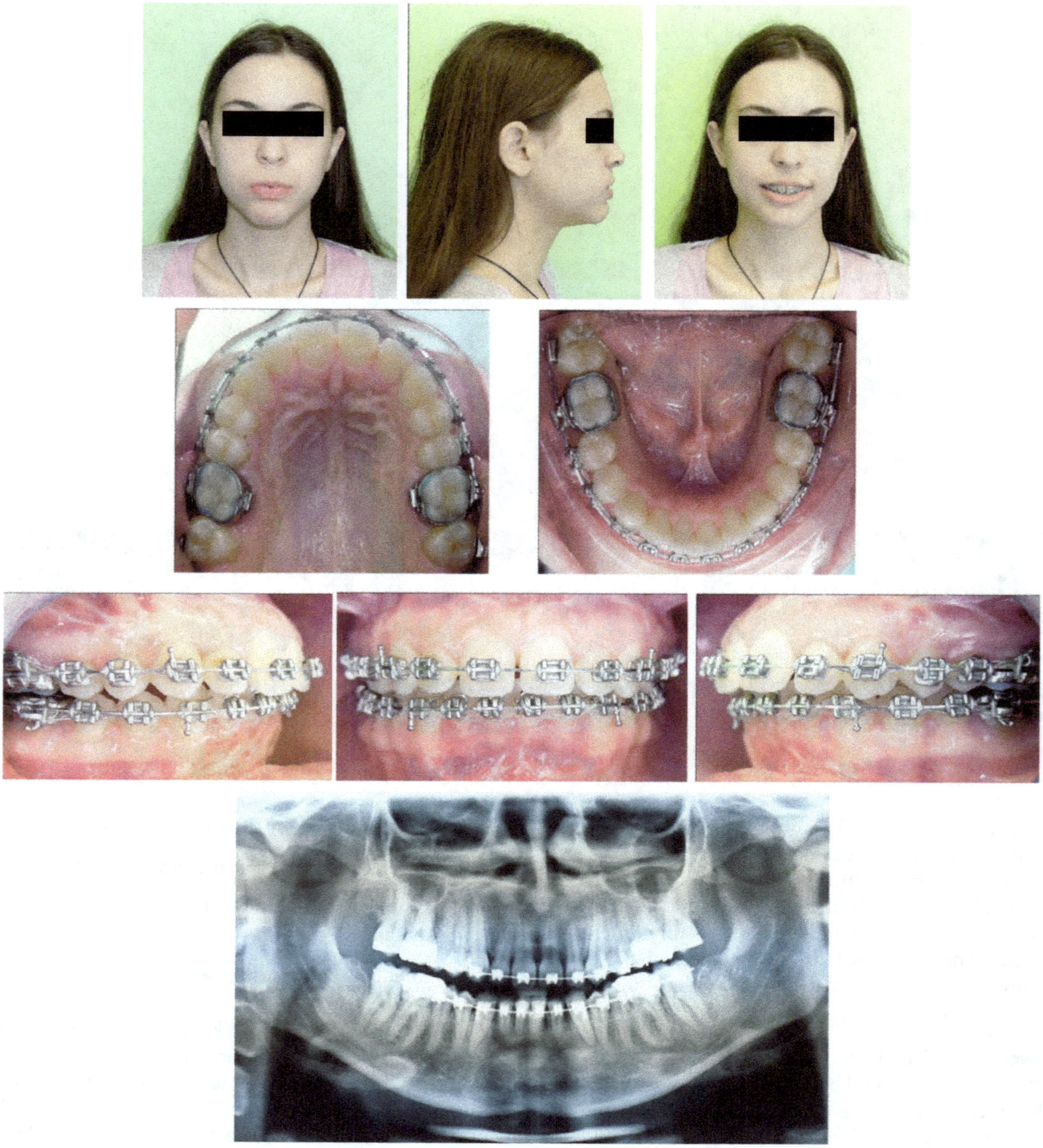

Figure 5: Extraoral photographs (T2), intraoral photographs (T2), and orthopantomogram (T2); T2=treatment progress (18 months).

regarding the extent of lengthening, and sufficient time for the callus to mature before frame or nail removal [20].

The use of proper appliances, careful surgery and follow-up, and cooperation between the surgical and orthodontic teams are the key to success in this demanding approach.

Discomfort, apical trauma, and local infections are the main disadvantages of TMD, as reported in the literature [4, 21].

Lip and cheek irritation, as well as speech and eating difficulties are commonly related to osteodistraction devices. Gingival recession, gingivitis, and irritation of the mucosa often represent soft tissue complications [22, 23].

Concerning the present case, several treatment alternatives were explored. Nevertheless, dental compensation could not be achieved because severe crowding in the lower arch cannot be properly fixed with Interproximal Enamel Reduction (IPR) and inclination of the mandibular incisors. As an alternative, the extraction of one mandibular central incisor could be considered.

Therefore, TMD was the best option for mandibular expansion and arch form improvement.

Concerning the upper arch, the severe inclination of the maxillary incisors reduces the chances to solve the crowding only with IPR.

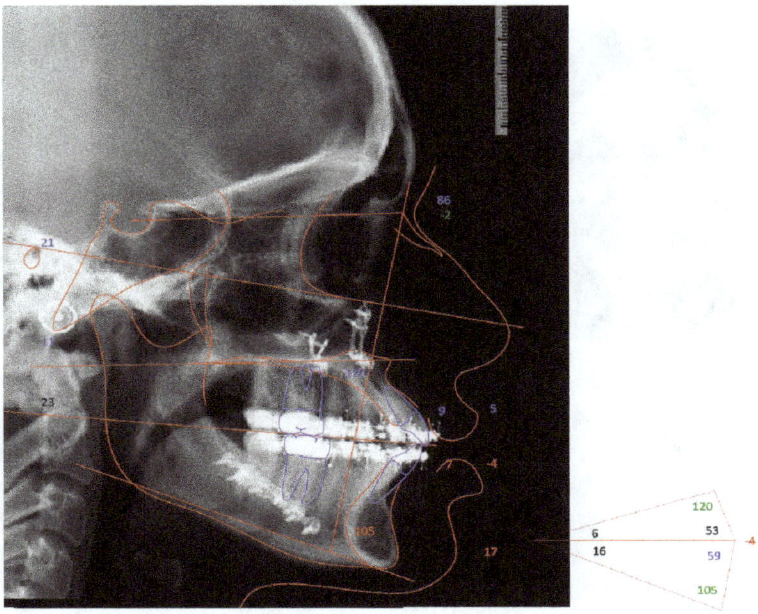

FIGURE 6: Cephalometric tracing (T2); T2=treatment progress (18 months).

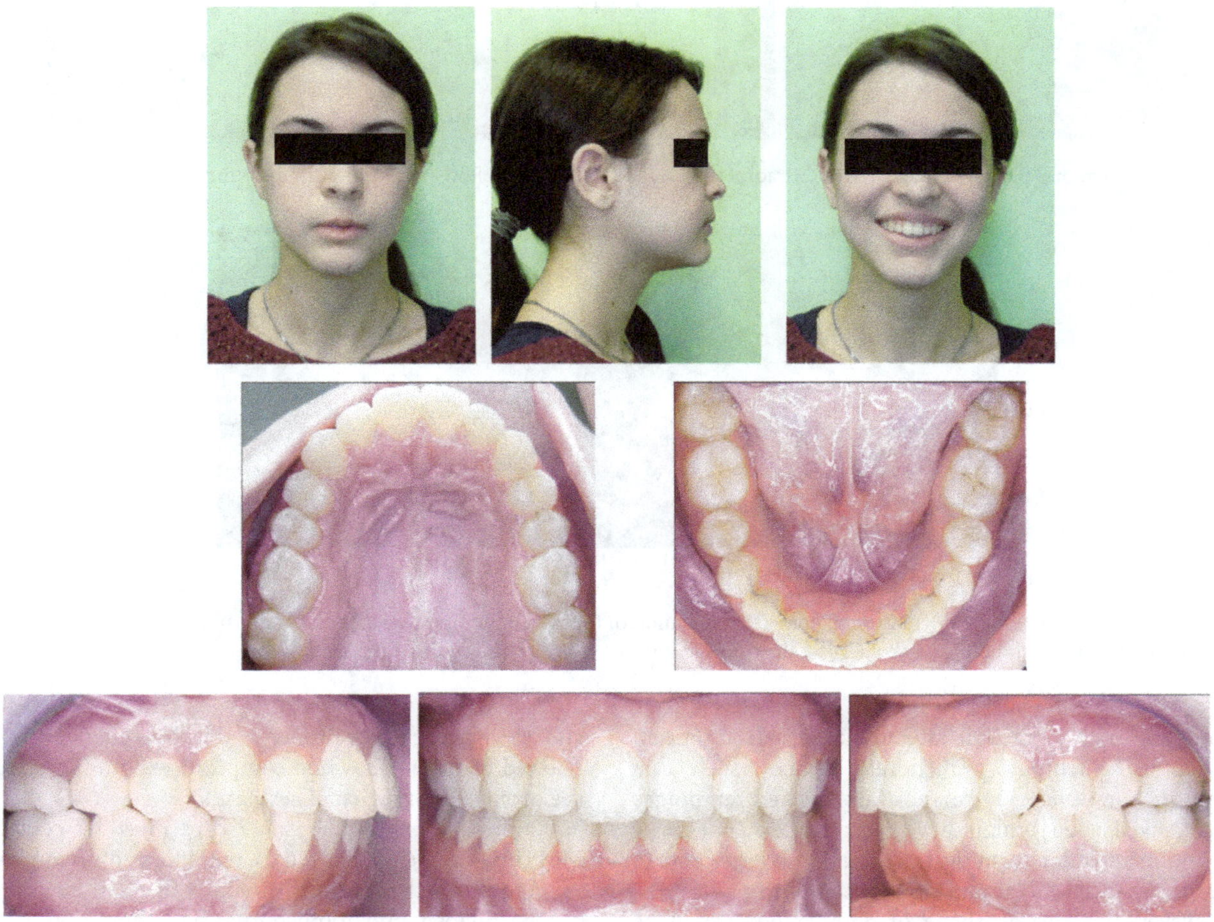

FIGURE 7: Extraoral photographs (T3) and intraoral photographs (T3); T3=posttreatment (36 months).

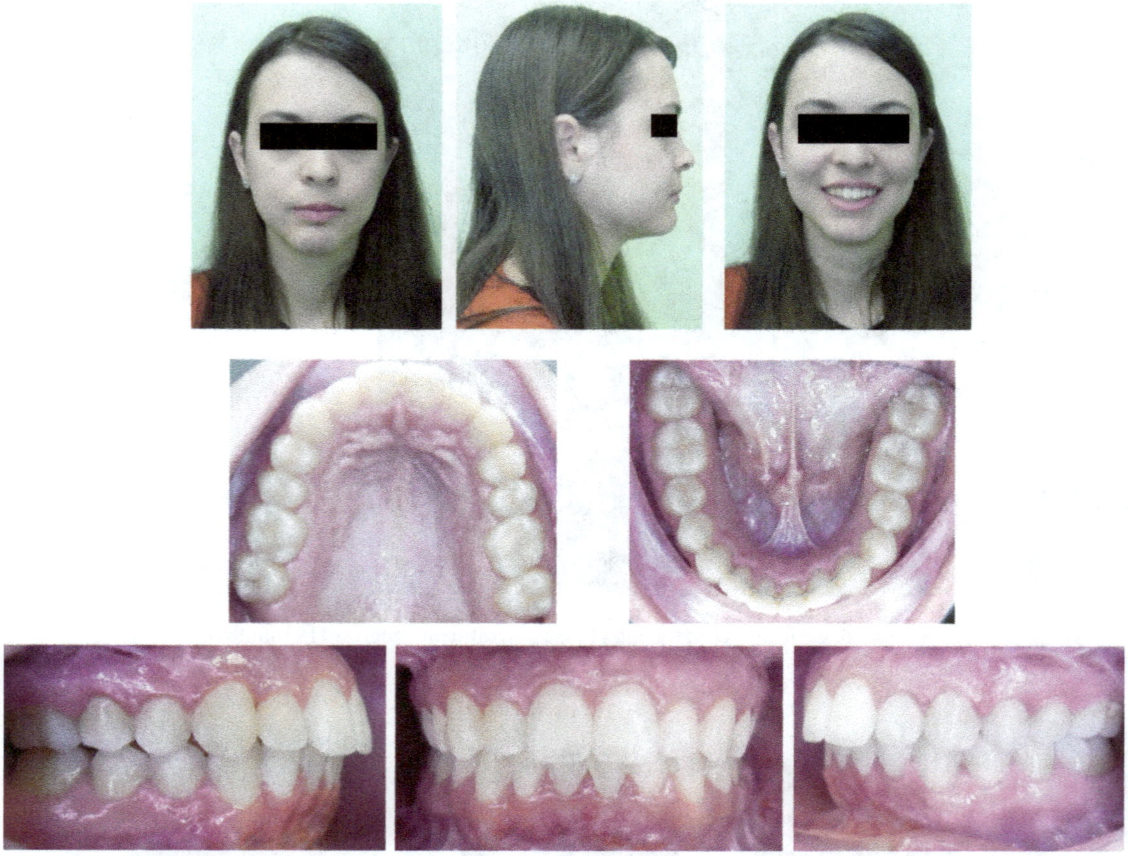

FIGURE 8: Extraoral photographs (T4) and intraoral photographs (T4); T4=follow-up (30 months after the end of the treatment).

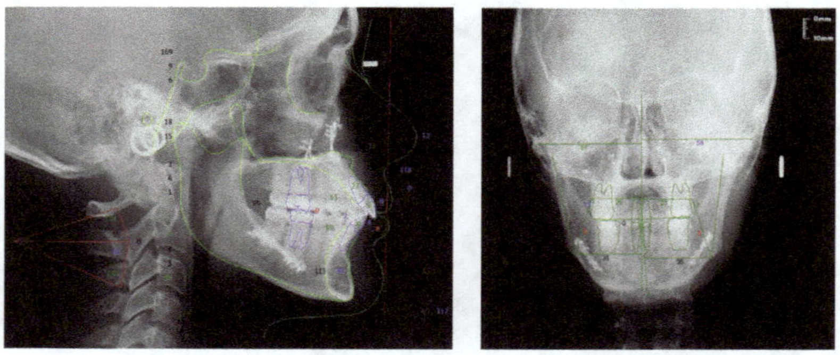

(a) (b)

FIGURE 9: Cephalometric tracing (T4): (a) cephalometric evaluation of the lateral radiograph of the skull and (b) cephalometric evaluation of the posteroanterior radiograph of the skull; T4=follow-up (30 months after the end of the treatment).

Anterior tooth retraction after molar distalization and retraction using temporary anchorage devices (such as a zygoma anchor device [24] or palatally located temporary anchorage device [25]) might have been an alternative treatment option in order to mitigate the severe overjet and to secure an enhanced molar and canine relationship.

However, the narrow shape of both arches would be left unaltered.

Therefore, SARPE was the best option for maxillary arch expansion and arch form improvement.

Extraction of two bicuspids in both arches was aimed at obtaining sufficient space to correct the severe crowding and to increase OVJ properly; this treatment option was rejected because this would compromise both the occlusion, the profile, and the dental aesthetics.

Overall, even though some care must be considered, MMTOD can be recognized as a safe form of treatment.

As regards the type of distractors that can be used, they can be divided into tooth-borne, bone-borne, and hybrid devices, mainly differing from the position of the fixation points and the stiffness of the appliance.

Tooth-borne devices induce less parallel expansion than bone-borne distractors because they apply their vector above the center of resistance: this difference implies an increase of anterior mandible widening when using the tooth-borne devices as compared when using the bone-borne and hybrid distractors.

The parallel expansion of the hemimandibles [26] leads to bone regeneration both at the basal and alveolar level, and it is crucial to reduce relapse.

Ideally, a basal bone widening would decrease the long-term relapse [27, 28].

The rigidity of a distractor defines the parallel movement of segments and the quantity of micromotion between segments.

The choice of bone-borne appliances is preferable because of a biomechanical advantage (vector applied close to the center of resistance) and a clinical advantage (smaller loss of anchorage and less skeletal relapse both during and after expansion and lower incidences of cortical fenestration and buccal root compared to tooth-borne distractors [29]; reduced risk of craniomandibular disorders minimizing lateral displacement of the condyle [30]).

In this case, the enlargement of the transversal diameter was obtained from the canines to the first and second premolars leading to a "fan-shaped" maxilla.

The symphyseal osteodistraction demonstrated parallel movements along the lower jaw, leading to a "square-shaped" mandible.

The slight bimaxillary advancement was deemed necessary to achieve completely the aesthetic goals of the treatment completely, with operational control of facial height and projection.

We decided to increase the facial projections with a slight undercorrection of the facial height in order to leave the patient's face slightly long from a qualitative standpoint, with the elimination of the lip strain and an attractive smile with the elimination of buccal corridors because of the previous maxillomandibular transversal expansion.

The Hawley retainer for the upper arch was selected to promote postorthodontic settling of the posterior occlusion of the patient [31]; this is a bonded retainer for the lower arch because of the slightly better stability over removable retainers and more acceptability to wear. A multistranded stainless steel wire was preferred over a fiber-reinforced composite retainer because of the absence of aesthetic concerns or allergy to metals [32].

The follow-up showed satisfactory long-term stability even though significant skeletal relapse was reported in the literature [33].

4. Conclusions

The Maxillomandibular Transverse Osteodistraction technique associated with orthognathic surgery described here could obtain both functional and aesthetic results in patients with reduced maxillary and mandibular transverse dimensions and severe dental crowding.

Abbreviations

MSDO: Mandibular symphyseal distraction osteogenesis
MMD: Mandibular midline (osteo-) distraction
TMSD: Transmandibular symphyseal (osteo-) distraction
SARPE: Surgically assisted rapid palatal expansion
SARME: Surgically assisted rapid maxillary expansion
MMTOD: Maxillomandibular transverse osteodistraction
CCE: Common childhood exanthemas
TMJ: Temporomandibular joint
OVJ: Overjet
OVB: Overbite
TPD: Transpalatal distractor
TMD: Transmandibular distractor
BSSO: Bilateral sagittal split osteotomy
IPR: Interproximal enamel reduction.

Authors' Contributions

Turatti G. and Bruni A. equally contributed to this work.

References

[1] P. Gandini, A. Schiavi, D. Camassa, and M. Manuelli, "Statistical survey of malocclusion in school age children," *Mondo Ortodontico*, vol. 14, no. 1, pp. 73–78, 1989.

[2] M. Bayram, M. Ozer, S. Arici, and A. Alkan, "Nonextraction treatment with rapid maxillary expansion and mandibular symphyseal distraction osteogenesis and vertical skeletal dimensions," *The Angle Orthodontist*, vol. 77, no. 2, pp. 266–272, 2007.

[3] S. Malkoç, S. Üşümez, and H. J. A. J. Işeri, "Long-term effects of symphyseal distraction and rapid maxillary expansion on pharyngeal airway dimensions, tongue, and hyoid position," *American Journal of Orthodontics and Dentofacial Orthopedics*, vol. 132, no. 6, pp. 769–775, 2007.

[4] M. Y. Mommaerts, Y. J. E. Spaey, P. E. G. S. Correia, and G. R. J. Swennen, "Morbidity related to transmandibular distraction osteogenesis for patients with developmental deformities," *Journal of Cranio-Maxillofacial Surgery*, vol. 36, no. 4, pp. 192–197, 2008.

[5] C. Burstone, "Precision lingual arches. Active applications," *Journal of Clinical Orthodontics*, vol. 23, no. 2, pp. 101–109, 1989.

[6] P. D. McDougall, J. A. McNamara, and J. M. Dierkes, "Arch width development in Class II patients treated with the Frankel appliance," *American Journal of Orthodontics*, vol. 82, no. 1, pp. 10–22, 1982.

[7] M. Weinberg and C. Sadowsky, "Resolution of mandibular arch crowding in growing patients with Class I malocclusions treated nonextraction," *American Journal of Orthodontics and Dentofacial Orthopedics*, vol. 110, no. 4, pp. 359–364, 1996.

[8] L. Pascon, C. Bazert, and E. Bardinet, "Contribution of mandibular symphyseal distraction osteogenesis to our therapeutic strategies," *Journal of Dentofacial Anomalies and Orthodontics*, vol. 19, no. 3, p. 305, 2016.

[9] G. J. C. D. H. Sperber, *Facial Skeleton*, BC Decker Inc., Ontario, Canada, 2001.

[10] J. W. King, J. C. Wallace, D. L. Winter, and J. A. Niculescu, "Long-term skeletal and dental stability of mandibular symphyseal distraction osteogenesis with a hybrid distractor," *American Journal of Orthodontics and Dentofacial Orthopedics*, vol. 141, no. 1, pp. 60–70, 2012.

[11] C. Guerrero, W. Bell, G. Contasti, and A. Rodriguez, "Mandibular widening by intraoral distraction osteogenesis," *British Journal of Oral and Maxillofacial Surgery*, vol. 35, no. 6, pp. 383–392, 1997.

[12] A. Haas, "Long-term posttreatment evaluation of rapid palatal expansion," *The Angle Orthodontist*, vol. 50, no. 3, pp. 189–217, 1980.

[13] G. Brown, *The Surgery of Oral and Facial Diseases and Malformations*, Kimpton, London, 1938.

[14] N. J. Betts, R. L. Vanarsdall, H. D. Barber, K. Higgins-Barber, and R. J. Fonseca, "Diagnosis and treatment of transverse maxillary deficiency," *The International Journal of Adult Orthodontics and Orthognathic Surgery*, vol. 10, pp. 75–96, 1995.

[15] L. Suri and P. Taneja, "Surgically assisted rapid palatal expansion: a literature review," *American Journal of Orthodontics and Dentofacial Orthopedics*, vol. 133, no. 2, pp. 290–302, 2008.

[16] J. W. King and J. C. Wallace, "Unilateral Brodie bite treated with distraction osteogenesis," *American Journal of Orthodontics and Dentofacial Orthopedics*, vol. 125, no. 4, pp. 500–509, 2004.

[17] W. R. Proffit, R. P. White, and D. M. Sarver, *Contemporary Treatment of Dentofacial Deformity*, Mosby, 2003.

[18] F. A. Bianchi, G. Gerbino, M. Corsico et al., "Soft, hard-tissues and pharyngeal airway volume changes following maxillo-mandibular transverse osteodistraction: computed tomography and three-dimensional laser scanner evaluation," *Journal of Cranio-Maxillofacial Surgery*, vol. 45, no. 1, pp. 47–55, 2017.

[19] G. A. Ramieri, M. C. Spada, M. Austa, S. D. Bianchi, and S. Berrone, "Transverse maxillary distraction with a bone-anchored appliance: dento- periodontal effects and clinical and radiological results," *International Journal of Oral and Maxillofacial Surgery*, vol. 34, no. 4, pp. 357–363, 2005.

[20] Z. S. AI-Aql, A. S. Alagl, D. T. Graves, L. C. Gerstenfeld, and T. A. Einhorn, "Molecular mechanisms controlling bone formation during fracture healing and distraction osteogenesis," *Journal of Dental Research*, vol. 87, pp. 107–118, 2008.

[21] J. von Bremen, D. Schäfer, W. Kater, and S. Ruf, "Complications during mandibular midline Distraction," *The Angle Orthodontist*, vol. 78, no. 1, pp. 20–24, 2008.

[22] A. Alkan, M. Özer, B. Baş et al., "Mandibular symphyseal distraction osteogenesis: review of three techniques," *International Journal of Oral and Maxillofacial Surgery*, vol. 36, no. 2, pp. 111–117, 2007.

[23] T. Gunbay, M. C. Akay, A. Aras, and M. Gomel, "Effects of transmandibular symphyseal distraction on teeth, bone, and temporomandibular joint," *Journal of Oral and Maxillofacial Surgery*, vol. 67, no. 10, pp. 2254–2265, 2009.

[24] M. A. Cornelis and H. J. de Clerck, "Maxillary molar distalization with miniplates assessed on digital models: a prospective clinical trial," *American Journal of Orthodontics and Dentofacial Orthopedics*, vol. 132, no. 3, pp. 373–377, 2007.

[25] M. Nienkemper, B. Wilmes, A. Pauls, S. Yamaguchi, B. Ludwig, and D. Drescher, "Treatment efficiency of mini-implant-borne distalization depending on age and second-molar eruption," *Journal of Orofacial Orthopedics / Fortschritte der Kieferorthopädie*, vol. 75, pp. 118–132, 2014.

[26] G. Raoul, T. Wojcik, and J. Ferri, "Outcome of mandibular symphyseal distraction osteogenesis with bone-borne devices," *Journal of Craniofacial Surgery*, vol. 20, no. 2, pp. 488–493, 2009.

[27] R. Conley and H. Legan, "Mandibular symphyseal distraction osteogenesis: diagnosis and treatment planning considerations," *The Angle Orthodontist*, vol. 73, pp. 3–11, 2003.

[28] M. Del Santo, C. A. Guerrero, P. H. Buschang, J. D. English, M. L. Samchukov, and W. H. Bell, "Long-term skeletal and dental effects of mandibular symphyseal distraction osteogenesis," *American Journal of Orthodontics and Dentofacial Orthopedics*, vol. 118, no. 5, pp. 485–493, 2000.

[29] M. Mommaerts, "Transpalatal distraction as a method of maxillary expansion," *British Journal of Oral and Maxillofacial Surgery*, vol. 37, no. 4, pp. 268–272, 1999.

[30] M. Y. Mommaerts, R. Polsbroek, G. Santler, P. E. G. S. Correia, J. V. S. Abeloos, and N. Ali, "Anterior transmandibular osteodistraction: clinical and model observations," *Journal of Cranio-Maxillofacial Surgery*, vol. 33, no. 5, pp. 318–325, 2005.

[31] E. M. Bauer, R. Behrents, D. R. Oliver, and P. H. Buschang, "Posterior occlusion changes with a Hawley vs Perfector and Hawley retainer: a follow-up study," *The Angle Orthodontist*, vol. 80, no. 5, pp. 853–860, 2010.

[32] A. Lucchese, M. Manuelli, L. Bassani et al., "Fiber reinforced composites orthodontic retainers," *Minerva Stomatologica*, vol. 64, no. 6, pp. 323–333, 2015.

[33] G. Rossini, B. Vinci, R. Rizzo, T. M. D. Pinho, and A. Deregibus, "Mandibular distraction osteogenesis: a systematic review of stability and the effects on hard and soft tissues," *International Journal of Oral and Maxillofacial Surgery*, vol. 45, no. 11, pp. 1438–1444, 2016.

32

Facial Emphysema following Closure of Oroantral Fistulae

Muhammad Aiman Mohd Nizar[1] **and Syed Nabil**[2]

[1]*Department of Diagnostic and Bioscience Craniofacial, Faculty of Dentistry, Universiti Kebangsaan Malaysia, Malaysia*
[2]*Department of Oral and Maxillofacial Surgery, Faculty of Dentistry, The National University of Malaysia, Malaysia*

Correspondence should be addressed to Syed Nabil; dr_syednabil@yahoo.com.my

Academic Editor: Eugenio Maiorano

Subcutaneous emphysema (SE) is a swelling which develops due to air entrapped underneath the subcutaneous tissue and facial planes causing distention of the overlying skin. SE can develop due to trauma, surgery, or infection. The diagnosis of SE is mostly based on clinical findings of crepitation upon palpation of the swelling. Once diagnosed, SE is usually managed by close observation and in some cases may require surgical decompression and antibiotic prophylaxis. We report a rare case of SE of the left malar which developed following closure of oroantral communication using the buccal fat pad.

1. Introduction

Oroantral communication (OAC) is a condition where a connection exists between the maxillary sinus and the oral cavity, which, over time, will be lined by epithelium to form an oroantral fistula (OAF). The condition occurs commonly in upper posterior maxillary teeth extractions, especially ones with preexisting periapical abnormalities or when the roots are widely divergent [1]. Other reported causes of OAC include implant surgery, enucleation of cysts and tumors, maxillary orthognathic osteotomies, osteomyelitis, trauma, and various maxillary pathologic entities [1].

There are few treatment options for oroantral communication, including buccal advancement flap, plasma-rich fibrin and buccal fat pad (BFP), or a combination thereof. The BFP was mentioned for the first time by Heister in 1727 and was known as "glandula molaris" [2]. It was later described in detail by Marie-François-Xavier Bichat in 1802 [2]. It has been documented to provide a good clinical outcome when used for the closure of OAC [3]. Dolanmaz et al. reported that all of the 75 patients who underwent OAC closure with pedicled BFP in their series had successful outcomes [3].

Pedicled BFP is an established treatment option for OAF closure. Its richness of vascularity, low donor-site morbidity, simple surgical procedure, and proximity to the recipient site are the main advantages of this technique [4]. The familiar complications following this procedure include partial breakdown of the flap, especially in the closure of large maxillary defect, excessive scarring, and infection [5]. Emphysema, which develops as a result of air being pushed subcutaneously, is rarely anticipated with the use of BFP [6]. The authors report a rare case of subcutaneous emphysema at the left malar region that developed in the early postoperative period following closure of OAF using BFP.

2. Case Report

A 45-year-old man visited our clinic with the complaint of a persistent hole in the 27-socket area. He explained that he had had tooth 27 extracted five years earlier and subsequently noted an opening at the socket which had never closed. He recalled that the extraction procedure itself had been uncomplicated. Subsequently, he had occasionally developed symptoms of chronic sinusitis such as nasal congestion and nasal discharge, but he had never sought treatment for it. There was also an occasional fluid discharge from the opening, but it never troubled him too much. Otherwise, he had no underlying medical illnesses. Upon examination, it was noted that there was a fistula of 1.5 cm × 1 cm in the area of the extracted 27. Tooth 16 was present, but 18 was missing. No fluid discharge was seen. Further investigation with cone beam CT confirmed an oroantral fistula measuring 9.4 mm × 7.7 mm (Figures 1 and 2). The sinus lining was noticeably thickened.

He underwent closure of the oroantral fistula under local anesthesia. A buccal mucoperiosteal flap was elevated around the fistula. Subsequently, the periosteum under the flap was incised to give access to the BFP. The BFP was mobilized and advanced to cover the fistula. Thereafter, the buccal mucoperiosteal flap was advanced over the BFP to achieve two-layered closure of the fistula. The advancing flaps were approximated with vertical mattress suturing. Bleeding was minimal throughout the procedure, and he was discharged with antibiotics, antihistamine, and nonsteroidal anti-inflammatory analgesia. He was advised on nasal precautions including instructions to sneeze with the mouth open and avoid blowing the nose, forceful spitting, and use of straws.

Around 2 hours postoperative, he contacted the clinic to inform us that he had a sudden facial swelling that developed over a few seconds (Figure 3). The swelling occurred immediately after he tried to clear his throat. There was no associated pain or bleeding during the development of swelling. He was asked to come back to the clinic immediately. Upon examination of the swelling, crepitation was felt on palpation. Intraorally, the surgical wound was intact, and no indication of bleeding was noted. Diagnosis of emphysema was made on the basis of the sudden progression of swelling after a trigger and clinical findings. He was reassured, and reemphasis was placed on the sinus precaution. Besides the already prescribed medications, no additional intervention was made. The swelling was slightly reduced 8 hours after its initial appearance (Figure 4). Otherwise, he was well with minimal bleeding and pain.

Upon review, 3 days later, the swelling was significantly reduced (Figure 5). At 7 days postoperative, the swelling had completely resolved (Figure 6). He was well throughout the postoperative period. Upon examination of the intraoral wound, no dehiscence was seen, and the oroantral fistula was completely closed. He was followed up again a few weeks later, and no reoccurrence of swelling or OAF was seen.

3. Discussion

Subcutaneous emphysema (SE) is a swelling that develops as a result of air being forced underneath the tissue and facial planes and is characterized by a crepitus sound upon palpation [7]. It could be of iatrogenic, incidental (patient factor), traumatic, or pathological cause [8]. It could be misinterpreted as a hypersensitivity reaction (angioedema), cellulitis, or necrotizing fasciitis [9]. In this case, the left malar SE developed following surgery using BFP for the closure of OAF when the patient tried to clear his throat. It is likely that the increase in intranasal pressure and subsequently in the maxillary sinus allowed air to escape through the sinus defect and travel to the subcutaneous tissue via the mucoperiosteal opening created to access the BFP. Roccia et al. explained that the increasing pressure inside the upper airways can lead the air to be forced into the surrounding tissues through mucoperiosteal tears resulting from the defects of the paranasal air sinuses and takes the path of least resistance between the loose connective tissues [10]. A study measuring the intranasal pressure in adults during nose blowing, sneezing, and coughing using fluid dynamic simulations concluded that the high intranasal pressures generated by nose blowing would propel viscous fluid into paranasal sinuses [11]. Therefore, it is possible that the act of clearing the throat with a closed mouth might also cause increased pressure in the paranasal sinuses.

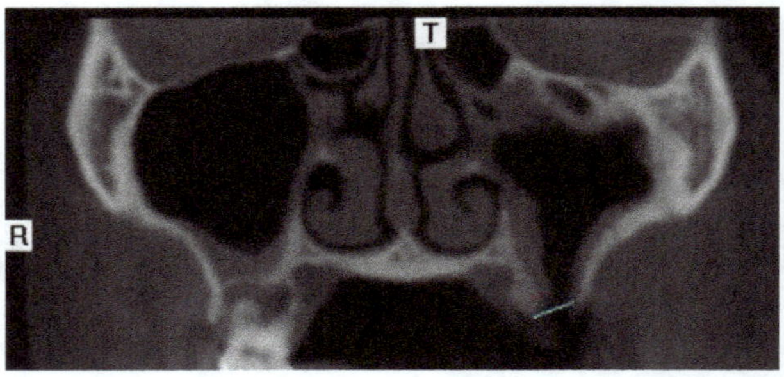

Figure 1: Cone beam computed tomography (CBTC) showing the oroantral communication in coronal view.

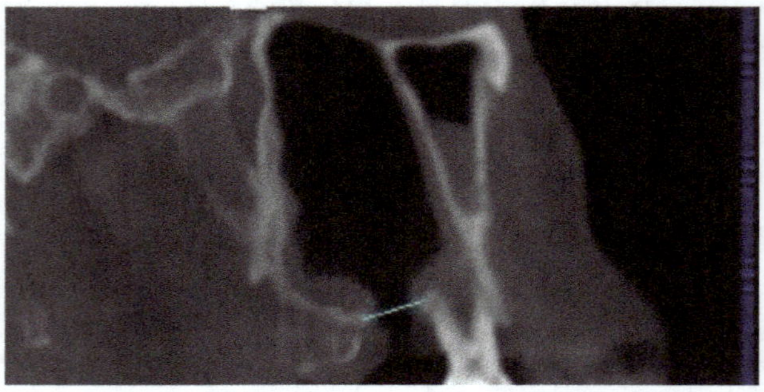

Figure 2: Cone beam computed tomography (CBTC) showing the oroantral communication in sagittal view.

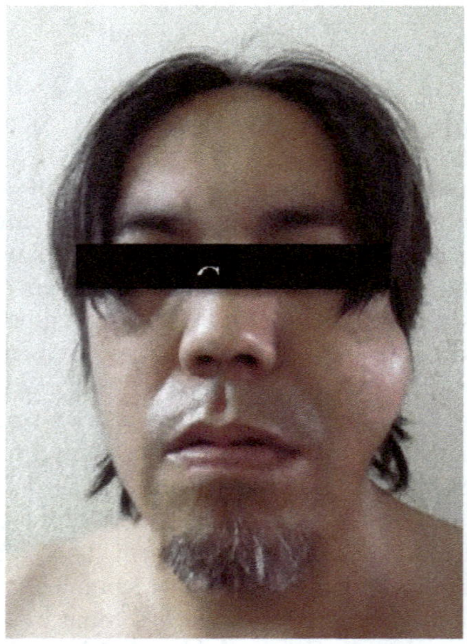

Figure 3: Immediately after swelling developed at the left malar region (around 2 hours postoperatively).

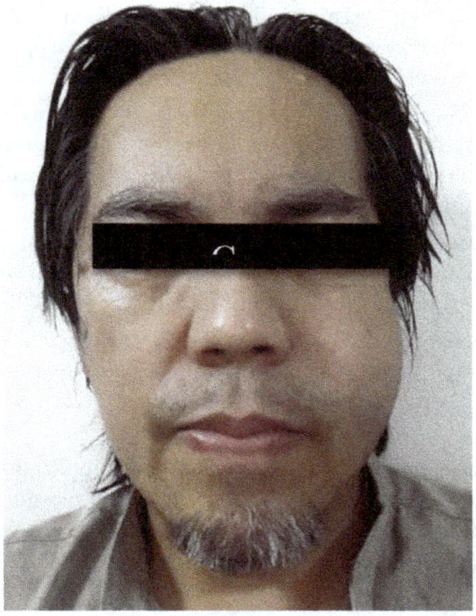

FIGURE 4: Postoperative 8 hours shows resolving of the left malar swelling.

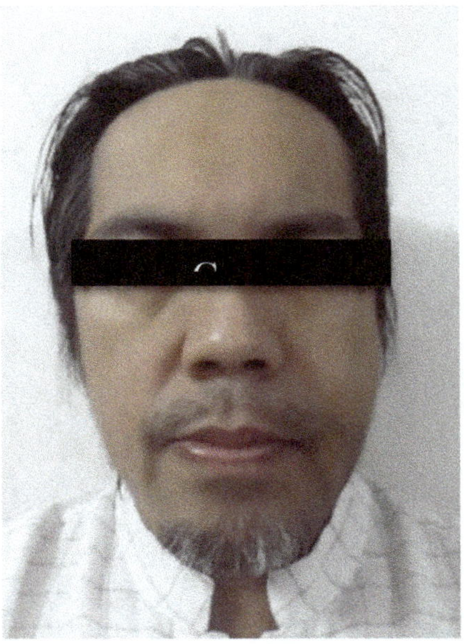

FIGURE 5: Postoperative day 3 shows that residual left malar swelling remains.

SE usually is self-limiting and does not require treatment, but observation is crucial [8]. Occasionally, subcutaneous emphysema can cause infection [7, 12]. Antibiotics are therefore commonly prescribed in SE. The rationale for antibiotic prescription is that air introduced subcutaneously could be nonsterile [7]. A broad-spectrum-coverage antibiotic can be used to cover the more common head, neck, sinus, and skin microflora. Systemic steroids, meanwhile, can be used to reduce soft-tissue edema [13]. Rarely, an extensive SE may need multiple stab incisions to decompress the emphysema [8]. Subcutaneous emphysema could also be fatal in the case where the emphysema travels to the lateral pharyngeal space and may reach the mediastinum by dissecting the visceral

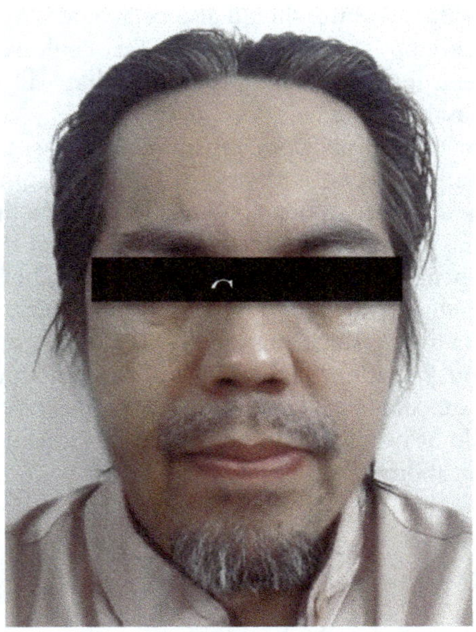

FIGURE 6: Postoperative day 7 shows that the swelling is completely resolved.

space and causing pneumomediastinum, which is characterized by Hamman's sign—a friction rub sound upon cardiac auscultation [13]. In our reported case, the patient was prescribed antibiotics following surgery, and this was continued following the development of emphysema. However, no steroids were prescribed as the swelling was quite localized.

SE following a surgery of closure of the oroantral fistula using a pedicel BFP is very rare [14]. In the only previously reported case, swelling of the left cheek developed a few seconds after the patient sneezed two hours after the surgery. The swelling was associated with crepitus upon palpation. In that reported case, after a course of antibiotics, the emphysema completely resolved after 14 days. Similarly, in our case, two hours postoperative, a swelling developed at the left malar after the patient tried to clear his throat. Crepitation was felt on palpation of the swelling. We prescribed antibiotics, antihistamines, and nonsteroidal anti-inflammatory analgesia, and the swelling completely resolved after 10 days. Between these two cases, there are similarities in terms of onset, clinical presentation, management, and the final outcome. This suggests predictability in the causes of such occurrences, making prevention possible. More importantly, both had an uneventful recovery with conservative management; therefore, they should not discourage the clinician from utilizing BFP for similar OAF cases.

Here, we would like to emphasize that the postoperative instructions given to the patient should be very clear regarding the sinus precautions as it appears that in both cases, adherence to these instructions would have prevented the development of postoperative subcutaneous emphysema. These precautions include sneezing and coughing with the mouth open, avoiding blowing or whistling, and avoiding doing the Valsalva maneuver. Use of a straw and smoking are also prohibited. This will help to prevent an increase in nasal and intraoral pressure which may lead to subcutaneous emphysema. Strenuous physical activity, which will increase intrasinusoidal pressure, should also be avoided. Apart from that, there are options for medication that could reduce the risk of sneezing, such as antihistamines that will keep the patient's nasal dry and nasal decongestant.

In conclusion, subcutaneous emphysema is a possible complication following a closure of oroantral communication as reported here. This complication occurs due to air escaping the paranasal sinuses via an opening at the socket into the subcutaneous tissue of the malar area. The breached periosteum due to the harvesting of BFP is a crucial factor in allowing air to go subcutaneously. A crepitus sensation and sound upon palpation of the swelling is a pathognomonic feature of subcutaneous emphysema. Postoperative instructions should be explained very clearly to the patient to avoid this complication.

Consent

Written consent was obtained from the patient involved in this report.

References

[1] H. Dym and J. C. Wolf, "Oroantral communication," *Oral and maxillofacial surgery*, vol. 24, no. 2, pp. 239–247, 2012.

[2] U. G. Marzano, "Lorenz Heister's 'molar gland'," *Plastic and Reconstructive Surgery*, vol. 115, no. 5, pp. 1389–1393, 2005.

[3] D. Dolanmaz, H. Tuz, S. Bayraktar, M. Metin, E. Erdem, and T. Baykul, "Use of pedicled buccal fat pad in the closure of oroantral communication: analysis of 75 cases," *Quintessence International (Berlin, Germany: 1985)*, vol. 35, no. 3, pp. 241–246, 2004.

[4] J. Singh, K. Prasad, R. M. Lalitha, and K. Ranganath, "Buccal pad of fat and its applications in oral and maxillofacial surgery: a review of published literature (February) 2004 to (July) 2009," *Oral Surgery, Oral Medicine, Oral Pathology, Oral Radiology, and Endodontics*, vol. 110, no. 6, pp. 698–705, 2010.

[5] A. D. Rapidis, C. A. Alexandridis, E. Eleftheriadis, and A. P. Angelopoulos, "The use of the buccal fat pad for reconstruction of oral defects: review of the literature and report of 15 cases," *Journal of Oral and Maxillofacial Surgery*, vol. 58, no. 2, pp. 158–163, 2000.

[6] A. Hassani, S. Shahmirzadi, and S. Saadat, "Applications of the buccal fat pad in oral and maxillofacial surgery," *A Textbook of Advanced Oral and Maxillofacial Surgery*, vol. 3, p. 3417, 2016.

[7] W. S. McKenzie and M. Rosenberg, "Iatrogenic subcutaneous emphysema of dental and surgical origin: a literature review," *Journal of Oral and Maxillofacial Surgery*, vol. 67, no. 6, pp. 1265–1268, 2009.

[8] S. M. Balaji, "Subcutaneous emphysema," *Journal of Maxillofacial and Oral Surgery*, vol. 14, no. 2, pp. 515–517, 2015.

[9] B. F. Brasileiro, A. L. Cortez, L. Asprino et al., "Traumatic subcutaneous emphysema of the face associated with paranasal sinus fractures: a prospective study," *Journal of Oral and Maxillofacial Surgery: Official Journal of the American Association of Oral and Maxillofacial Surgeons*, vol. 63, no. 8, pp. 1080–1087, 2005.

[10] F. Roccia, A. Griffa, A. Nasi, and N. Baragiotta, "Severe subcutaneous emphysema and pneumomediastinum associated with minor maxillofacial trauma," *The Journal of Craniofacial Surgery*, vol. 14, no. 6, pp. 880–883, 2003.

[11] J. M. Gwaltney Jr., J. O. Hendley, C. D. Phillips, C. R. Bass, N. Mygind, and B. Winther, "Nose blowing propels nasal fluid into the paranasal sinuses," *Clinical Infectious Diseases*, vol. 30, no. 2, pp. 387–391, 2000.

[12] A. Shudo, "Buccal abscess derived from subcutaneous emphysema caused by the Valsalva maneuver after oral surgery with pedicled buccal fat pad grafting," *Oral Surgery*, 2021.

[13] N. Patel, S. K. Lazow, and J. Berger, "Cervicofacial subcutaneous emphysema: case report and review of literature," *Journal of Oral and Maxillofacial Surgery*, vol. 68, no. 8, pp. 1976–1982, 2010.

[14] R. Metin and U. Tatli, "An unexpected complication after use of pedicled buccal fat pad for closure of oroantral fistulae: emphysema," *Journal of dentistry and oral sciences*, vol. 1, no. 3, pp. 1–8, 2019.

33

Mouthwash with Active Oxygen (blue®m) Reduces Postoperative Inflammation and Pain

Bruna Marca Mattei,[1] **Soraia A. W. Imanishi**,[1] **Grasieli de Oliveira Ramos**,[1] **Paloma Santos de Campos**,[2] **Suyany Gabriely Weiss**,[3] **and Tatiana Miranda Deliberador**[4]

[1]*Universidade do Oeste de Santa Catarina (UNOESC), Joaçaba, Santa Catarina, Brazil*
[2]*Universidade Federal do Rio Grande do Sul (UFRGS), Porto Alegre, Rio Grande do Sul, Brazil*
[3]*School of Health Sciences, Department of Dentistry, Universidade Positivo, Curitiba, Paraná, Brazil*
[4]*Latin American Institute of Dental Research and Education (ILAPEO), Curitiba, Paraná, Brazil*

Correspondence should be addressed to Tatiana Miranda Deliberador; tdeliberador@gmail.com

Academic Editor: Adrian Kasaj

The aim of this case series was to evaluate the effects of blue®m mouthwash on oral surgical wounds. Eleven patients underwent bilateral preprosthetic surgery and were instructed to apply the product only to the right side of the surgery. In this way, the right side corresponds to the test side and the left side (place without applying any type of solution) to the control side. After seven days of using the product (3 times a day), the following parameters were evaluated by means of a visual analogue scale: pain, changes in taste, and acceptance by the patient. Then, the level of tissue inflammation was assessed, by the number of pixels, using ImageJ® software. The main results show that the blue®m mouthwash was widely accepted by patients, reducing their pain. The number of inflammation pixels was lower on the test side ($p < 0.05$), indicating improved healing. It is suggested that blue®m mouthwash positively influences tissue healing reducing pain and the postsurgical inflammatory process; however, randomized clinical trials should be done to prove this clinical observation.

1. Introduction

Chlorhexidine (CHX) is considered the gold standard in the antiseptic treatment of the oral mucosa, due to its broad antibacterial spectrum [1, 2]; it is recommended in postsurgical follow-ups, since mechanical hygiene control could cause trauma to the surgical wound, rupture of the suture, and loss of the ability to keep tissues in position [3, 4]. However, studies have shown that CHX has a cytotoxic effect on gingival fibroblasts [5, 6], gingival epithelial cells [7], periodontal ligament cells [8], cultured alveolar bone cells [9], and osteoblastic cells [10]. It has also been demonstrated to interfere with tissue regeneration processes [10]. From the search for a mouthwash that minimized the undesirable effects with the use of CHX, new lines of research are needed, among them, the treatment with active oxygen [11].

A team of dental surgeons led by Dr. Peter Blijdorp in the Netherlands developed a product based on active oxygen (blue®m) with the intention of putting all the desirable properties of mouthwashes in just one product. blue®m mouthwash has in its composition sodium perborate, the enzyme glucose oxidase derived from honey, xylitol, and lactoferrin [12]. Applications in dentistry vary from use in inflammation of gums and ulcers, peri-implantitis, and after oral surgery to a substitute for hypochlorite sodium during irrigation of root canals [13]. Inclusion in everyday hygienic oral care of toothpaste and mouthwash blue®m reduced the severity of inflammatory changes and improved the hygienic condition of the oral cavity in cardiology patients suffering from periodontal disease [14]. A randomized controlled clinical trial showed that toothpaste containing active oxygen and lactoferrin has comparable antiplaque and antigingivitis efficacies with triclosan-containing toothpaste [15]. Previous in vitro studies from the team have demonstrated that blue®m at higher concentrations provided inhibitory halo of Porphyromonas gingivalis similar to chlorhexidine digluconate [16] and human keratinocyte cell line demonstrated a greater proliferation rate when exposed to lower concentrations of blue®m mouthwash [17]. Nevertheless, more studies are needed to evaluate patient experience and the effects on wound healing.

Wound healing is an extremely complex process, which requires a variety of cells to increase its metabolic activity, resulting in oxygen demand [18]. The application of topical oxygen to the wound has been shown to promote healing through several processes, including antibacterial activities, neovascularization, collagen production, epithelialization, phagocytosis (encompassing microorganisms, cells, or debris by macrophages or neutrophils), and degradation of necrotic tissue wound [19]. Topical Oral Oxygen Therapy (OOT) is aimed at accelerating the healing process by ensuring neovascularization, removing toxins, stimulating the formation of new blood cells, increasing the production of stem cells, and eradicating bacteria [20]. OOT with blue®m can be a substitute for CHX in postsurgical care, not showing the disadvantages observed with the use of CHX, especially in relation to the cytotoxic effect on gingival cells [12].

The local use of active oxygen as support for wound healing and tissue regeneration may be a tendency to replace the use of CHX, but it inspires parsimony, due to the small number of clinical monitoring cases reported or clinical trials in the literature. It is hypothesized that the use of the mouthwash will improve healing thus reducing postoperative pain. Hence, the aim of this case series is to evaluate the effects of blue®m mouthwash (OOT) in postoperative oral surgery care.

2. Case Series Report

2.1. Ethical Aspects. This study was approved by the Ethics and Research Committee on Human Beings at UNOESC under the number 2.031.509 CAAE: 65808817.3.0000.5367. Each patient received and signed an informed consent form and an image use term. The work was conducted in compliance with the Declaration of Helsinki.

2.2. Inclusion Criteria. A sample of 14 patients of both sexes, aged between 54 and 74 years old, who underwent preprosthetic surgeries at Universidade do Oeste de Santa Catarina (UNOESC), Joaçaba, São Paulo, Brazil, was selected.

2.3. Exclusion Criteria. The exclusion criteria involved patients that used drugs that could directly interfere with the tissue response, such as anticoagulants and antiplatelet agents, patients who have been on antibiotic or anti-inflammatory therapy in the past three months, diabetics, smokers, and individuals who have reported a history of hypersensitivity to any mouthwash. Also, irradiated patients, pregnant women, and patients who presented lesions such as candidiasis or lichen were considered exclusion criteria.

2.4. Study Design. The patients were submitted to preprosthetic surgery to remove hyperplasia of the maxillary posterior and anterior ridge. Infiltrative anesthesia was performed in the anterior border region using 4% articaine with epinephrine 1 : 100,000. Two parallel linear incisions were made, along the upper or lower alveolar ridge, extending along the excessive fibrous tissue over the ridge. The two incisions were found at the base (deepest region), forming a wedge of fibrous tissue. After making the incisions, the fibrous tissue was carefully removed with the aid of a Molt detacher. The continuous scalloped suture was performed with 4-0 silk thread. The surgeries were performed by different operators.

After preprosthetic surgery, each patient was prescribed acetaminophen 750 mg and received 50 ml of the test antiseptic (blue®m mouthwash) together with 15 units of flexible rods with cotton tips. In the postoperative period, the patient was instructed to apply the solution over the entire length of the region, only on the right side up to the midline (below the nose), with the aid of flexible rods three times a day (upon waking up, after lunch, and before bedtime), for a week. The left side served as a control. Patients were instructed not to rinse their mouths with water or other mouthwashes and neither to eat for 30 minutes after applying the solution.

2.5. Follow-Up. The postoperative evaluation was performed 7 days after the surgery, at the time of suture removal (Figure 1). An intraoral physical examination was performed to assess the healing of the surgical wound. Pain was measured using the visual analogue scale (VAS). Patients were asked about changes in taste, the occurrence of adverse effects, and whether they would use the antiseptic again. After removing the suture, the operated area was dried with gauze and photographic records were made. All recordings were performed with a cell phone camera (iPhone 6, Apple®, California, USA) with the aid of retractors (Lip Retractor Expandex—Indusbello®, Paraná, Brazil). The patient was positioned lying down for all sites operated on the upper arch and seated for all surgical sites on the lower arch. All data collections were performed by the same researcher.

2.6. Photographic Analysis. The photos of the healing surgical wound were analyzed using the ImageJ® program, developed by Wayne Rasband of the Research Services Branch, National Institute of Mental Health (Bethesda, Maryland, USA), which is a domain Java image processor and image analyzer software inspired in NIH Image for the Apple Macintosh. The repertoire of functions of this software can be expanded by means of several ready-made plugins, available on the Internet, or by developing new ones.

Areas of inflammation (red), considered a less healed oral tissue, and areas of healthy tissue (pink), considered with a better healing tissue, were selected. A saturation pattern was set for all images to equalize the contrast by 0.5%. Through the threshold color plugin available on the Internet, the selection of colors given in pixel shapes was carried out. The area of interest was defined, whether covered with healthy tissue or granulation/inflammation. The number of red pixels (Figure 2) and pink pixels was obtained after appropriate adjustment of the scale, where the software turns

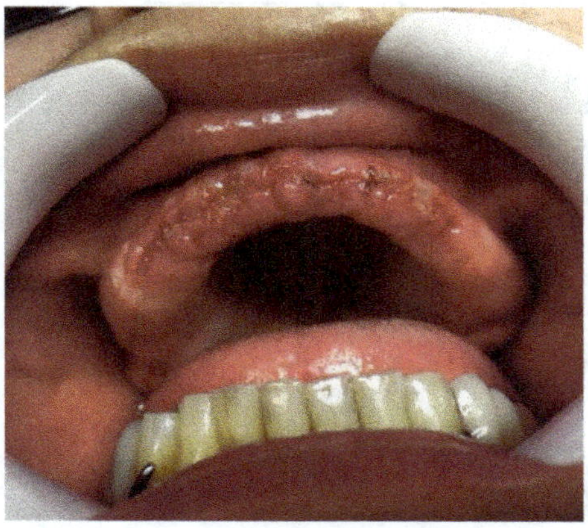

Figure 1: 7-day postoperative period. Image used for analyzing pixels.

the areas that satisfy the chosen pattern to black and the other areas to white.

2.7. Statistical Analysis. All analyses were performed with a significance level of 0.05 using the Bioestat® Program version 5.3. Pain values (test side and control side) were compared using the ANOVA test. The healing images were subjected to the ANOVA test of paired samples.

3. Results

There were 14 patients in the study, 8 were women and 11 were men, and 81% of them were over 60 years old. Three were excluded: one because he was unable to attend the follow-up on the 7th day to remove the suture and for the photographic record and the other two because they had used antiseptic throughout the length of the surgery. Therefore, the study evaluated 11 patients.

Regarding the minimum pain measured by patients (categorized by pain intensity numbers 0 and 1), it was more often reported on the test side than on the control side (Figure 3). The most severe pain (categorized by pain intensity numbers 7 and 8) was reported more frequently on the control side ($p < 0.05$), as shown in Figure 4. It is possible to see in the adjusted curve of the graph that the average pain intensity is lower for the test side.

There were no patient-reported changes in taste, nor was there any adverse effect. Everyone replied that they would use the product again.

The control and test sides analyzed by the ImageJ® program showed statistical significance ($p < 0.05$) in relation to the number of red pixels (Figure 5) but did not show statistical significance ($p > 0.05$) when analyzed in relation to the number of pink pixels. More than 90% of the patients had a lower index of red pixels on the test side, while only 72% of patients presented with a lower index of red pixels on the control side.

4. Discussion

Postoperative pain and the presence of inflammation are common symptoms after oral surgeries. In this series of cases, we opted to prescribe for patients the topical application of a new mouthwash (blue®m) that has a slow release of oxygen, with the hypothesis that, on the side that the product was applied, the patient would feel less pain and have a lesser inflammatory process. Our results showed that the hypothesis can be accepted. The mouthwash effects seem to reduce postoperative pain and inflammation.

Some people have difficulty controlling plaque build-up by only conventional tooth cleaning. Oral surgery usually requires the use of chlorhexidine mouthwashes, in addition to conventional tooth cleaning, to avoid injuries, drop of sutures, or even patient's inability. Chlorhexidine is an effective chemical method of plaque control, used for the treatment of several periodontal conditions, such as gingivitis [21, 22]. However, the use of chlorhexidine is associated with a variety of local side effects such as brown staining of the teeth and oral tissues [23], altered taste perception [23–25], supragingival calculus accumulation [25, 26], and oral mucosal lesions [23, 25]. Thus, the search for mouthwash as effective as chlorhexidine with fewer side effects has become relevant. blue®m products have oxygen as an active ingredient, and it was demonstrated that toothpaste containing active oxygen and lactoferrin has comparable antiplaque and antigingivitis efficacies with triclosan-containing toothpaste [15]. It is also known that oxygen application is involved in several stages of the healing process, such as reepithelialization, angiogenesis, and collagen synthesis [20]. Therefore, the present case series is aimed at evaluating the effects of blue®m mouthwash in postoperative oral surgery care.

This split-mouth model using test and control sides in the same patient was based on many intraoral studies in humans and also in animal studies. This methodological aspect was similar to that used by Laureano Filho et al. [27] and Marlière et al. [28], which allowed qualifying the patient as a control group for himself. In this way, it was possible to control individual variations (eating habits, metabolism, hygiene, and personal behavior) in addition to variations in the surgical procedure itself (operator, duration, type of anesthetic, and technique). However, it is still necessary to consider a bias in our study, which is the possible interference of prostheses in the postsurgical period. We believe that in two cases (in which the most severe pain occurred precisely on the test side), it was not due to the ineffectiveness of the antiseptic but because perhaps there was interference from the prosthesis. Still, in relation to this bias, there are reports that the resilient material used as a temporary reshaper also affected the healing of soft tissues [29].

Despite the presence of the product having reached a statistical difference, the pain intensities reported between the test and control sides should be more discrepant. One answer to this inconsistency would be the inappropriate choice of the method of collecting pain measurement in elderly patients. According to Gold and Roberto [30], the Visual Analogue Scale (VAS) requires a higher level of cognitive function; therefore, it may be inappropriate for patients with low levels of education and with cognitive changes. Considering that our patients really had difficulty in quantifying the intensity of pain, we corroborate that, for elderly people with a low level of formal education, perhaps the best

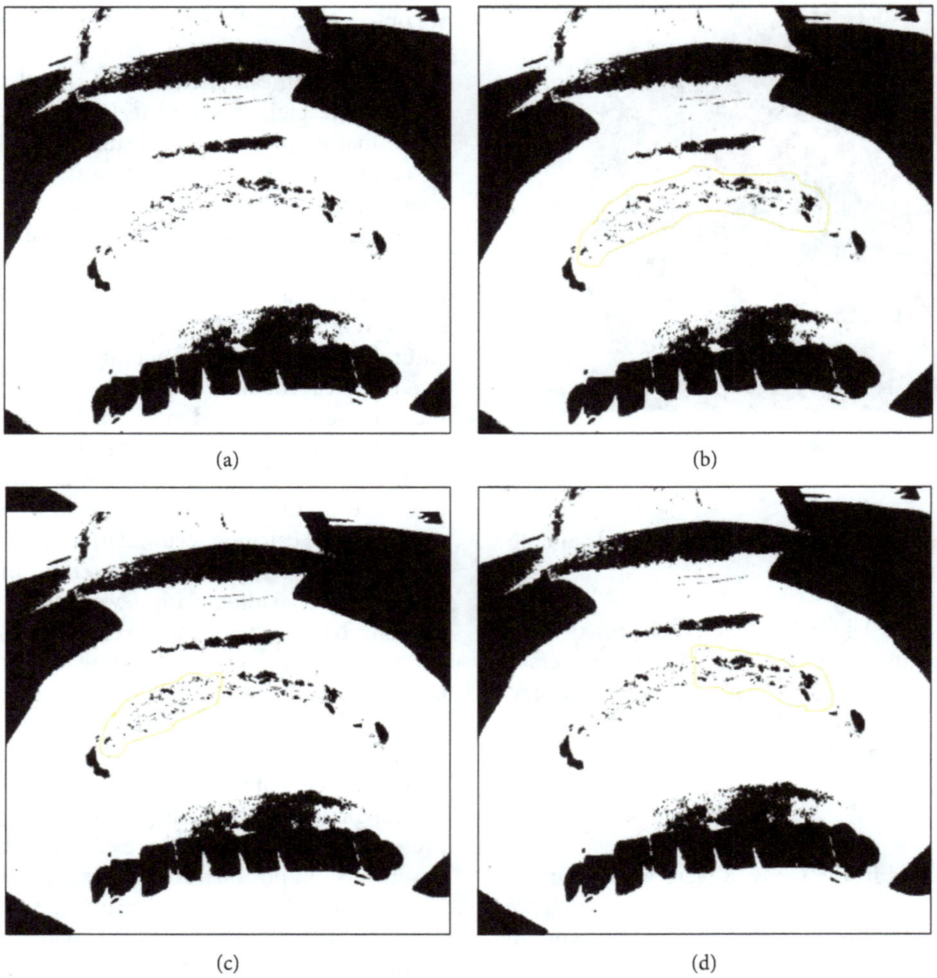

FIGURE 2: Analysis of images using the ImageJ® program for red pixels. (a) Image obtained after the appropriate adjustment of the red color scale; the software turns the area of interest to black and the other areas to white. (b) Segmentation of the total area of interest to obtain the total amount of red pixels. (c) Segmentation of the right area (test side) to obtain red pixels. (d) Segmentation of the left region (control side) to obtain red pixels in this area.

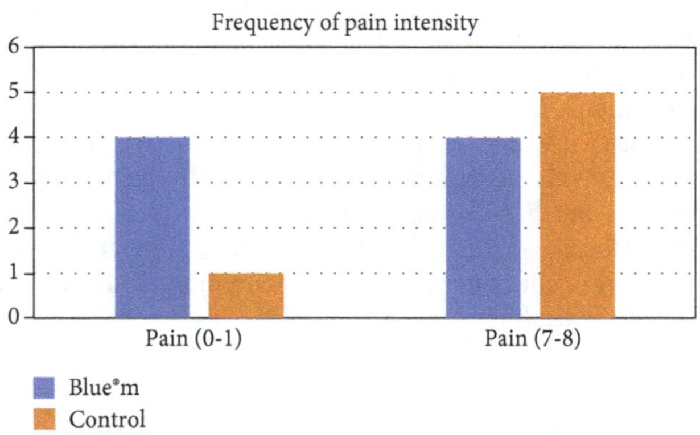

FIGURE 3: Frequency of pain by stratification of pain intensity.

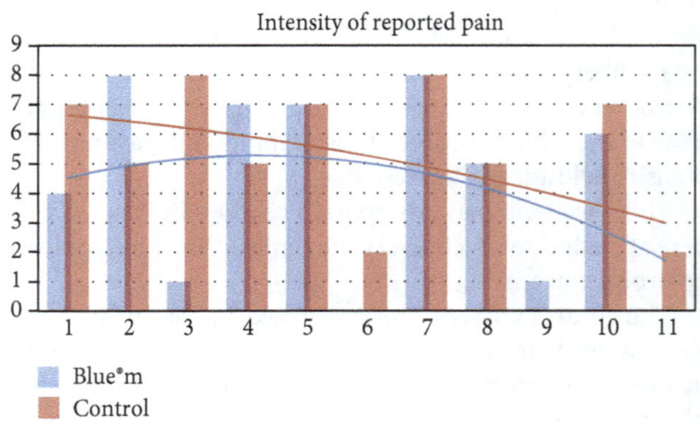

FIGURE 4: Intensity of reported pain between the control and test sides. ANOVA, $p = 0.0233$.

method of measuring pain is the face scale, as proposed by the same authors.

It is known that there are many difficulties in performing clinical analysis of tissue healing. So, in this series of cases, we chose to use a methodology that was able to make the comparison between the test and control sides using an objective program (ImageJ®). This methodology had already been carried out in medical studies and is now beginning to be introduced in dentistry [31–33].

The analysis of healing by ImageJ® revealed that sites treated with blue®m showed a higher frequency of less

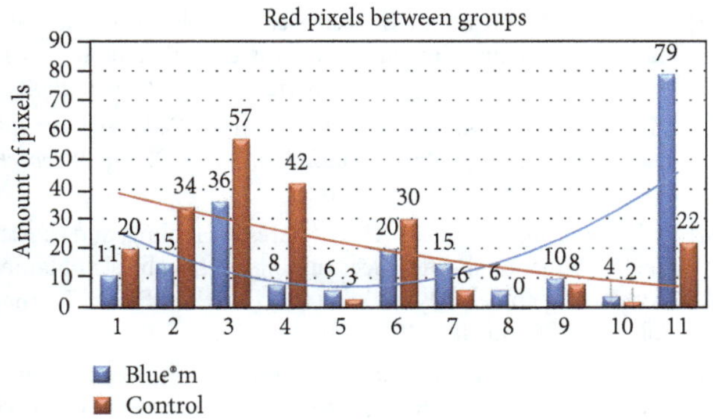

Figure 5: Comparison of the number of red pixels between the control and test sides. ANOVA: two-paired samples. $p < 0.05$.

inflamed sites (fewer red pixels). However, there was no difference when analyzing the number of more healed sites (pink pixels). The work of Pansani et al. [34] clarifies this issue. It has been reported that the individual's age factor alters the synthesis and proliferation of fibroblasts but has no influence on their inflammatory activity. Therefore, fibroblasts from older individuals maintain the capacity of the inflammatory response similar to what occurs in fibroblasts from young individuals. Thus, in the studied sample, regardless of age, the product appears to have reduced inflammation. In the improvement of healing, no difference was observed between the sides; one of the justifications is the time period of only 7 days of the analyses.

Photographic monitoring is used to monitor and illustrate the different degrees of severity of skin lesions. Benson et al. [35] used photographic images to monitor dental treatment using the Pro-Plus® software. In this manuscript, the authors were concerned with reducing the reflection produced in photography with the aid of specific devices, demonstrating that it influences the results of image analysis, and therefore, there is a need for standardization in image capture. In our study, the photographic records were made only with ambient light and avoiding shadows, which may explain the lack of pixel difference between the test and the control sides.

The results of the present study prove to be promising. Therefore, studies on new mouthwash alternatives are necessary to reduce any harmful effect on oral tissues, especially during the postsurgical healing phase, aiding in healing and decreasing the morbidity of oral surgeries.

5. Conclusion

Within the limits of this study, blue®m mouthwash seems to reduce postoperative pain as well as clinical signs of inflammation.

References

[1] H. Loe and C. Rindom Schiott, "The effect of mouthrinses and topical application of chlorhexidine on the development of dental plaque and gingivitis in man," *Journal of Periodontology*, vol. 5, no. 2, pp. 79–83, 1970.

[2] S. Jenkins, M. Addy, and R. G. Newcombe, "Dose response of chlorhexidine against plaque and comparison with triclosan," *Journal of Clinical Periodontology*, vol. 21, no. 4, pp. 250–255, 1994.

[3] F. C. Batista, J. Batista, L. Eraldo, and B. R. Fronza, "Características microscópicas de superfície e biocompatibilidade dos fios de sutura mais utilizados na cirurgia bucal," *Revista Brasileira de Cirurgia e Implantodontia*, vol. 9, no. 35, pp. 243–249, 2002.

[4] A. Aranega, T. Okamoto, and E. G. Jardim Junior, "Clorexidina e fio de sutura: influência da antissepsia com clorexidina sobre a contaminação bacteriana em suturas com fio de poliéster. Estudo microbiológico e histomorfológico em ratos," *Revista Gaúcha de Odontologia*, vol. 47, no. 2, pp. 71–74, 1999.

[5] S. Boisnic, L. Ben Slama, M. C. Branchet-Gumila, M. Watts, and G. D'Arros, "Wound healing effect of Eludril® in a model of human gingival mucosa," *Revue de Stomatologie et de Chirurgie Maxillo-faciale*, vol. 107, no. 6, pp. 431–435, 2006.

[6] A. J. Mariotti and D. A. Rumpf, "Chlorhexidine-induced changes to human gingival fibroblast collagen and non-collagen protein production," *Journal of Periodontology*, vol. 70, no. 12, pp. 1443–1448, 1999.

[7] H. Babich, B. J. Wurzburger, Y. L. Rubin, M. C. Sinensky, and L. Blau, "An *in vitro* study on the cytotoxicity of chlorhexidine digluconate to human gingival cells," *Cell Biology and Toxicology*, vol. 11, no. 2, pp. 79–88, 1995.

[8] Y. C. Chang, F. M. Huang, K. W. Tai, and M. Y. Chou, "The effect of sodium hypochlorite and chlorhexidine on cultured human periodontal ligament cells," *Oral Surgery, Oral Medicine, Oral Pathology, Oral Radiology, and Endodontics*, vol. 92, no. 4, pp. 446–450, 2001.

[9] C. T. Cabral and M. H. Fernandes, "*In vitro* comparison of chlorhexidine and povidone-iodine on the long-term proliferation and functional activity of human alveolar bone cells," *Clinical Oral Investigations*, vol. 11, no. 2, pp. 155–164, 2007.

[10] M. Gianelli, F. Chellini, M. Margheri, P. Tonelli, and A. Tani, "Effect of chlorohexidine digluconate on different cell types: a molecular and ultrastructural investigation," *Toxicology In Vitro*, vol. 2, pp. 308–317, 2008.

[11] *Oxigen enriched water and oral oxygen terapy*, A. Pakdaman, Germany, 1985, February 2017, http://www.bluemcare.com/pt/beneficios-do-bluem/publicacoes.

[12] April 2020, https://www.swallowdental.co.uk/catalogues/Bluem-Compendium.pdf.

[13] P. W. KRIJNEN, "Healing oxygen: healing action applied in dentistry," 2011, April 2020, https://static.webshopapp.com/shops/035143/files/056054158/dutch-journal-dentistry-tandartspraktijk-healing-o.pdf?_ga=1.179714342.323417379.1487907128.

[14] I. M. Makeeva and N. V. Tambovtseva, "Applying toothpaste and mouthwash BLUEM in complex oral care in patients with coronary heart disease," *Stomatologiia (Mosk)*, vol. 93, no. 3, pp. 18–20, 2014.

[15] E. J. Cunha, C. M. Auersvald, T. M. Deliberador et al., "Effects of active oxygen toothpaste in supragingival biofilm reduction: a randomized controlled clinical trial," *International Journal of Dentistry*, vol. 2019, Article ID 3938214, 7 pages, 2019.

[16] T. M. Deliberador, S. G. Weiss, F. Rychuv et al., "Comparative analysis *in vitro* of the application of blue oral gel versus chlor-

hexidine on *Porphyromonas gingivalis*: a pilot study," *Advances in Microbiology*, vol. 10, no. 4, pp. 194–201, 2020.

[17] B. Mattei, S. Imanishi, G. Ramos, P. Campos, S. Weiss, and T. Deliberador, "Mouthwash with active oxygen (blue) induces keratinocytes proliferation," *Open Journal of Stomatology*, vol. 10, no. 6, pp. 107–114, 2020.

[18] S. Schreml, R. M. Szeimies, L. Prantl, S. Karrer, M. Landthaler, and P. Babilas, "Oxygen in acute and chronic wound healing," *The British Journal of Dermatology*, vol. 163, no. 2, pp. 257–268, 2010.

[19] D. R. Knighton, T. K. Hunt, H. Scheuenstuhl, B. J. Halliday, Z. Werb, and M. J. Banda, "Oxygen tension regulates the expression of angiogenesis factor by macrophages," *Science*, vol. 221, no. 4617, pp. 1283–1285, 1983.

[20] D. E. Eisenbud, "Oxygen in wound healing: nutrient, antibiotic, signaling molecule, and therapeutic agent," *Clinics in Plastic Surgery*, vol. 39, no. 3, pp. 293–310, 2012.

[21] P. James, H. V. Worthington, C. Parnell et al., "Chlorhexidine mouthrinse as an adjunctive treatment for gingival health," *Cochrane Database of Systematic Reviews*, vol. 3, article CD008676, 2017.

[22] L. F. N. P. da Costa, C. D. S. F. Amaral, D. D. S. Barbirato, A. T. T. Leão, and M. F. Fogacci, "Chlorhexidine mouthwash as an adjunct to mechanical therapy in chronic periodontitis: a meta-analysis," *Journal of the American Dental Association (1939)*, vol. 148, no. 5, pp. 308–318, 2017.

[23] M. Addy, "Chlorhexidine compared with other locally delivered antimicrobials. A short review," *Journal of Clinical Periodontology*, vol. 13, no. 10, pp. 957–964, 1986.

[24] M. G. Marinone and E. Savoldi, "Chlorhexidine and taste. Influence of mouthwashes concentration and of rinsing time," *Minerva Stomatologica*, vol. 49, no. 5, pp. 221–226, 2000.

[25] D. A. Strydonck, D. E. Slot, U. Velden, and F. Weijden, "Effect of a chlorhexidine mouthrinse on plaque, gingival inflammation and staining in gingivitis patients: a systematic review," *Journal of Clinical Periodontology*, vol. 39, no. 11, pp. 1042–1055, 2012.

[26] I. D. Mandel, "Antimicrobial mouthrinses: overview and update," *Journal of the American Dental Association (1939)*, vol. 125, no. 2, pp. 2–10, 1994.

[27] J. R. Laureano Filho, I. B. Camargo, A. C. B. Firmo, and E. D. Oliveira e Silva, "Evaluation of laser therapy in edema, pain and trismus reductipon after removal of inferior third molars:preliminary results," *Revista de Cirurgia e Traumatologia Buco Maxilo Facial*, vol. 8, no. 1, pp. 47–56, 2008.

[28] D. A. A. Marlière, L. F. Lanini, T. C. Bittencourt, and N. M. S. P. Assis, "Combination therapeutic dexamethasone and meloxicam in inflammatory controlafter third molars surgery," *Revista de Cirurgia e Traumatologia Buco Maxilo Facial*, vol. 15, no. 4, pp. 15–24, 2015.

[29] C. Chaves, C. E. Vergani, D. Thomas et al., "Biological effects of soft denture reline materials on L929 cells in vitro," *Journal of Tissue Engineering*, vol. 5, 2014.

[30] D. T. Gold and K. A. Roberto, "Correlates and consequences of chronic pain in older adults," *Geriatric Nursing*, vol. 21, no. 5, pp. 270–273, 2000.

[31] C. A. Damante, S. L. Greghi, A. C. Sant'ana, and E. Passanezi, "Clinical evaluation of the effects of low-intensity laser (GaAlAs) on wound healing after gingivoplasty in humans," *Journal of Applied Oral Science*, vol. 12, no. 2, pp. 133–136, 2004.

[32] R. Schara, I. Sersa, and U. Skaleric, "T1 relaxation time and magnetic resonance imaging of inflamed gingival tissue," *Dentomaxillofacial Radiology*, vol. 38, no. 4, pp. 216–223, 2009.

[33] M. Cáceres, A. Oyarzun, and P. C. Smith, "Defective wound-healing in aging gingival tissue," *Journal of Dental Research*, vol. 93, no. 7, pp. 691–697, 2014.

[34] T. N. Pansani, F. G. Basso, D. G. Soares, J. Hebling, and C. A. S. Costa, "Functional differences in gingival fibroblasts obtained from young and elderly individuals," *Brazilian Dental Journal*, vol. 27, no. 5, pp. 485–491, 2016.

[35] P. E. Benson, A. A. Shah, and D. R. Willmot, "Measurement of white lesions surrounding orthodontic brackets: captured slides vs digital camera images," *The Angle Orthodontist*, vol. 75, no. 2, pp. 226–300, 2005.

34

High Submandibular Anteroparotid Approach for Open Reduction and Internal Fixation of Condylar Fracture

Kamichika Hayashi[1] **Takeshi Onda,**[1] **Hirona Honda,**[1] **Mitsuru Takata,**[2] **Hiroyuki Matsuda,**[2] **Hidetoshi Tamura,**[2] **and Masayuki Takano**[1]

[1]*Department of Oral and Maxillofacial Surgery, Tokyo Dental College, Tokyo, Japan*
[2]*Oral and Maxillofacial Surgery, Kameda General Hospital, Chiba, Japan*

Correspondence should be addressed to Kamichika Hayashi; hayashikamichika@tdc.ac.jp

Academic Editor: Alberto Delbem

Aim. There are several techniques for the treatment of mandibular condylar fractures. This is the first report of the high submandibular anteroparotid approach for open reduction and internal fixation of condylar fracture. *Materials and Methods.* A 41-year-old woman fell indoors and injured her face. She was referred to our department for detailed examination and treatment of a suspected mandibular fracture. X-ray and computed tomography showed a right mandibular condylar base fracture and lateral dislocation of the fracture fragment. Open reduction and internal fixation procedures were performed for a right mandibular condylar fracture under general anesthesia. The mandibular ramus was reached by approaching from the inferior margin of the mandible, delaminating the masseter fascia posteriorly, and bypassing the anterior margin of the parotid gland. Once the fractured bone was reached, reduction and fixation were performed. *Results.* We have achieved good results by the high submandibular anteroparotid approach, which is minimally invasive and simple, to reduce and fix condylar fractures. With this approach, no facial artery or retromandibular vein was encountered, and the mental stress for the surgeon was minimal. Postoperative wound infection, parotid gland complications such as parotitis and salivary fistula, facial nerve dysfunction such as facial paralysis, and esthetic disorders such as scarring were not observed. *Conclusions.* Although it is necessary to examine more cases in the future, the high submandibular anteroparotid approach may be useful as a new approach for open reduction and internal fixation of condylar fractures.

1. Introduction

The treatment policy for mandibular condylar fractures is based on local factors, such as the fracture site and the presence or absence of concurrent fractures, and patient characteristics such as age, general condition, and social background [1, 2]. There is no consensus on the treatment for mandibular condylar fractures [3–5]. In adult mandibular condylar neck and base fractures, surgical therapy is reported to have a better functional prognosis than nonsurgical therapy [6–9].

The approaches to surgery can be categorized mainly as intraoral and extraoral. The intraoral approach is performed using an intraoral mucosal incision. Extraoral approaches include the Al-Kayat approach performed using a preauricular incision and the retromandibular approach and submandibular approaches (the Risdon approach) performed using skin incisions. The choice of surgery should be based on the fracture site (head, neck, and base of the mandibular condyle) and mode (crack, displacement, metastasis, or dislocation) [10]. Both approaches consider the course of the facial nerve. Recently, the clinical usefulness of the retromandibular approach [11–13], the downward and curvilinear extension of the preauricular skin crease incision [14–16], and the high perimandibular transmasseteric approach (HPTM) [17–20] have been recognized. These approaches facilitate the expansion of the operative field for mandibular condylar neck and base fractures and minimize the risk of postoperative facial nerve dysfunction.

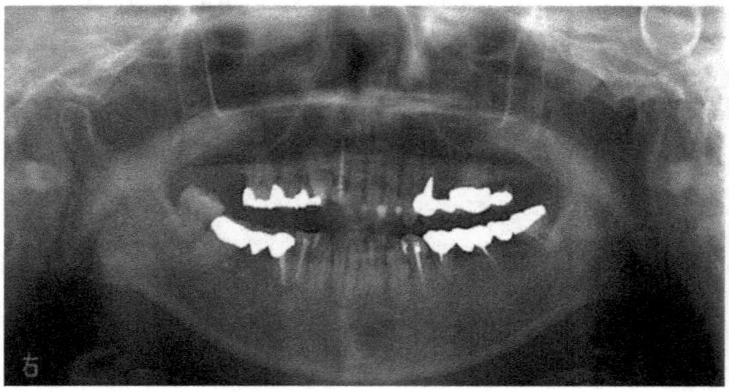

(a)

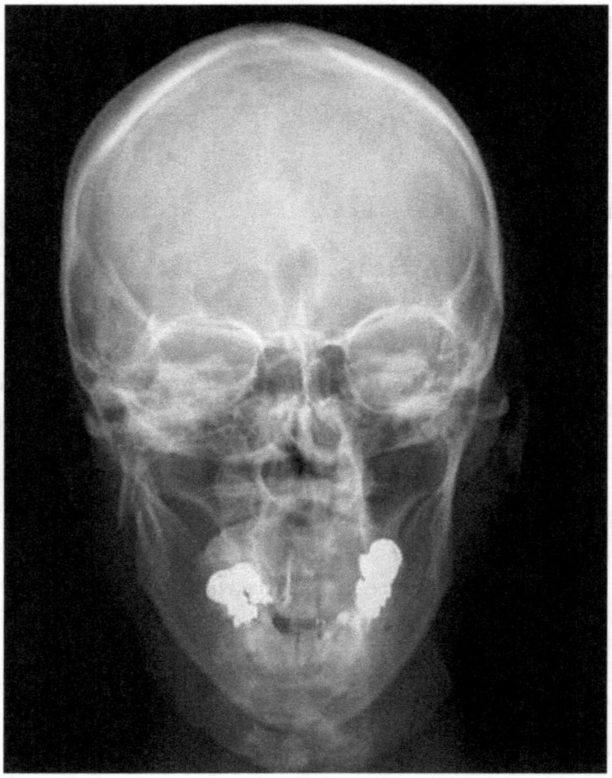

(b)

Figure 1: (a) Panoramic X-ray at the first visit. A right mandibular condylar base fracture is observed. (b) A simple head X-ray at the first visit (P-A). A fracture of the right mandibular condyle and external displacement of the bone fragment are observed.

We applied a high submandibular anteroparotid approach involving a skin incision in the inferior margin of the mandible to the delamination of the masseter fascia in the posterior direction, by bypassing the anterior margin of the parotid gland to reach the mandible and obtained good results. A summary of a case is presented along with a literature review.

2. Case Presentation

The patient was a 41-year-old woman with a height of 166 cm and a weight of 58 kg. In January 2019, she fell indoors and injured her face and visited a hospital for medical treatment. Her chief complaint was trismus. A close examination of the head at the head and neck surgery department showed no abnormal findings. She was referred to our department for detailed examination and medical treatment for a suspected mandibular fracture. Her first visit to our department was on the following day. Her family history was unremarkable. Facial findings on the first visit included mild swelling and reddening in the right preauricular region. The intraoral finding was displacement of the median line of the mandible to the right. The right molar was also in early contact, and the left molar had an open bite. Trismus was observed, and her mouth opening capacity was 10 mm between the upper and lower central incisors. A panoramic radiograph showed a right mandibular condylar base fracture (subcondylar fracture, Lindahl's classification [21]) (Figure 1(a)). An X-ray of the head (P-A) showed a right mandibular condylar dislocation fracture (displacement fracture, Maclennan's classification [22]) (Figure 1(b)). Computed tomography (CT) imaging showed a right mandibular condylar base fracture and lateral dislocation of the fracture fragment (Figure 2). No fractures were observed elsewhere. No fractures of the teeth and of the alveolar bones of the upper and lower jaws were seen. Amoxicillin 750 mg/day was prescribed for 3 days to prevent infection, and acetaminophen 500 mg was prescribed for pain on an as-needed basis. Because she hoped for early functional recovery, open reduction and internal fixation, rather than a nonsurgical approach, were chosen. The patient was consulted on the treatment policy.

Nine days after the first visit, open reduction and internal fixation procedures were performed on the right mandibular condylar fracture under general anesthesia. During surgery, 1 g of cefmetazole sodium was administered to prevent surgical site infection. The skin incision was designed to be 5 mm caudal to the inferior margin of the mandible and 5 to 7 mm posterior to the posterior margin of the mandible to include the mandibular angle. The incision line extended more posteriorly than Wilk's skin incision [17, 18]. Thus, an incision line with a total length of approximately 5 cm was made (Figure 3(a)). Subsequently, a subcutaneous cut of approximately 2 cm was made in the skin along the platysma fascia. Delamination was performed between the subcutaneous and platysma fascia. The platysma was located and incised to the depth of the masseter fascia; the incision was 1 cm

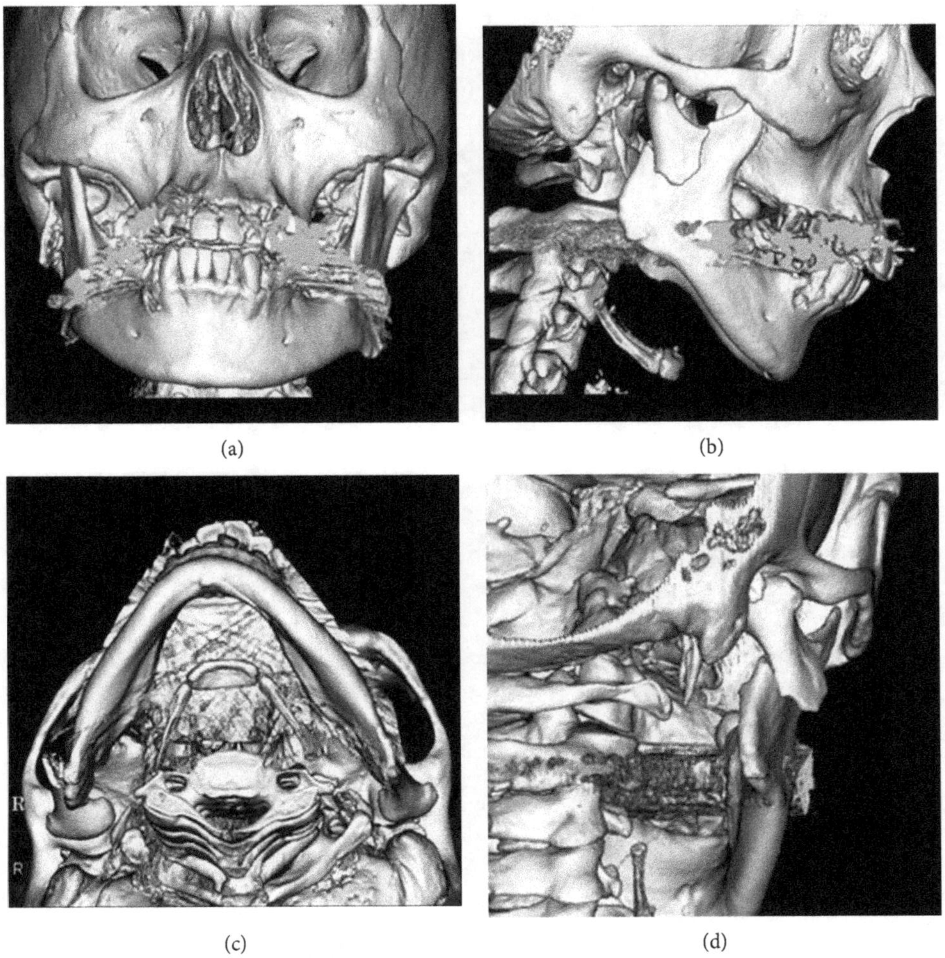

Figure 2: 3D-constructed CT image at the first visit. (a) Front. (b) Right side. (c) Axial. (d) 45 degrees behind to the right. CT imaging shows a right mandibular condylar base fracture and lateral dislocation of the fracture fragment. No fractures are observed except for those of the mandible. No fractures of the alveolar bones of the upper and lower jaws are also observed. No tooth fracture is observed.

cranial from the mandibular margin in the anterior direction and 2 cm cranial from the mandibular margin in the posterior direction. Wilk and Biotchane [17, 18] made an incision up to the masseter muscle; however, in the present case, an incision was made only in the platysma muscle, and the masseter fascia was delaminated approximately 2 cm further cranially along the masseter fascia. The platysma was thin, with the masseter fascia immediately inside the platysma (Figure 3(b)). A buccal muscle branch that was running along the masseter fascia was found and retracted cranially to avoid injuring it. Next, the masseter fascia was delaminated towards the posterior margin of the ramus. While proceeding with the delamination towards the posterior margin of the ramus, the parotid gland was encountered, and delamination was performed between the parotid gland and the masseter fascia using a Metzenbaum scissor. A muscle retractor was applied to the anterior margin of the parotid gland to slight traction of the parotid tissue backward. The posterior margin of the parotid gland was located by inserting a reverse warping muscle retractor at the posterior margin of the ramus followed by a gentle displacement of the parotid gland posteriorly. A periosteal incision was made in the posterior margin of the ramus by a round-edged knife. Next, the periosteum on the medial and lateral surfaces of the ramus was delaminated by a periosteal elevator, and the fracture site was reached. A muscle retractor was inserted on the anterior side, and the masseter muscle was slightly extruded anteriorly to permit the localization and observation of the fractured site. A protector was inserted inside the mandibular ramus; a hole of approximately 2 cm was drilled from the lateral side on the caudal side of the fracture line by a steel bar. A 0.5-mm-diameter metal wire was passed through the hole (Figure 3(c)). An assistant attempted to reduce the fractured fragment by pulling the metal wire and the ramus downward (Figure 3(d)). After reducing the fractured fragment, plate fixation was performed. A MatrixMANDIBLE Subcondylar Strut Plate (Depuy Synthes, Switzerland), developed for mandibular condylar fractures was used for the fixation (Figure 3(e)) [23]. The surgeon manually confirmed the patient's jaw movements. The surgeon manually opened and closed the patient's jaw. In addition, the surgeon manually moved the patient's jaw from side to side. And after confirming the absence of occlusion, a periosteal suture was placed with an absorbable thread. The platysma was also sutured, followed by the dermis. The skin was sutured with a nonabsorbable thread. Finally, Dual-Top anchor screws

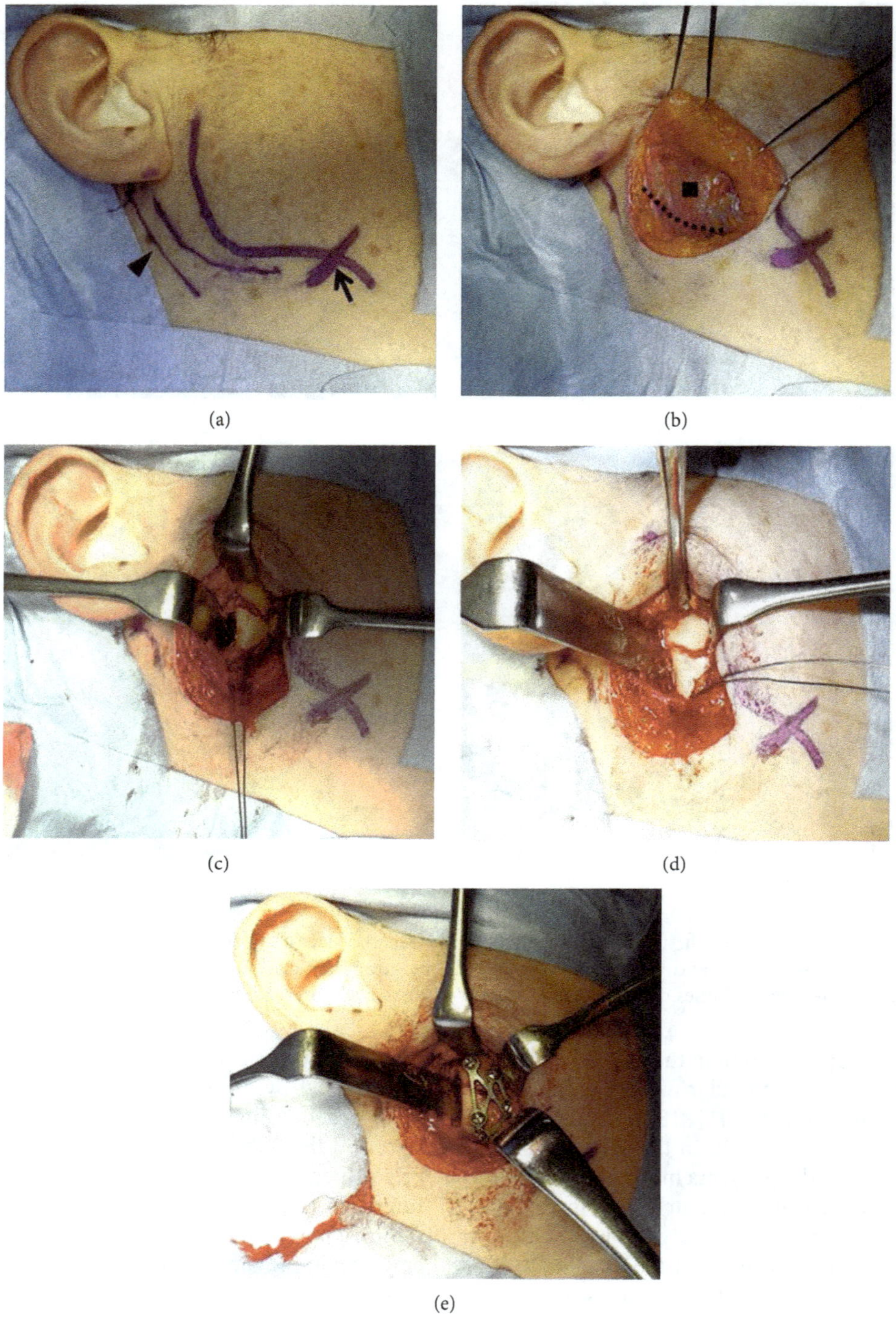

Figure 3: (a) Black arrow: facial artery; black triangle: sternocleidomastoid muscle. The skin incision line, the outline of the mandible, the sternocleidomastoid muscle, and the facial artery are traced using gentian violet. The planned skin incision is 0.5 mm caudally from the mandibular margin and 5 to 7 mm posteriorly from the posterior margin of the ramus to include the mandibular angle. An incision line with a total length of approximately 5 cm is made. (b) Black dotted line: platysma incision line; black square: masseter muscle. The platysma fascia is incised, approximately 2 cm subcutaneously, and the flap is raised. Once the platysma is located, it is incised to the depth of the masseter fascia such that the incision is 1 cm cranial from the mandibular margin in the anterior direction and 2 cm cranial from the mandibular margin in the posterior direction. In women, the platysma is thin, and the masseter fascia lies immediately inside the platysma. (c) A reverse warping muscle retractor is applied to the posterior margin of the ramus to gently extrude the parotid gland backward, and the masseter muscle is pulled slightly forward with the muscle retractor to expand the operative field. The periosteum is delaminated from the posterior margin of the ramus using a raspatorium, and the fracture site is located. A 0.5-mm-diameter metal wire for pulling the mandibular ramus is passed through caudally to approximately 2 cm of the fracture line. (d) By pulling the metal wire downward, the ramus is pulled sufficiently downward, and reduction is achieved. (e) After reduction, the fragment is fixed using a MatrixMANDIBLE Subcondylar Strut Plate.

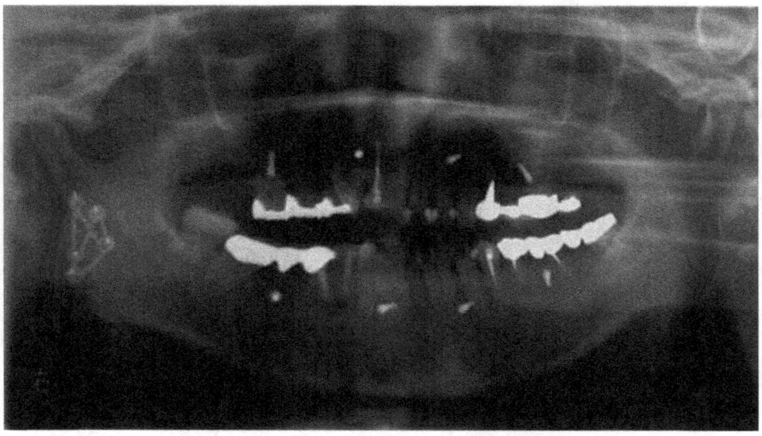

(a)

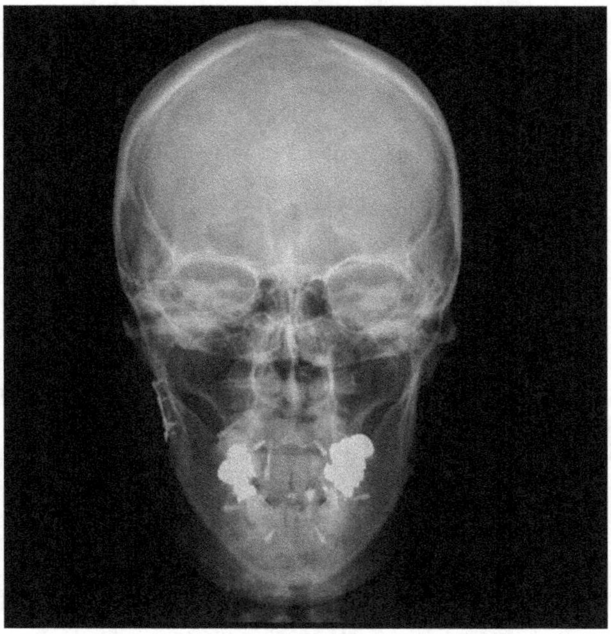

(b)

Figure 4: (a) Panoramic X-ray on the day after the surgery. The right mandibular condylar fracture is reduced and fixed. (b) Head X-ray (PA) on the day after surgery. The bone fragment that was displaced externally is reduced and fixed.

(Jeil Medical Corporation, Korea) were placed in the maxilla and mandible for postoperative intermaxillary traction, and that completed the procedure. There were no abnormalities during the surgical procedure.

Cefmetazole sodium 2 mg/day was administered for 48 hours after surgery to prevent postoperative infection, and acetaminophen 1000 mg was prescribed for pain on an as-needed basis. The reduction and fixation were confirmed on panoramic and head X-rays (P-A) a day after the surgery (Figures 4(a) and 4(b)). No postoperative dysfunction such as facial paralysis was observed. From the day after surgery, elastic was used for intermaxillary fixation to control mouth opening. Two weeks after the surgery, the intermaxillary fixation was released. She started self-opening exercises involving daily horizontal movements of the lower jaw forward and to the left and right and vertical movements involving opening and closing of the mouth. Approximately one month after the surgery, her mouth opening capacity recovered to 30 mm between the upper and lower central incisors. By 2 months after the surgery, her mouth opening capacity had recovered to 40 mm. Three months after the surgery, she recovered and had no interference with her daily life. No facial deformity, wound infection, or scarring was observed.

3. Discussion

Mandibular fractures are the most common facial fractures. Mandibular condylar fractures are the most prevalent of mandibular fractures, accounting for 25-50% of all jaw fractures [24, 25]. Treatment policies for condylar fractures vary from institution to institution, and no gold standard for treatment has been determined [3, 4]. Recently, open reduction and internal fixation surgery have been recommended for adult condylar fractures from the perspective of functional recovery [7–9, 26–29]. When applying open reduction and internal fixation surgery for a condylar fracture, the

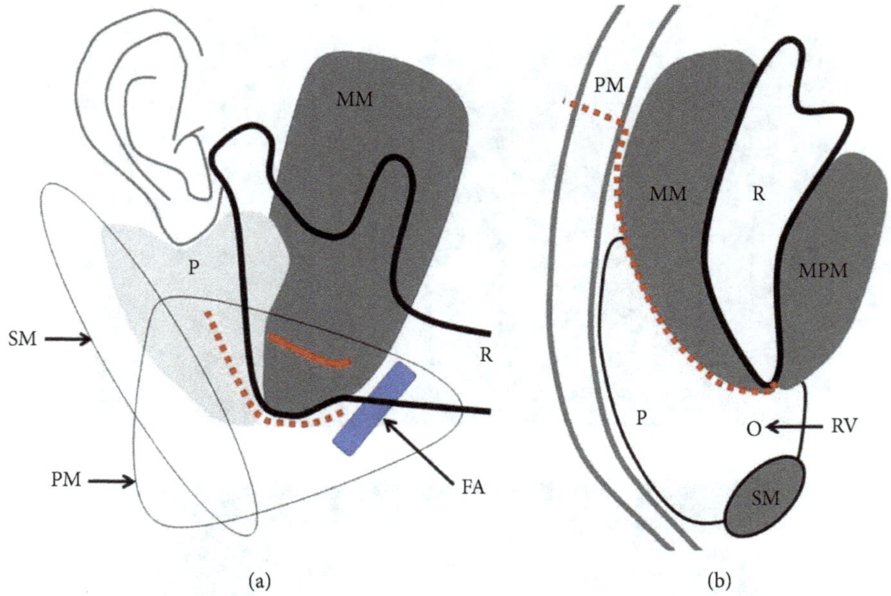

FIGURE 5: (a) FA: facial artery; MM: masseter muscle; P: parotid glands; PM: platysma; R: mandibular bone; SM: sternocleidomastoid muscle; red dotted line: skin incision line; red line: platysma incision line. (b) MM: masseter muscle; P: parotid glands; MPM: medial pterygoid muscle; PM: platysma; R: mandibular bone; RV: retromandibular-vein; SM: sternocleidomastoid muscle; Red dotted line: the approach route.

approaches to the condyle are generally classified as intraoral and extraoral. The intraoral approach is associated with superior aesthetics and a low risk of nerve damage; however, it is only applicable to a limited number of cases. When it is used, it is difficult to expand the operative field, and the narrow field of view makes it difficult to reach the fracture site and operate [30]. Therefore, the intraoral approach can be applied only to condylar base fractures that are fissure fractures or just slightly lateral displacement/dislocation fractures. It should not be applied otherwise. Moreover, due to its difficulty, its duration is longer than that of the extraoral approach [31]. Recently, an intraoral approach using an endoscope has been reported; however, its use has not been widespread because an endoscope is required [32]. The extraoral approaches include the following, ordered from the cranial to the caudal and depending on the position of the skin incision: the Al-Kayat approach [33], preauricular skin crease incision extended downward in a curvilinear manner [14], the retromandibular approach [11, 12], HPTM [18], and the Risdon approach [34]. These approaches also have advantages and disadvantages. Which approach to the fractured site to select has not been determined [10, 31, 35–38].

In open reduction and internal fixation surgery for mandibular condylar fractures, the greatest concern is a facial nerve disorder. Surgeons need to consider the course of the facial nerve when approaching the articular process [39]. The facial nerves form the parotid plexus on the masseter muscle. An anastomosis of the buccal and zygomatic branches is seen in 70 to 100% of cases, whereas temporal branches and ramuses are isolated peripheral branches with few nerve anastomoses [40]. Temporal branches and ramuses may be involved in postoperative dysfunction following excessive traction and compression associated with the surgery. The traffic between the marginal ramus and branches of other facial nerves is as low as 0-16% [20, 40]. There is a high risk of persistent postoperative nerve palsy occurring in the temporal branch with the Al-Kayat approach [33] and in the marginal ramus with the Risdon approach [32]. Recently, the retromandibular approach (RMRP) [11–13, 41], preauricular skin crease incision extended downward in a curvilinear manner [14–16], retromandibular transparotid approach (RMTP) [15, 42–45], retroparotid transmasseteric approach (RPTM), and transmasseteric anteroparotid approach (TMAP) [46, 47] and the HPTM [18] have been commonly used for mandibular condylar neck and base fractures.

In the high submandibular anteroparotid approach, a skin incision is made immediately below the inferior margin of the mandible into the platysma on the cranial side of the marginal ramus of the facial nerve; this minimizes the risk of directly injuring the marginal ramus. As the distance to the articular process is short, and the amount of tissue that is pulled cranially when expanding the operative field is small, the risk of damage to the mandibular bifurcation following intraoperative traction and compression is low. In the high submandibular anteroparotid approach, it is easy to identify the buccal branch that runs along the masseter fascia, and it should be protected by retracting it cranially or caudally when it is exposed. Even if the buccal branch is injured, the likelihood of anastomoses with other nerve branches is high, and postoperative facial nerve disorders are therefore unlikely. In addition, the skin incision immediately below the mandibular margin in the high submandibular anteroparotid approach is inconspicuous and hidden within the mandibular margin. Since the skin traction during surgery is minimal, postoperative scarring is also minimal. This is an approach that allows adequate expansion of the operative field, and optimal reduction and fixation can be performed without extensive pulling of the surrounding tissue. Wilk's approach was improved by dissecting only the platysma and advancing the masseter fascia posteriorly, thereby bypassing the anterior margin of the parotid gland to reach the posterior margin of the ramus. With this improved approach, no facial artery or retromandibular vein was encountered, and the mental stress for the surgeon was minimal [46, 47]. (Figures 5(a) and 5(b)).

In patients with developed parotid glands and a large amount of fat, the soft tissues expand, which makes it difficult to expand the operative field. In addition, it is difficult to distinguish the boundary between the anterior margin of the parotid gland and adipose tissue in a patient with parotid atrophy from fatty degeneration due to aging. The high submandibular anteroparotid approach has these drawbacks, and it may take time to learn.

In the present case, the mandibular condylar fracture was fixed with an adequate operative field permitted by the high submandibular anteroparotid approach. Postoperative surgical site infection, parotid gland complications such as parotitis and salivary fistula, facial nerve dysfunction such as facial paralysis, and esthetic disorders such as scarring were not observed. Although it is necessary to examine more cases in the future, the high submandibular anteroparotid approach may be useful as a new approach for open reduction and internal fixation of condylar fractures.

4. Conclusion

Open reduction and internal fixation procedures were performed for a right mandibular condylar fracture. The ramus was reached by approaching from the inferior margin of the mandible, delaminating the masseter fascia posteriorly, and bypassing the anterior margin of the parotid gland. Once the fractured bone was reached, reduction and fixation were performed. Satisfactory results were obtained. After the surgery, no functional impairment was observed.

Consent

Fully informed consent was obtained from the patient for the use of clinical information relating to this case.

Acknowledgments

The authors would like to thank the staff of Kameda General Hospital Dental Center for editing this manuscript.

References

[1] N. Zachariades, M. Mezitis, C. Mourouzis, D. Papadakis, and A. Spanou, "Fractures of the mandibular condyle: a review of 466 cases. Literature review, reflections on treatment and proposals," *Journal of Cranio-Maxillo-Facial Surgery*, vol. 34, no. 7, pp. 421–432, 2006.

[2] E. Al-Moraissi and E. Ellis 3rd., "Surgical treatment of adult mandibular condylar fractures provides better outcomes than non-surgical approach: a systematic review and meta-analysis," *Journal of Oral and Maxillofacial Surgery*, vol. 73, no. 3, pp. 482–493, 2015.

[3] M. I. Nussbaum, D. M. Laskin, and A. M. Best, "Closed versus open reduction of mandibular condylar fractures in adults: a meta-analysis," *Journal of Oral and Maxillofacial Surgery*, vol. 66, no. 6, pp. 1087–1092, 2008.

[4] U. Eckelt, M. Schneider, F. Erasmus et al., "Open versus non-surgical approach of fracture of the mandibular condylar process. A prospective randomized multi-centre study," *Journal of Cranio-Maxillo-Facial Surgery*, vol. 34, no. 5, pp. 306–314, 2006.

[5] R. R. Bos, R. P. Ward Booth, and L. G. de Bont, "Mandibular condyle fractures: a consensus," *The British Journal of Oral & Maxillofacial Surgery*, vol. 37, no. 2, pp. 87–89, 1999.

[6] L. A. Assael, "Open versus closed reduction of adult mandibular condyle fractures: an alternative interpretation of the evidence," *Journal of Oral and Maxillofacial Surgery*, vol. 61, no. 11, pp. 1333–1339, 2003.

[7] A. K. Danda, M. R. Muthusekhar, V. Narayanan, M. F. Baig, and A. Siddareddi, "Open versus non-surgical approach of unilateral subcondylar and condylar neck fractures: a prospective, randomized clinical study," *Journal of Oral and Maxillofacial Surgery*, vol. 68, no. 6, pp. 1238–1241, 2010.

[8] V. Singh, A. Bhagol, M. Goel, I. Kumar, and A. Verma, "Outcomes open versus non-surgical approach of mandibular subcondylar fractures: a prospective randomized study," *Journal of Oral and Maxillofacial Surgery*, vol. 68, no. 6, pp. 1304–1309, 2010.

[9] M. Schneider, F. Erasmus, K. L. Gerlach et al., "Open reduction and internal fixation versus non-surgical approach and mandibulomaxillary fixation of fractures of the mandibular condylar process: a randomized, prospective, multicenter study with special evaluation of fracture level," *Journal of Oral and Maxillofacial Surgery*, vol. 66, no. 12, pp. 2537–2544, 2008.

[10] J. Handschel, T. Rüggeberg, R. Depprich et al., "Comparison of various approaches for the treatment of fractures of the mandibular condylar process," *Journal of Cranio-Maxillo-Facial Surgery*, vol. 40, no. 8, pp. e397–e401, 2012.

[11] E. Ellis and J. Dean, "Rigid fixation of mandibular condyle fractures," *Oral Surgery, Oral Medicine, and Oral Pathology*, vol. 76, no. 1, pp. 6–15, 1993.

[12] C. Chossegros, F. Cheynet, J. L. Blanc, and Z. Bourezak, "Short retromandibular approach of subcondylar fractures: clinical and radiologic long-term evaluation," *Oral Surgery, Oral Medicine, Oral Pathology, Oral Radiology, and Endodontics*, vol. 82, no. 3, pp. 248–252, 1996.

[13] A. Spinzia, R. Patrone, E. Belli et al., "Open reduction and internal fixation of extracapsular mandibular condyle fractures: a long-term clinical and radiological follow-up of 25 patients," *BMC Surgery*, vol. 14, no. 1, 2014.

[14] A. W. Wilson, M. Ethunandan, and P. A. Brennan, "Transmasseteric antero-parotid approach for open reduction and internal fixation of condylar fractures," *The British Journal of Oral & Maxillofacial Surgery*, vol. 43, no. 1, pp. 57–60, 2005.

[15] A. Vesnaver, M. Gorjanc, A. Eberlinc, D. A. Dovsak, and A. A. Kansky, "The periauricular transparotid approach for open

reduction and internal fixation of condylar fractures," *Journal of Cranio-Maxillo-Facial Surgery*, vol. 33, no. 3, pp. 169–179, 2005.

[16] R. Gali, S. K. Devireddy, K. R. Venkata, S. R. Kanubaddy, C. Nemaly, and M. Dasari, "Preauricular transmasseteric anteroparotid approach for extracorporeal fixation of mandibular condyle fractures," *Indian journal of plastic surgery*, vol. 49, no. 1, pp. 59–65, 2016.

[17] A. Wilk and I. Biotchane, "Osteosynthesis of subcondylar fracture using a rectangular 3-dimensional stabilization plate," *Revue de Stomatologie et de Chirurgie Maxillo-Faciale*, vol. 98, pp. 40–44, 1997.

[18] A. Wilk, "High perimandibular approach/modified Risdon-Strasbourg approach," in *Fractures of the Mandibular Condyle*, J. Kleinhenz and C. Meyer, Eds., pp. 143–154, Quintessence Verlag, London, 2009.

[19] J. C. Lutz, P. Clavert, R. Wolfram-Gabel, A. Wilk, and J. L. Kahn, "Is the high submandibular transmassetric approach to the mandibular condyle safe for the inferior buccal branch?," *Surgical and Radiologic Anatomy*, vol. 32, no. 10, pp. 963–969, 2010.

[20] J. C. Lutz, P. Clavert, R. Wolfram-Gabel, A. Wilk, and J. L. Kahn, "Is the high submandibular transmasseteric approach to the mandibular condyle safe for the inferior buccal branch?," *Surgical and Radiologic Anatomy*, vol. 32, no. 10, pp. 963–969, 2010.

[21] L. Lindahl, "Condylar fractures of the mandible. I: classification and relation to age, occlusion, and concomitant injuries of the teeth and teeth supporting structures, and fractures of the mandibular body," *International Journal of Oral and Maxillofacial Surgery*, vol. 6, pp. 12–21, 1977.

[22] W. D. Maclennan, "Consideration of 180 cases of typical fractures of the mandibular condylar process," *British Journal of Plastic Surgery*, vol. 5, pp. 122–128, 1995.

[23] R. Cortelazzi, M. Altacera, M. Turco, V. Antonicelli, and M. Benedittis, "Development and clinical evaluation of MatrixMANDIBLE Subcondylar Plate System," *Craniomaxillofacial Trauma and Reconstruction*, vol. 8, no. 2, pp. 94–99, 2015.

[24] A. C. Salgarelli, A. Anesi, P. Bellini et al., "How to improve retromandibular transmasseteric anteroparotid approach for mandibular condylar fractures: our clinical experience," *International Journal of Oral and Maxillofacial Surgery*, vol. 42, no. 4, pp. 464–469, 2013.

[25] P. N. Afrooz, M. R. Bykowski, I. B. James, L. N. Daniali, and J. A. Clavijo-Alvarez, "The epidemiology of mandibular fractures in the United States, part 1: a review of 13,142 cases from the US National Trauma Data Bank," *Journal of Oral and Maxillofacial Surgery*, vol. 73, no. 12, pp. 2361–2366, 2015.

[26] F. L. Merlet, F. Grimaud, R. Pace et al., "Outcomes of functional treatment versus open reduction and internal fixation of condylar mandibular fracture with articular impact: a retrospective study of 83 adults," *Journal of stomatology, oral and maxillofacial surgery*, vol. 119, no. 1, pp. 8–15, 2018.

[27] L. O. Ana, B. S. Belimda, and C. Ricardo, "Mandibular condyle fractures: a diagnosis with controversial treatment," *Cirugia y Cirujanos*, vol. 87, pp. 587–594, 2019.

[28] C. A. Landes and R. Lipphardt, "Prospective evaluation of pragmatic treatment rationale: open reduction and internal fixation of displaced and dislocated condyle and condylar head fractures and closed reduction of non-displaced, non-dislocated fractures part I: condyle and subcondylar fractures," *International Journal of Oral and Maxillofacial Surgery*, vol. 34, pp. 859–870, 2005.

[29] C. A. Landes and R. Lipphardt, "Prospective evaluation of pragmatic treatment rationale: open reduction and internal fixation of displaced and dislocated condyle and condylar head fractures and closed reduction of non-displaced, non-dislocated fractures part II: high condylar and condylar head fractures," *International Journal of Oral and Maxillofacial Surgery*, vol. 35, no. 2, pp. 115–126, 2006.

[30] T. Jensen, J. Jensen, S. E. Norholt, L. Lenkhansen, and P. Sevensson, "Open reduction and rigid fixation of mandibular condylar fractures by an intraoral approach: a long-term follow-up study of 15 patients," *Journal of Oral and Maxillofacial Surgery*, vol. 64, no. 12, pp. 1771–1779, 2006.

[31] S. M. Nam, Y. B. Kim, S. J. Lee, E. S. Park, and J. H. Lee, "A comparative study of intraoral versus retromandibular approach in the management of subcondylar fracture," *BMC Surgery*, vol. 19, no. 1, p. 28, 2019.

[32] I. Soichiro, Y. Norie, K. Koji, and S. Akira, "Endoscope-assisted transoral reduction and internal fixation of a mandibular subcondylar fracture with a 3D-shaped plate," *International Journal of Contemporary Medical Research*, vol. 4, no. 2, pp. 574–576, 2017.

[33] A. Al-Kayat and P. Bramley, "A modified prearicular approach to the temporomandibular joint and malar arch," *The British Journal of Oral Surgery*, vol. 17, no. 2, pp. 91–103, 1979.

[34] R. Alexander, J. Y. Su, and M. M. Stark, "An accurate approach for open reduction and internal fixation of high and low condylar process fractures," *Journal of Oral and Maxillofacial Surgery*, vol. 52, no. 8, pp. 808–812, 1994.

[35] M. Schneider, G. Lauer, and U. Eckelt, "Surgical treatment of fractures of the mandibular condyle: a comparison of long-term results following different approaches-functional, axiographical and radiological findings," *Journal of Cranio-Maxillo-Facial Surgery*, vol. 35, no. 3, pp. 151–160, 2007.

[36] K. G. Kempers, P. D. Quinn, and K. Silverstein, "Surgical approaches to mandibular condylar fractures: a review," *The Journal of Cranio-Maxillofacial Trauma*, vol. 5, no. 4, pp. 25–30, 1999.

[37] Z. Hunges, L. Jean-Christophe, Z. Simone, and W. Astrid, "Epidemiology and treatment outcome of surgically treated mandibular condyle fractures. A five years retrospective study," *Journal of Cranio-Maxillo-Facial Surgery*, vol. 42, pp. 879–884, 2014.

[38] S. B. Ritoban, D. Sumit, and G. Samiran, "Viability of tmap approach for condylar fractures: a case series and review of literature," *International Journal of Current Research*, vol. 11, no. 5, pp. 4027–4031, 2019.

[39] G. J. Knepil, A. N. Kanatas, and R. J. Loukota, "Classification of surgical approaches to the mandibular condyle," *The British Journal of Oral & Maxillofacial Surgery*, vol. 49, no. 8, pp. 664-665, 2011.

[40] A. Gosain, "Surgical anatomy of the facial nerve," *Clinics in Plastic Surgery*, vol. 22, no. 2, pp. 241–251, 1995.

[41] J. Kleinheinz, "Retromandibular approach," in *Fractures of the Mandibular Condyle*, J. Kleinheinz and C. Meyer, Eds., pp. 155–159, Quintessence Verlag, London, 2009.

[42] T. Kanno, S. Sukegawa, H. Tatsumi et al., "Does retromandibular transparotid approach for the open treatment of condylar fractures result in facial nerve injury?," *Journal of Oral and Maxillofacial Surgery*, vol. 74, no. 10, pp. 2019–2032, 2016.

[43] D. Weingart, "Transparotideal approach," in *Fractures of Mandibular Condyle*, J. Kleinheinz and C. Meyer, Eds., pp. 135–137, Quintessence Verlag, London, 2009.

[44] J. Klatt, P. Pohlenz, M. Blessmann et al., "Clinical follow-up examination of surgically treated fractures of the condylar process using the transparotid approach," *Journal of Oral and Maxillofacial Surgery*, vol. 68, no. 3, pp. 611–617, 2010.

[45] K. Tomar, "Efficacy of the retroparotid trans-masseteric approach via retromandibular incision in ORIF of subcondylar fractures: our institution experience," *Journal of maxillofacial and oral surgery*, vol. 17, no. 3, pp. 332–338, 2018.

[46] Y. Leiser, M. Peled, R. Braun, and N. I. Abu-El, "Treatment of low subcondylar fractures a 5 year retrospective study," *International Journal of Oral and Maxillofacial Surgery*, vol. 42, no. 6, pp. 716–720, 2013.

[47] J. Hou, L. Chen, T. Wang et al., "A new surgical approach to treat medial or low condylar fractures: the minor parotid anterior approach," *Oral Surgery, Oral Medicine, Oral Pathology, Oral Radiology*, vol. 117, no. 3, pp. 283–288, 2014.

35

Management of Intracanal Separated File Fragment in a Four-Rooted Mandibular Third Molar

Benoy Jacob, Anjaneyulu K., Aishwarya Ranganath, and Riluwan Siddique

Department of Conservative Dentistry and Endodontics, Saveetha Institute of Medical and Technical Sciences, Chennai, Tamil Nadu, India

Correspondence should be addressed to Benoy Jacob; benjacz733@hotmail.com

Academic Editor: Alberto Delbem

The success of endodontic therapy is attributed to complete arbitration of the bound entities concealed within the complexity and absolute disinfection of the root canal system, thus, deeming it mandatory to effectively negotiate and overcome the challenges posed by obstruction, either iatrogenic or anatomic. To achieve this, considerable depth of knowledge and expertise with reference to variations in root canal morphology and clinical mishap management is substantially as important as developing fine observation skills in conjunction with an appropriate armamentarium and a keen sense of determination, thereby enhancing one's clinical acumen by several folds. In the present case, following rubber dam isolation, the temporary restoration was removed, and the remaining carious dentin was excavated. Endodontic access cavity was refined and explored with a DG-16 probe, following which three separate canal orifices were identified in the pulp chamber floor (mesiobuccal, mesiolingual, and distal). On further observation under a surgical operating microscope and continuous exploration with the DG-16 probe, a fourth canal was found in the mesial aspect of the tooth (middle mesial). With instrumentation, it was confirmed that a fractured object was indeed present at the apical third of the mesiolingual root of tooth 38. Bypassing of the fractured fragment was initiated with a size 10 SS K-file coupled with copious irrigation with 3% sodium hypochlorite. In the present case report, four distinct canals comprising 3 mesial and 1 distal canal were recognized, and the fractured instrument in one of the canals was bypassed successfully.

1. Background

The root canal in all its glory is a relentless enigma unfolding itself during the endodontic treatment procedure. It is therefore pertinent to remember that a complete understanding of the bound entity is indeed an essentiality in order to achieve the most prolific of all outcomes [1]. A successful endodontic treatment is immeasurably attained through persistent chemo-mechanical cleansing of the root canal system [2]. The above statement is adjudged for the very fact that the interplay between an in-depth knowledge of tooth anatomy and root canal morphology conjoined with meticulous planning for the proposed treatment is often necessary to rid the root canal complexities of microorganisms and pulp tissue remnants [1]. Aberrations in anatomy are sizeably as important as the normal anatomy of the root canal system, thereby strengthening the need to acquire considerable depth of knowledge and expertise in this regard [1, 3].

The general prerequisites to be considered prior to the management of a complex anomaly often involve earlier discussed criteria as well as a definite focus on the pulp chamber floor, proper judgement, and use of sufficient armamentarium keeping in mind the biological anthropology of a tooth and its varied anatomy [4]. Apart from the usual and aberrant configurations concerning permanent first and second molar teeth, wide variations in the root canal morphology with respect to permanent third molars have also been studied and investigated upon [5]. Although in vitro studies, by clearing methods, have established the incidence of variations in the number of canals in mandibular third molars [6–9], however, there exists scarcity in clinical cases with advanced imaging modalities. This paper brings to the fore the case of a successful nonsurgical clinical aberrative and mishap management of a previously initiated four-rooted left mandibular third molar harbouring four root canals whose configuration of 3 mesial and 1 distal root was confirmed following CBCT evaluation, with a 1-year follow-up for the same.

2. Case Description

A 31-year-old Indian male patient reported to the Department of Conservative Dentistry and Endodontics with a chief complaint of spontaneous pain in the lower left back tooth region for the past 4 days. Medical history was noncontributory. The patient revealed a history of intermittent pain for 3 weeks which continued to increase in severity, aggravated while chewing food at the affected site, and relieved with medication. The patient gave a detailed history on the subjective symptoms and disclosed that the tooth had been treated 8 months back. On clinical examination, it was noticed that the patient had undergone extraction of teeth 36 and 37, and restoration was present in 38. Soft tissue examination revealed neither oedema nor tenderness to palpation. The tooth elicited moderate to severe tenderness on the application of finger pressure. Multiple parallax radiographs were taken to assess the condition of the tooth and its surrounding structures. The preoperative radiograph revealed radiopacity in the pulpal chamber and at the apical third of one of the roots (Figure 1). While the former was indicative of a restorative material, the latter on the other hand disclosed a fractured/separated instrument from the previously initiated therapy (Figure 1). Furthermore, the periapical region of the said tooth revealed a radiolucent area. Based on both clinical and radiographic findings, a diagnosis of previously initiated, symptomatic apical periodontitis, was confirmed. Nonsurgical endodontic therapy was proposed as the treatment of choice.

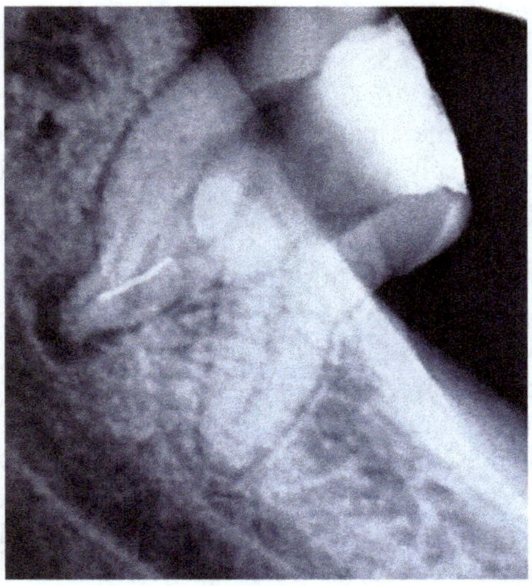

Figure 1: Preoperative radiograph.

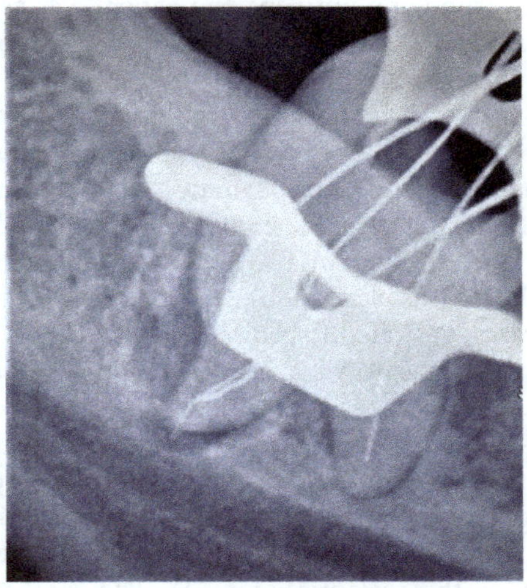

Figure 2: File bypass/working length.

The tooth was anaesthetised with 1.8 ml 2% lignocaine containing 1 : 200,000 epinephrine (Xylocaine; AstraZeneca Pharma India Ltd., Bangalore, India). Following rubber dam isolation, the temporary restoration was removed, and the remaining carious dentin was excavated. The endodontic access cavity was refined and explored with a DG-16 probe (Hu-Friedy, Chicago, IL, USA), following which three separate canal orifices were identified in the pulp chamber floor (mesiobuccal, mesiolingual, and distal). On further observation under a surgical operating microscope (Carl Zeiss OPMI Pico, Jena, Germany) and continuous exploration with the DG-16 probe, a fourth canal was found in the mesial aspect of the tooth (middle mesial). Once all four canals were scouted, the access was modified into a trapezoidal cavity using an Endo Z bur (Dentsply Maillefer, Baillagues, Switzerland) to obtain straight-line access of all four canals. Nickel-titanium (NiTi) ProTaper Gold SX orifice shapers (Dentsply Maillefer) were used for coronal enlargement followed by patency establishment using a size 10 stainless steel (SS) K-file (Dentsply Maillefer). With instrumentation, it was confirmed that a fractured object was indeed present at the apical third of the mesiolingual root of tooth 38. Bypassing of the fractured fragment was initiated with a size 10 SS K-file coupled with copious irrigation with 3% sodium hypochlorite. The size 10 K-file was implemented mesially along the inner curvature of the target site to bypass the fragment lodged within the curvature. Following each attempt, the file was removed, inspected, cleaned, and engaged again with a gentle push-pull and/or watch winding motion. On inspection, if a file was distorted, it was immediately replaced with a new size 10 K-file and instrumented repeatedly as described above till the resistance was bypassed, after which a size 15 SS K-file was introduced and worked in a similar fashion. Subsequent radiographs were taken to understand the extent of bypassing of the fractured fragment achieved with the size 15 K-file. Once the fractured file was bypassed completely (Figure 2), sequentially larger files (size 20 K-files) were introduced seamlessly till the size 25 SS K-files working their way to the apex, as described earlier. It is to be noted that the entire bypassing procedure was facilitated with a 3% sodium hypochlorite solution as a lubricant. Next, working length determination was performed using an electronic apex locator (Root ZX; J Morita, Tokyo, Japan) and was established at 18 mm for the distal canal, 17 mm for the mesiolingual and mesiobuccal canals, and 16 mm for the middle mesial

>canal. Then, the remainder of the canals was apically prepared up to size 25 SS K-file, further shaping and finishing was achieved with ProTaper Gold (Dentsply Maillefer) NiTi rotary instrumentation (sequentially) using an electric motor (X-Smart, Dentsply Maillefer) along with subsequent recapitulation per sequence. Final cleansing of the canals was achieved with 17% EDTA solution (META BIOMED CO.LTD), intermediate flushing with normal saline followed by 3% sodium hypochlorite as the endmost irrigant. Canals were dried with absorbent paper points (Dentsply Sirona) after which a thick creamy mix of calcium hydroxide powder mixed with 3% sodium hypochlorite [10, 11] was incorporated into the canals with lentulospirals (Dentsply Maillefer). Cotton pellet was placed, and the access cavity was temporarily restored with Cavit. The patient was prescribed dolonex 20 mg tab DT twice daily for two days for relief of painful symptoms, and the next appointment was scheduled after two weeks.

At the second appointment, the patient was asymptomatic with resolution of signs and symptoms. After removal of the temporary restoration along with intracanal dressing, care was taken to flush out the remaining medicament from the canal system by way of copious saline irrigation and 3% sodium hypochlorite. Sonic agitation was executed using the EndoActivator® with a 25/04 noncutting polymer tip (Dentsply Specialities, Tulsa, OK, USA). Following irrigant delivery, the tip was placed 1 mm short of the working length for each canal, activated for 30 seconds, and then removed. Drying of the canals was made certain with absorbent paper points (Dentsply Sirona), following which the master cone fit was checked and confirmed on a radiograph (Figure 3). Obturation of the prepared canals was attained by the single cone gutta-percha (Dentsply Maillefer) technique with AH Plus resin-based sealer (Dentsply DeTrey, Konstanz, Germany) as the sealant (Figure 4). The tooth was then restored with a Filtek Z350XT (3MESPE) posterior composite resin material. The patient was followed up at regular intervals. At 1-year follow-up, a radiograph was taken (Figure 5) and a CBCT scan was performed. CBCT (Dentsply Sirona, Orthophos XG 3D) was taken at standardized settings (90 kV, 6 mA, 5 $*$ 5.5 cm, 160 μm, 14 s). Reduction in size of the lesion was markedly visible at the 1-year follow-up period (Figure 5).

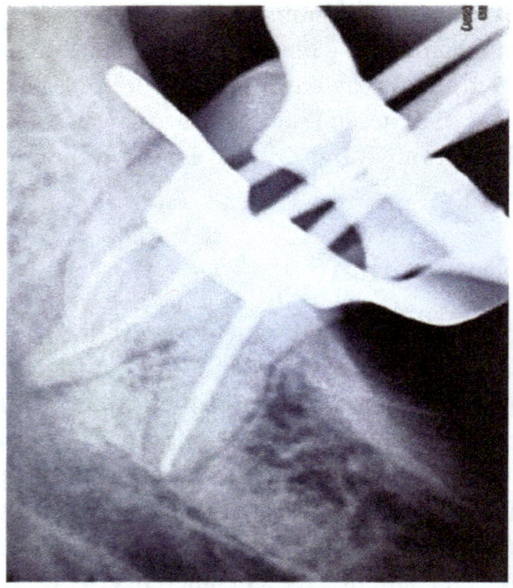

Figure 3: Master cone.

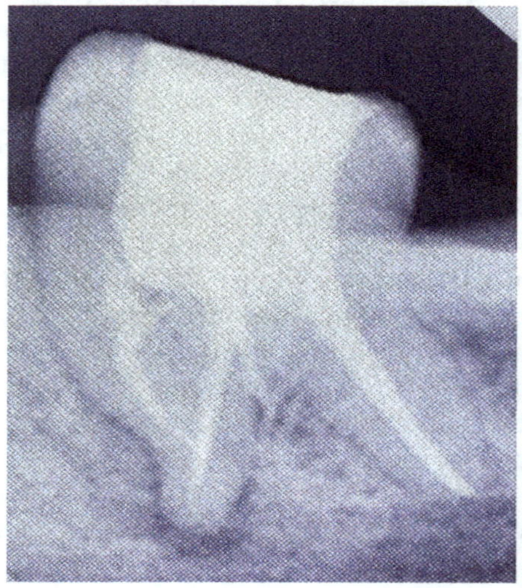

Figure 4: Postoperative radiograph.

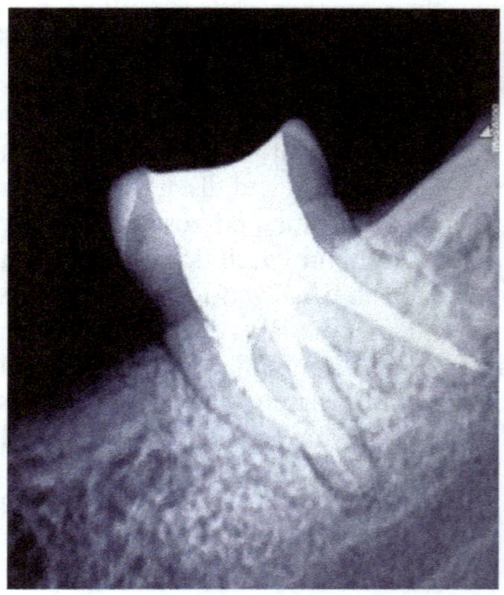

Figure 5: 1-year follow-up.

3. Discussion

The mandibular third molar is the last tooth to erupt into the oral cavity, usually between 17 and 21 years of age or at a later stage in life, partially erupt or perhaps not erupt at all [12]. Owing to its nonfunctional position, much credence has been given to early uprooting of the third molar tooth to rid the patient and operator of the diverse problems in dealing with it [13, 14]. However, current practice asserts "to serve, save and protect" the functional tooth at any cost, and the best way to save it is "to not lose it at all" in the first place. The retention of the third molar in clinical situations wherein the opposing tooth is either present or missing does not hold significance in this case as the abutting second molar was absent. Therefore, in the present case, root canal therapy was perpetrated to conserve the tooth in question, consequently serving as a prudent abutment for a possible prosthesis [13]. Most importantly, despite being treated upon earlier by another practitioner, the patient reported continuous nagging pain partly because of it and partly due to the patient's inability to return to the previous practitioner for the remainder of the treatment. The patient's desire to retain the said tooth was prioritized and primarily taken into consideration.

The mandibular third molar is indeed a cut above the rest with reference to anatomical variation [15]. Barring a few infrequently reported anatomical occurrences, the solitary or binary variants entombing one to four canals are observed to be the most recurrent [6, 7, 16]. Silberman et al., 2009, reported a peculiar case of a three-rooted mandibular right third molar tooth encasing 5 canals (4 mesial, 1 distal), for which endodontic therapy was successfully accomplished [17]. Apart from the above published clinical case, two studies incorporating in vitro clearing methods confirmed the presence of 5 canals in similar teeth [6, 7]. Plotino, in 2008, was the first to report a rare clinical case wherein three mesial canals including a distal canal were identified in a four-rooted mandibular third molar tooth [18]. Most conspicuously, Sinha and Sinha, 2014, in their case report, described the management of a mandibular third molar housing 5 canals, thus, contributing to the literature significantly [19]. Periapical radiograph was the imaging modality of choice in both the above-described case reports. In the present case report, CBCT was not opted for at first as the canal orifices could be detected with the aid of a dental operating microscope (Carl Zeiss OPMI Pico, Jena, Germany) and a champagne bubble test. Moreover, the orifices first identified/located were almost equidistant from one another, in accordance with the laws of symmetry as proposed by Krasner and Rankow, 2004 [4].

At 1 year follow-up, it was decided that a CBCT scan should be done to highlight the unique four-rooted variation of the mandibular third molar, encasing four distinct canals [20, 21]. Additionally, an advanced radiographic modality regarding such an anomaly has not been employed in previously published case reports. Moreover, the extent of healing of the lesion involving the teeth could also be assessed with CBCT in addition to a conventional radiograph. According to the guidelines put forward by the American Association of Endodontics (AAE), CBCT scan with a small field of view is recommended in clinical research trials for diagnostic accuracy [22]. Furthermore, in the present case, much credence had been given to achieving a sterile environment, enforcing a stringent disinfection protocol pertaining to irrigant delivery, its activation, and placement of a suitable intracanal medicament. Time and again, the judicious application of calcium hydroxide as an interappointment medication for effectively controlling microbial activity in the root canal system has been authenticated. Interestingly, Hamed et al., 2014, concluded in their research that the combined antibacterial effect of the mixture of calcium hydroxide and sodium hypochlorite as intracanal medicament was superlative against both gram-positive and gram-negative bacteria in comparison to calcium hydroxide when used alone. The notable findings from the above-stated were in conformity with those produced in a study effectuated by Farhad et al., 2012 [23].

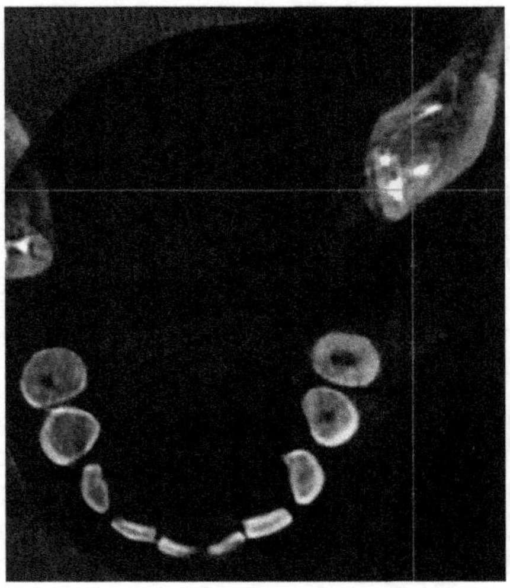

FIGURE 6: CBCT axial view (postoperative).

The most common site of occurrence of separated instruments has often been reported in mandibular molars. The aforesaid statement is reckoned from the fact that compelling evidence has been accorded for the same, as disclosed by Shen et al., 2004, Cujé et al., 2010, and Nevares et al., 2012 [24–26]. Interestingly, fractured instruments are claimed to not be the direct cause of recontamination emanating from the root canal complexity [27]. Furthermore, on a riveting note, it was affirmed in a systematic review by Panitvisai et al., 2010, that there was no statistically significant difference in healing rates between teeth with and without retained instrument fragment [28]. However, when a periradicular lesion is present, it becomes even more obligatory that the fragment is either removed or bypassed, thus, envisaging acceptable/satisfactory/complete healing of the infected tooth [26]. The success of endodontic therapy depends on complete disinfection of the root canal system, and its outcome solely depends upon the depth at which an irrigant effectively penetrates [29], thus, deeming it mandatory to effectively negotiate and overcome the challenges posed by obstructions, either iatrogenic or anatomic, within the root canal pathways. Various factors influence the outcome of the treatment in case of fractured fragments, namely, the root canal anatomy, presence of curvature, the position of the fractured instrument, and the ability of the operator to negotiate or retrieve the foreign object [30].

In routine dental practice, by and large, it is uncommon to frequently come across retained instrument fragments in the root canals of endodontically initiated and/or treated teeth with a low rate of incidence being reported for the same. However, during a serendipitous encounter, adept knowledge, and dexterous proficiency in this regard succour to assess the limitations in hand and opt for the best suitable technique coupled with existing and/or emerging technologies available, capable of ensuring a better prognosis for the tooth in question, as evinced in the present case report. With reference to root canal aberrancies, "there's more to it than meets the eye," as the root canal is an incessant conundrum unto itself. Having said that, the acronym "KODAC"-sound knowledge (K) of aberrant anatomy, keen observation (O) skills for locating shrouded canals, ever-zealous sense of determination (D), indispensable armamentarium (A) for scouting, enduring commitment (C) to follow-up such cases, holds significant credibility in the long-term successful management of complex root canal anatomies and mishaps of iatrogenic/anatomical origin.

4. Conclusion

Existing literature reveals that the greatest percentage of instrument fracture is witnessed in the apical third of the root canal, probably due to inadequate patency and canal width [31–33]. At this juncture, negotiating the file can be considered initially as attempts to retrieve the fractured instrument may further result in the reduction of root dentin at the apical third, transportation, ledge formation, or perhaps even perforation [34, 35]. In the present case report, the fractured instrument was bypassed successfully.

In the present case report, from a clinical and radiographic point of view, four distinct canals were recognized. Following a CBCT examination, 3 mesial and 1 distal canal (3 M and 1D) were clearly discernible (Figure 6). General inevitable discrepancies must be expected owing to certain anatomical anomalies such as those involving a tooth which has become rotated, subsequently contributing to confounding yet perceivable anatomical complexities by employing 3-dimensional diagnostic imaging modalities for diagnostic precision. Adding on to the existing literature, the present case report deals with a patient of Indian origin, thus, emphasizing the additional importance of attaining familiarity with variations in root canal anatomy and complexities of diverse ethnicities.

References

[1] F. J. Vertucci, "Root canal morphology and its relationship to endodontic procedures," *Endodontic Topics*, vol. 10, no. 1, pp. 3–29, 2005.

[2] A. BYSTRÖM and G. SUNDQVIST, "Bacteriologic evaluation of the efficacy of mechanical root canal instrumentation in endodontic therapy," *European Journal of Oral Sciences*, vol. 89, no. 4, pp. 321–328, 1981.

[3] F. S. Weine, H. J. Healey, H. Gerstein, and L. Evanson, "Canal configuration in the mesiobuccal root of the maxillary first molar and its endodontic significance," *Oral Surgery, Oral Medicine, and Oral Pathology*, vol. 28, no. 3, pp. 419–425, 1969.

[4] P. Krasner and H. J. Rankow, "Anatomy of the pulp-chamber floor," *Journal of Endodontia*, vol. 30, no. 1, pp. 5–16, 2004.

[5] I. A. Ahmad, M. M. Azzeh, A. M. Zwiri, M. A. S. A. Haija, and M. M. Diab, "Root and root canal morphology of third molars in a Jordanian subpopulation," *Saudi Endodontic Journal*, vol. 6, no. 3, p. 113, 2016.

[6] S. J. Sidow, L. A. West, F. R. Liewehr, and R. J. Loushine, "Root canal morphology of human maxillary and mandibular third molars," *Journal of Endodontia*, vol. 26, no. 11, pp. 675–678, 2000.

[7] S. Sert, G. Şahinkesen, F. T. Topçu, Ş. E. Eroğlu, and E. A. Oktay, "Root canal configurations of third molar teeth. A comparison with first and second molars in the Turkish population," *Australian Endodontic Journal*, vol. 37, no. 3, pp. 109–117, 2011.

[8] K. Gulabivala, A. Opasanon, Y.-L. Ng, and A. Alavi, "Root and canal morphology of Thai mandibular molars," *International Endodontic Journal*, vol. 35, no. 1, pp. 56–62, 2002.

[9] M. Kuzekanani, J. Haghani, and H. Nosrati, "Root and canal morphology of mandibular third molars in an Iranian population," *J Dent Res Dent Clin Dent Prospects.*, vol. 6, no. 3, pp. 85–88, 2012.

[10] S. J. Hamed, A. L.-Y. IK, N. T. Ali, and M. A. Al-Feron, "Antibacterial activity of calcium hydroxide combined with chlrohexidine or sodium hypochlorite against gram positive and gram negative bacteria," *J Nat Sci Res*, vol. 4, 2014.

[11] Z. Mohammadi, S. Shalavi, A. Moeintaghavi, and H. Jafarzadeh, "A review over benefits and drawbacks of combining sodium hypochlorite with other endodontic materials," *The Open Dentistry Journal*, vol. 11, no. 1, pp. 661–669, 2017.

[12] S. J. Nelson, *Wheeler's Dental Anatomy*, Physiology and Occlusion-E-Book, Elsevier Health Sciences, 2014.

[13] D. Normando, "Third molars: to extract or not to extract?," *Dental Press Journal of Orthodontics*, vol. 20, no. 4, pp. 17-18, 2015.

[14] RC S, *Woelfel's Dental Anatomy: Its Relevance to Dentistry*, Wolters Kluwer, Lippincott Williams& Wilkins, 2007.

[15] S. J. Nelson, *Physiology, and Occlusion*, St. Louis, Mo, Saunders Elsevier, 2010.

[16] D. M. Guerisoli, R. A. de SOUZA, M. D. de Sousa Neto, R. G. Silva, and J. D. Pecora, "External and internal anatomy of third molars," *Brazilian Dental Journal*, vol. 9, no. 2, pp. 91–94, 1998.

[17] A. Silberman, C. Heilborn, and N. Cohenca, "Endodontic therapy of a mandibular third molar with 5 canals: a case report," *Quintessence Int*, vol. 40, no. 6, 2009.

[18] G. Plotino, "A mandibular third molar with three mesial roots: a case report," *Journal of Endodontia*, vol. 34, no. 2, pp. 224–226, 2008.

[19] D. J. Sinha and A. A. Sinha, "An endodontic management of mandibular third molar with five root canals," *Saudi Endod J.*, vol. 4, no. 1, p. 36, 2014.

[20] Z. K. Dalili, M. Taramsari, N. F. Khosravi, and M. Kanani, "Accuracy of cone-beam computed tomography in comparison with standard method in evaluating root canal morphology: an in vitro study," *Iran Endod J*, vol. 13, no. 2, pp. 181–187, 2018.

[21] B. Gümrü and B. Tarçın, "Imaging in endodontics: an overview of conventional and alternative advanced imaging techniques," *Journal of Marmara University Institute of Health Sciences*, vol. 3, no. 1, 2013.

[22] M. I. Fayad, M. Nair, M. D. Levin et al., "AAE and AAOMR joint position statement: use of cone beam computed tomography in endodontics 2015 update," *Oral Surgery, Oral Medicine, Oral Pathology, Oral Radiology*, vol. 120, no. 4, pp. 508–512, 2015.

[23] A. R. Farhad, B. Barekatain, M. Allameh, and T. Narimani, "Evaluation of the antibacterial effect of calcium hydroxide in combination with three different vehicles: an in vitro study," *Dental Research Journal*, vol. 9, no. 2, 2012.

[24] Y. Shen, B. Peng, and G. S. Cheung, "Factors associated with the removal of fractured NiTi instruments from root canal systems," *Oral Surgery, Oral Medicine, Oral Pathology, Oral Radiology, and Endodontology*, vol. 98, no. 5, pp. 605–610, 2004.

[25] J. Cujé, C. Bargholz, and M. Hülsmann, "The outcome of retained instrument removal in a specialist practice," *International Endodontic Journal*, vol. 43, no. 7, pp. 545–554, 2010.

[26] G. Nevares, R. S. Cunha, M. L. Zuolo, and C. E. da Silveira Bueno, "Success rates for removing or bypassing fractured instruments: a prospective clinical study," *Journal of Endodontia*, vol. 38, no. 4, pp. 442–444, 2012.

[27] S. Simon, P. Machtou, P. Tomson, N. Adams, and P. Lumley, "Influence of fractured instruments on the success rate of endodontic treatment," *Dental Update*, vol. 35, no. 3, pp. 172–179, 2008.

[28] P. Panitvisai, P. Parunnit, C. Sathorn, and H. H. Messer, "Impact of a retained instrument on treatment outcome: a systematic review and meta-analysis," *Journal of Endodontia*, vol. 36, no. 5, pp. 775–780, 2010.

[29] M. Haapasalo, Y. Shen, W. Qian, and Y. Gao, "Irrigation in endodontics," *Dental Clinics of North America*, vol. 54, no. 2, pp. 291–312, 2010.

[30] M. Hülsmann and I. Schinkel, "Influence of several factors on the success or failure of removal of fractured instruments from the root canal," *Dental Traumatology*, vol. 15, no. 6, pp. 252–258, 1999.

[31] M. T. Ankrum, G. R. Hartwell, and J. E. Truitt, "K3 Endo, ProTaper, and ProFile systems: breakage and distortion in severely curved roots of molars," *Journal of Endodontia*, vol. 30, no. 4, pp. 234–237, 2004.

[32] M. K. Iqbal, M. R. Kohli, and J. S. Kim, "A retrospective clinical study of incidence of root canal instrument separation in an endodontics graduate program: a PennEndo database study," *Journal of Endodontia*, vol. 32, no. 11, pp. 1048–1052, 2006.

[33] J. Wu, G. Lei, M. Yan, Y. Yu, J. Yu, and G. Zhang, "Instrument separation analysis of multi-used ProTaper universal rotary system during root canal therapy," *Journal of Endodontia*, vol. 37, no. 6, pp. 758–763, 2011.

[34] A. Kapalas and T. Lambrianidis, "Factors associated with root canal ledging during instrumentation," *Dental Traumatology*, vol. 16, no. 5, pp. 229–231, 2000.

[35] N. J. Souter and H. H. Messer, "Complications associated with fractured file removal using an ultrasonic technique," *Journal of Endodontics*, vol. 31, no. 6, pp. 450–452, 2005.

Permissions

All chapters in this book were first published by Hindawi Publishing Corporation; hereby published with permission under the Creative Commons Attribution License or equivalent. Every chapter published in this book has been scrutinized by our experts. Their significance has been extensively debated. The topics covered herein carry significant findings which will fuel the growth of the discipline. They may even be implemented as practical applications or may be referred to as a beginning point for another development.

The contributors of this book come from diverse backgrounds, making this book a truly international effort. This book will bring forth new frontiers with its revolutionizing research information and detailed analysis of the nascent developments around the world.

We would like to thank all the contributing authors for lending their expertise to make the book truly unique. They have played a crucial role in the development of this book. Without their invaluable contributions this book wouldn't have been possible. They have made vital efforts to compile up to date information on the varied aspects of this subject to make this book a valuable addition to the collection of many professionals and students.

This book was conceptualized with the vision of imparting up-to-date information and advanced data in this field. To ensure the same, a matchless editorial board was set up. Every individual on the board went through rigorous rounds of assessment to prove their worth. After which they invested a large part of their time researching and compiling the most relevant data for our readers.

The editorial board has been involved in producing this book since its inception. They have spent rigorous hours researching and exploring the diverse topics which have resulted in the successful publishing of this book. They have passed on their knowledge of decades through this book. To expedite this challenging task, the publisher supported the team at every step. A small team of assistant editors was also appointed to further simplify the editing procedure and attain best results for the readers.

Apart from the editorial board, the designing team has also invested a significant amount of their time in understanding the subject and creating the most relevant covers. They scrutinized every image to scout for the most suitable representation of the subject and create an appropriate cover for the book.

The publishing team has been an ardent support to the editorial, designing and production team. Their endless efforts to recruit the best for this project, has resulted in the accomplishment of this book. They are a veteran in the field of academics and their pool of knowledge is as vast as their experience in printing. Their expertise and guidance has proved useful at every step. Their uncompromising quality standards have made this book an exceptional effort. Their encouragement from time to time has been an inspiration for everyone.

The publisher and the editorial board hope that this book will prove to be a valuable piece of knowledge for researchers, students, practitioners and scholars across the globe.

List of Contributors

M. S. Nivedhitha and Aishwarya Ranganath
Department of Conservative Dentistry and Endodontics, Saveetha Institute of Medical and Technical Sciences, No. 162, Poonamalle High Road, Chennai, 600077 Tamil Nadu, India

Benoy Jacob
Department of Conservative Dentistry and Endodontics, Saveetha Institute of Medical and Technical Sciences, No. 162, Poonamalle High Road, Chennai, 600077 Tamil Nadu, India
Department of Conservative Dentistry and Endodontics, Saveetha Institute of Medical and Technical Sciences, Chennai, Tamil Nadu, India

Ashwag Yagoub Aloyouny
Basic Dental Sciences Department, College of Dentistry, Princess Nourah Bint Abdulrahman University, Riyadh, Saudi Arabia

Laïla Azzahim, Nisrin Bassim and Faïza Abdallaoui
Faculty of Dentistry of Rabat, Mohamed V University, Rabat, Morocco

Yoshio Ohyama
Department of Oral and Maxillofacial Surgery, Shizuoka City Shizuoka Hospital, 10-93, Outemachi, Aoi-ku, Shizuoka-shi, Shizuoka 420-8690, Japan

Masaru Ogawa and Satoshi Yokoo
Department of Oral and Maxillofacial Surgery, and Plastic Surgery, Gunma University Graduate School of Medicine, 3-39-15, Showamachi, Maebashi-Shi, Gunma 371-8511, Japan

Hitoshi Sato, Yuji Kurihara, Sunao Shiogama, Kotaro Saka, Yuya Kurasawa, Masakatsu Itose, Atsutoshi Yaso and Tatsuo Shirota
Department of Oral and Maxillofacial Surgery, School of Dentistry, Showa University, 2-1-1 Kitasenzoku, Ota-ku,Tokyo 145-8515, Japan

Hai Anh Trinh
Multidisciplinary Dental Biomaterials Science Program, Graduate School, Chulalongkorn University, Bangkok 10330, Thailand

Van Viet Dam
Department of Implantology, Hanoi National Hospital of Odonto-Stomatology, Hanoi 100000, Vietnam

Wijit Banlunara
Department of Pathology, Faculty of Veterinary Science, Chulalongkorn University, Bangkok 10330, Thailand

Polkit Sangvanich
Department of Chemistry, Faculty of Science, Chulalongkorn University, Bangkok 10330, Thailand

Pasutha Thunyakitpisal
Department of Anatomy, Multidisciplinary Dental Biomaterials Science Program, Research Unit of Herbal Medicine, Biomaterial and Material for Dental Treatment, Faculty of Dentistry, Chulalongkorn University, Bangkok 10330, Thailand

Saikrishna Ananthapadmanabhan and Anthony Noor
Department of Otolaryngology, Nepean Hospital, Kingswood, NSW 2747, Australia

Niranjan Sritharan
Department of Otolaryngology, Westmead Hospital, Westmead, NSW 2145, Australia

Neeta Patel, Akshayraj Langaliya, Aravind Kumbhar, Aarshvi Shah, Himani Bhatt, Drashti Panchal, Sharan Shah and Jinali Shah
AMC Dental College and Hosptial, Bhalakhiya Mill Compound, Opp. Anupam Cinema, Ahmedabad 380008, India

Aastha Buch
Government Dental College and Hospital, Civil Hospital Campus, Asarwa, Ahmedabad 380016, India

Shikha Kanodia
Faculty of Dental Sciences, Dharmsinh Desai University, Nadiad 387001, India

Irna Sufiawati
Department of Oral Medicine, Faculty of Dentistry, Padjajaran University, Indonesia

Ani Megawati
Oral Medicine Residency Program, Faculty of Dentistry, Padjadjaran University, Indonesia

Muhammad Al Farisyi
Oral Medicine Clinic, Kota Prabumulih General Hospital, South Sumatra, Indonesia

I. Nyoman Gede Juwita Putra
Department of Oral Medicine, Faculty of Dentistry, Mahasaraswati University, Indonesia

Sarang Suresh Hotchandani, Feroze Ali Kalhoro, Priya Rani Harjani and Mahwish Memon
Department of Operative Dentistry, Liaquat University of Medical & Health Sciences, Jamshoro, Pakistan

Saede Atarbashi-Moghadam and Ali Lotfi
Department of Oral and Maxillofacial Pathology, School of Dentistry, Shahid Beheshti University of Medical Sciences, Tehran, Iran

Mohammad Mehdizadeh
Department of Oral and Maxillofacial Surgery, School of Dentistry, Qom University of Medical Sciences, Qom, Iran

Fazele Atarbashi-Moghadam
Department of Periodontics, School of Dentistry, Shahid Beheshti University of Medical Sciences, Tehran, Iran

Soukaina El Kharroubi, Sofia Drouri, Bouchra Doumari, Sara Dhoum and Hafsa El Merini
Department of Conservative Dentistry and Endodontics, School of Dentistry, Hassan II University of Casablanca, Morocco

Venkata Ramanand Oruganti, Shylaja Sanjeevareddygari, Sharath Kumar Reddy Eppalapalli and Raghu Vamshi Vishwakarma
Department of Oral Pathology, SVS Institute of Dental Sciences, Mahabubnagar, Telangana, India

Manay Srinivas Munisekhar
Oral Pathology Division, Department of Preventive Dentistry, College of Dentistry, Jouf University, Sakaka, Al Jouf, Saudi Arabia

Kiran Kumar Ganji
Periodontics Division, Department of Preventive Dentistry, College of Dentistry, Jouf University, Sakaka, Al Jouf, Saudi Arabia

Rahul Halkai and Kiran R. Halkai
Department of Conservative Dentistry and Endodontics, Al-Badar Dental College and Hospital, Kalaburgi, Karnataka, India

Caterina Buffone
School of Dentistry, Magna Graecia University of Catanzaro, Italy

Amerigo Giudice and Leonzio Fortunato
School of Dentistry, Magna Graecia University of Catanzaro, Italy
Department of Health Sciences, Magna Graecia University of Catanzaro, Italy

Francesco Bennardo
Department of Health Sciences, Magna Graecia University of Catanzaro, Italy

Francesca Maria Plutino
Istituto Clinico De Blasi, Reggio Calabria, Italy

Seba Abraham, Bhagyalekshmi Mallika, Arunima Reshma and ReejaMol Mohammed Kassim
Department of Endodontics, Faculty of Dentistry, Mansoura University, Mansoura, Egypt

Ahmed Elhakim and Tarek Mohamed Abd El-Wahab
PMS College of Dental Science and Research, India

Maria S. Abbasi and Adil Bin Irfan
Department of Prosthodontics, Altamash Institute of Dental Medicine, Karachi 75500, Pakistan

Naseer Ahmed
Department of Prosthodontics, Altamash Institute of Dental Medicine, Karachi 75500, Pakistan
PhD Scholar Prosthodontics Unit University Sains Malaysia, School of Dental Sciences, Health Campus, 16150 Kubang Kerian, Kelantan, Malaysia

Samar Al-Saleh, Tariq Abduljabbar and Fahim Vohra
Department of Prosthetic Dental Science, College of Dentistry, King Saud University, 60169, Riyadh 11545, Saudi Arabia

Matheus Francisco Barros Rodrigues and Layla Louise de Amorim Rocha
Dentistry Course, Faculdade Cathedral, Boa Vista 69307-053, Brazil

Rodrigo da Franca Acioly and Daniel do Carmo Carvalho
Department of Oral and Maxillofacial Surgery and Traumatology, Hospital Geral de Roraima, Boa Vista 69305-455, Brazil

Cristofe Coelho Lopes da Rocha
Infrastructure Department, Instituto Federal, Boa Vista 69303-340, Brazil

Alisha Rewari
Department of Prosthodontics, SGT University, India

Nupur Dabas, Reshu Sanan, Shefali Phogat and Sumit Singh Phukela
Department of Prosthodontics, Faculty of Dental Sciences, SGT University, India

Monika Vigarniya
Shaheed Hasan Khan Mewati Government Medical College, India

H. C. Baranwal, Nidhi Singh, Neeraj Kumar, Riya Garg, Jyoti Yadav and Richik Tripathi
Faculty of Dental Sciences, IMS, BHU, Varanasi, India

Neelam Mittal, Vijay Parashar and Prasad Suresh Patel
Faculty of Dental Sciences, Institute of Medical Sciences, Banaras Hindu University, Varanasi, Up, India

V. Anuradha and Preeti Satish
HOSMAT Hospital, Magrath Road, Richmond Road, Bangalore 560025, India
Department of Oral and Maxillofacial Surgery, M R Ambedkar Dental College and Hospital, Bangalore, India

Satish Kumaran Pugazhendi
Department of Oral and Maxillofacial Surgery, M R Ambedkar Dental College and Hospital, Bangalore, India
Annasawmy Mudaliar General Hospital, Pulkeshi Nagar, Bangalore 560005, India

Ravi Sachidananda
People Tree Hospital, Tumkur Road, Goraguntepalya, Bangalore 560022, India

Romir Navaneetham
Oral and Maxillofacial Surgery, Vydehi Dental College, EPIP Area, Whitefield, Bangalore 560066, India

Yuya Kurasawa, Hitoshi Sato and Toshikazu Shimane
Department of Oral and Maxillofacial Surgery, Division of Oral Oncology, Showa University, School of Dentistry, Tokyo, Japan

Ryogo Katada, Takanobu Inada and Tatsuo Shirota
Department of Oral and Maxillofacial Surgery, Showa University, School of Dentistry, Tokyo, Japan

Nuha Abdel-Rahman Elmubarak
Department of Restorative Dentistry, National Ribat University, Khartoum, Sudan

Koki Takamatsu, Takashi Moriya, Arisa Yasuda, Takaaki Kamatani and Tatsuo Shirota
Department of Oral and Maxillofacial Surgery, School of Dentistry, Showa University, Tokyo, Japan

Hitoshi Sato
Department of Oral and Maxillofacial Surgery, School of Dentistry, Showa University, Tokyo, Japan
Department of Oral Oncology, School of Dentistry, Showa University, Tokyo, Japan

P. Stylianou, N. Soldatos, N. Angelov and R. Weltman
Department of Periodontics and Dental Hygiene, School of Dentistry, University of Texas, Health Science Center at Houston, Houston, TX, USA

E. K. Edmondson
Private Practice, San Antonio, TX, USA

Amerigo Giudice, Francesco Liborio, Fiorella Averta, Selene Barone and Leonzio Fortunato
School of Dentistry, Department of Health Sciences, Magna Graecia University of Catanzaro, Catanzaro, Italy

Alessandro Antonelli, Fiorella Averta, Federica Diodati, Danila Muracaz and Amerigo Giudice
School of Dentistry, Department of Health Sciences, "Magna Graecia" University of Catanzaro, Italy

Ylenia Brancaccio
School of Dentistry, Magna Graecia University of Catanzaro, Italy
School of Dentistry, Department of Health Sciences, "Magna Graecia" University of Catanzaro, Italy

Chiara Mignogna
Interdepartmental Service Center, "Magna Graecia" University of Catanzaro, Italy

Erol Cansiz
Istanbul University, Faculty of Dentistry, Department of Oral and Maxillofacial Surgery, Turkey

Emine Deniz Gozen and Murat Yener
Istanbul Cerrahpasa University, Medical Faculty, Department of Otorhinolaryngology, Turkey

Aliaa Abdelmoniem Bedeir Eita
Faculty of Dentistry, Oral Medicine, Periodontology, Diagnosis and Radiology Department, Alexandria University, Alexandria, Egypt

G. Turatti and M. Giordano
Odontostomatology OU, Martini Hospital, Via Tofane 71, Turin 10141, Italy

Muhammad Aiman Mohd Nizar
Department of Diagnostic and Bioscience Craniofacial, Faculty of Dentistry, Universiti Kebangsaan Malaysia, Malaysia

A. Bruni
CIR Dental School, Department of Surgical Sciences, Università degli Studi di Torino, Via Nizza 230, Turin 10126, Italy
Department of Mechanical and Aerospatial Engineering (DIMEAS), Politecnico di Torino, C.so Duca degli Abruzzi 24, Turin 10129, Italy

M. Savoini and G. Gerbino
Division of Maxillofacial Surgery, Department of Surgical Sciences, Università degli studi di Torino, Città della Salute e delle Scienza Hospital, Corso A.M. Dogliotti 14, Turin 10126, Italy

Syed Nabil
Department of Oral and Maxillofacial Surgery, Faculty of Dentistry, The National University of Malaysia, Malaysia

Bruna Marca Mattei, Soraia A. W. Imanishi and Grasieli de Oliveira Ramos
Universidade do Oeste de Santa Catarina (UNOESC), Joaçaba, Santa Catarina, Brazil

Paloma Santos de Campos
Universidade Federal do Rio Grande do Sul (UFRGS), Porto Alegre, Rio Grande do Sul, Brazil

Suyany Gabriely Weiss
School of Health Sciences, Department of Dentistry, Universidade Positivo, Curitiba, Paraná, Brazil

Tatiana Miranda Deliberador
Latin American Institute of Dental Research and Education (ILAPEO), Curitiba, Paraná, Brazil

Kamichika Hayashi, Takeshi Onda, Hirona Honda and Masayuki Takano
Department of Oral and Maxillofacial Surgery, Tokyo Dental College, Tokyo, Japan

Mitsuru Takata, Hiroyuki Matsuda and Hidetoshi Tamura
Oral and Maxillofacial Surgery, Kameda General Hospital, Chiba, Japan

Anjaneyulu K., Aishwarya Ranganath and Riluwan Siddique
Department of Conservative Dentistry and Endodontics, Saveetha Institute of Medical and Technical Sciences, Chennai, Tamil Nadu, India

Index

A

Active Oxygen, 181-183, 185-186

Adrenaline, 32, 75

Allografts, 26, 29, 159

Alloplasts, 26, 29

Ameloblastoma, 73, 76-77

Anteroparotid Approach, 187, 192-194

B

Basal Cells, 47, 50, 75

Biodentine, 109, 111, 113-114

Blood Clot, 6, 29

Bone Regeneration, 8, 26, 175

C

Cell Differentiation, 73, 75-76

Cellular Damage, 41, 164

Chlorhexidine, 7, 15-16, 27, 154, 181-183, 185-186

Condylar Fracture, 187-188, 191, 193

Connective Tissue, 1, 62-64, 74-75, 87, 89, 91, 97, 106, 138, 143-145, 150

Cortical Bone, 18, 21, 74, 87

Corticosteroid, 47-49, 52-53, 140, 147, 156, 170

Cytoplasm, 73, 75, 79

Cytotoxic Effect, 181-182

D

Dentin Formation, 6, 131

Depression, 45-51, 53, 164

Dysgeusia, 149, 161, 163-165

E

Electric Pulp Testing, 2, 38

Endodontic Etiology, 37-38, 43

Endodontics, 1-2, 4, 6-8, 24-25, 36, 43-44, 54-55, 60, 67-68, 71, 73, 93, 96, 114-115, 117, 135, 140, 156, 180, 185, 193, 196-197, 199-201

F

Facial Nerve, 118-119, 187, 192-194

G

Gingiva, 37, 45, 52, 55-58, 68, 78-79, 81, 83, 85, 87-89, 91-92, 142-143, 149, 151-156

Granular Cells, 75-77

H

Hyperkeratosis, 49-50, 153, 155

I

Immature Roots, 2-3

Incisional Biopsy, 20, 45, 47, 55, 77, 90, 146, 150

Inflammatory Cells, 2, 48, 74

Intraosseous Lipoma, 62, 64-66

L

Labial Mucosa, 45, 47-48, 51-52, 83

Leiomyoma, 78, 80, 84-86

Lingual Plates, 74, 90

Local Flaps, 157, 159

Lymphadenopathy, 10, 55

Lymphoid Tissue, 9-11

M

Mandibular Alveolus, 87, 89, 92

Maxillary Sinus, 17-19, 26-29, 31-36, 55-58, 177-178

N

Nasal Cavity, 15, 32, 34, 60, 122-123

O

Odontogenic Maxillary Sinusitis, 17, 19, 31, 35-36

Odontogenic Tumor, 20-21, 73-76

Oral Lichen Planus, 45, 53, 146, 148, 155

Orocutaneous Fistula, 157, 159

Oropharyngeal Candidiasis, 9-10

Osteogenic Properties, 15, 26

Osteotomes, 75, 125, 170

P

Palatine Tonsil, 9-12

Paraesthesia, 35, 37-39, 41-44, 62, 88

Parosmia, 161-164

Pathogenesis, 11, 45, 50, 53, 61, 71, 73, 146, 164

Pathophysiology, 17, 135, 164

Pedicled Flap, 157-158

Periapical Infection, 37-38, 43-44

Periapical Lesion, 1-3, 6-8, 13, 15-16, 44

Periodontal Disease, 27, 33, 68, 91, 145

Plasma Cell, 149-151, 155-156

Plexiform, 73-74, 77

Prelacrimal Window, 31-32, 34-35

Psychological Stress, 45, 49-51

R

Root Canal Therapy, 2, 55, 57, 198, 201

S
Salivary Glands, 78, 164
Segmental Resection, 21-22, 24, 90
Soft Tissues, 25, 158, 176, 183, 193
Styloid, 118-119, 121
Subcutaneous Emphysema, 177-180
Submandibular Gland, 157-160
Surgical Access, 31-32, 35
Surgical Treatment, 15, 19-20, 24, 60, 83, 102, 104, 193-194

T
Talon Cusp, 127-135
Temporomandibular Joint, 55, 136, 139-140, 175-176, 194
Tissue Healing, 93, 155, 181, 184
Tonsil, 9-12
Tooth Avulsion, 67, 71
Tumor Cells, 76, 81

U
Ulceration, 30, 41, 150, 153-154

V
Vertical Root Fracture, 109-110, 113-114

X
Xenografts, 26, 29

www.ingramcontent.com/pod-product-compliance
Lightning Source LLC
LaVergne TN
LVHW082229200926
848484LV00008B/2320